Case Studies in
PEDIATRIC
INTENSIVE CARE

Case Studies in

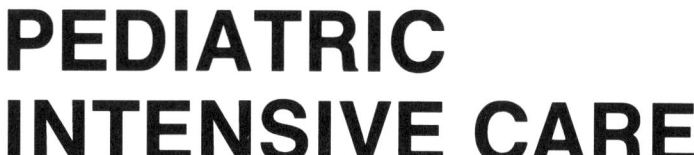

PEDIATRIC INTENSIVE CARE

Edited by

Mark C. Rogers, M.D.

Vice Chancellor for Health Systems
Executive Director, Duke University Hospital
Distinguished Professor of Anesthesiology and Pediatrics
Duke University
Durham, North Carolina
formerly
Distinguished Faculty Professor and Chairman
Department of Anesthesiology/Critical Care Medicine
Professor of Anesthesiology/Critical Care Medicine and
  Pediatrics
Associate Dean for Clinical Practice
The Johns Hopkins University School of Medicine
Baltimore, Maryland

Mark A. Helfaer, M.D.

Assistant Professor
Departments of Anesthesiology/Critical Care Medicine and
  Pediatrics
The Johns Hopkins University School of Medicine
Baltimore, Maryland

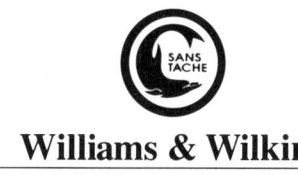

Williams & Wilkins

BALTIMORE • PHILADELPHIA • HONG KONG
LONDON • MUNICH • SYDNEY • TOKYO

A WAVERLY COMPANY

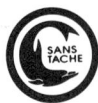

Editor: Timothy H. Grayson
Project Manager: Kathleen Courtney Millet
Copy Editor: Carol Zimmerman
Designer and Cover Designer: Wilma E. Rosenberger
Illustration Planner: Lorraine Wrzosek

Copyright © 1993
Williams & Wilkins
428 East Preston Street
Baltimore, Maryland 21202, USA

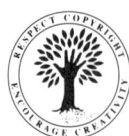

Accurate indications, adverse reactions, and dosage schedules for drugs are provided in this book, but it is possible that they may change. The reader is urged to review the package information data of the manufacturers of the medications mentioned.

Printed in the United States of America

Chapter reprints are available from the Publisher.

Library of Congress Cataloging-in-Publication Data

Case studies in pediatric intensive care / edited by Mark C. Rogers,
   Mark A. Helfaer.
      p.   cm.
   ISBN 0-683-07323-0
   1. Pediatric intensive care—Case studies.   I. Rogers, Mark
C. II. Helfaer, Mark A.   III. Title: Pediatric intensive care.
   [DNLM: 1. Intensive Care—in infancy & childhood—case
studies. WS 366 C337 1993]
RJ370.C38   1993
618.92′0025–dc20
DNLM/DLC
for Library of Congress   93-12263
                                                                  CIP

                                    93 94 95 96 97
                         1   2   3   4   5   6   7   8   9 10

*To all of our international colleagues
who make pediatric intensive care
both exciting and gratifying*

Preface

This book has been compiled with two goals in mind. First, it is directed to physicians in training. The hope is to expose young doctors to the interesting breadth and complexity of the patients who present to the Pediatric Intensive Care Unit (PICU). This is directed at any level of training. Starting pediatric interns can be exposed to a far greater number of cases than they would enjoy just by sequentially admitting their portion of the patients. Likewise, senior fellows will benefit from the experiences of a great number of PICUs around the world. They can be exposed to the diagnostic dilemmas as well as the variation of therapeutic inventions not only within their institutions but also variations around the country and around the world.

The second goal of *Case Studies in Pediatric Intensive Care* is to compile the experiences of PICUs around the world. In this age of international politics and international economics, intellectual pursuits such as medicine, and specifically, pediatric intensive care medicine, should also enjoy the benefits of internationalization. Attendees of the First World Congress of Pediatric Intensive Care in Baltimore could attest to how enlightening and invigorating the sharing of experiences and approaches to pediatric intensive care around the world was in an exciting field such as pediatric intensive care.

The reader can use *Case Studies in Pediatric Intensive Care* in two ways. First, the book can be used for self-testing using the Contents page to refer to random cases. Second, the Contents of Presentation/Diagnosis, located at the end of the text before the Index, can be used to locate cases by presentation in the PICU or by final diagnosis.

Our hope is that the compilations of these cases reflect the excitement, intellectual challenges, and innovation that have marked the explosion of interest in pediatric intensive care. We thank all our international colleagues for their contributions to this book and hope that they enjoy reading the experiences of their colleagues as much as we have.

Mark C. Rogers, M.D.
Mark A. Helfaer, M.D.

Acknowledgments

We would like to extend sincere appreciation for the tolerance, long hours, and perseverance of Trudy Campbell and Peggy Riley, without whom this and many other books would not have come to fruition. Our thanks also to Tim Grayson and Katey Millet at Williams & Wilkins for their excellent editorial support.

Contributors

David V. Anglin, M.D.
Department of Pediatrics
The Ohio State University School of Medicine
Chief, Section of Critical Care Medicine
Children's Hospital
Columbus, Ohio, USA

Andrew M. Atz, M.D.
Clinical Fellow
Department of Cardiology
Harvard Medical School
The Children's Hospital
Boston, Massachusetts, USA

Jose Baeza, M.D.
Associated Medical Director
Unidad Cuidados Intensivos
Hospital Luis Calvo Mackenna
Santiago, Chile

Paul R. Bakerman, M.D.
Associate Director, Pediatric Critical Care
Phoenix Children's Hospital
Phoenix, Arizona, USA

Olga Bandzakova, M.D.
Department of Anesthesiology and Resuscitation
Children's University Hospital
Bratislava, Slovakia

Steven D. Barnes, M.D.
Assistant Professor of Pediatrics and Anesthesiology
Rush Medical College
Associate Director, Pediatric Critical Care
Attending in Anesthesiology
Rush-Presbyterian-St. Luke's Medical Center
Chicago, Illinois, USA

Zohar Barzilay, M.D., F.C.C.M.
Associate Professor of Pediatrics
Tel-Aviv University
Sackler School of Medicine
Chairman, Division of Pediatrics
Director, Pediatric Intensive Care Unit
Chaim Sheba Medical Center
Tel Hashomer, Israel

Milan Beier, prim. M.D.
Department of Anesthesiology and
*   Resuscitation*
Children's University Hospital
Bratislava, Slovakia

Gary A. Bellus, M.D.
Fellow, Clinical Genetics
Department of Pediatrics
The Johns Hopkins University School of
*   Medicine*
Baltimore, Maryland, USA

Ondrej Benko, M.D.
Department of Anesthesiology and
*   Resuscitation*
Children's University Hospital
Bratislava, Slovakia

David W. Bernard, M.D.
Postdoctoral Fellow, Pediatric Emergency
*   Medicine*
Department of Pediatrics
The Johns Hopkins University School of
*   Medicine*
Baltimore, Maryland, USA

David H. Beyda, M.D.
Director, Pediatric Critical Care
Phoenix Children's Hospital
Phoenix, Arizona, USA

Wim Blom, Ph.D.
Division of Metabolic Diseases
Department of Pediatrics
Sophia Children's Hospital
University Hospital/Erasmus University
Rotterdam, The Netherlands

Nancy Braverman, M.D.
Fellow, Clinical Genetics
Department of Pediatrics

The Johns Hopkins University School of
*   Medicine*
Baltimore, Maryland, USA

Francisco Bruno, M.D.
Physician-in-Charge, Pediatric Intensive
*   Care Unit*
Hospital São Lucas de PUC and
*   Faculdade de Medicina PUC-RS*
Porto Alegre RS, Brazil

Jeffrey Burns, M.D.
Fellow, Pediatric Critical Care Medicine
Harvard Medical School
The Children's Hospital
Boston, Massachusetts, USA

Edward M. Burton, M.D.
Associate Professor and Chief of Pediatric
*   Radiology*
Department of Radiology
Medical College of Georgia
Augusta, Georgia, USA

Donna A. Caniano, M.D.
Associate Professor
Department of Surgery
The Ohio State University College of
*   Medicine*
Attending Surgeon
Children's Hospital
Columbus, Ohio, USA

G. Patricia Cantwell, M.D.
Assistant Professor of Clinical Pediatrics
Pediatric Critical Care Medicine
Department of Pediatrics
Associate Director, Emergency Medical
*   Skills Training Program, Medical*
*   Training and Simulation Laboratory*
University of Miami School of Medicine
Miami, Florida, USA

Coriene Catsman-Berrevoets, M.D.
Division of Pediatric Neurology
Department of Neurology
Sophia Children's Hospital
University Hospital/Erasmus University
Rotterdam, The Netherlands

Teerachai Chantarojanasiri, M.D.
Associate Professor of Pediatrics
Faculty of Medicine
Division of Pediatric Pulmonology and
    Critical Care
Department of Pediatrics
Ramathibodi Hospital
Mahidol University
Bangkok, Thailand

Edward E. Conway, Jr., M.D.
Assistant Professor of Pediatrics, Critical
    Care, and Anesthesiology
Director, Pediatric Critical Care
    Fellowship Program
The Children's Medical Center at
    Montefiore
Bronx, New York, USA

Jaime Cordero, M.D.
Assistant Professor of Pediatrics
Medical Director
Unidad Cuidados Intensivos
Hospital Luis Calvo Mackenna
Santiago, Chile

Sharon M. Dabrow, M.D.
Assistant Professor
Department of Pediatrics
University of Florida College of Medicine
Attending Physician, Pediatrics
Shands Hospital at the University of
    Florida
Gainesville, Florida, USA

Heidi J. Dalton, M.D.
Assistant Professor
Department of Pediatrics
Georgetown University Children's
    Medical Center
Washington, DC, USA

D. Lyn Davidson, M.D.
Assistant Professor of Pediatrics
University of South Alabama School of
    Medicine
Director, Pediatric Intensive Care Unit
USA Doctors Hospital
Mobile, Alabama, USA

Juan C. De Carlos, M.D.
Resident, Pediatric Intensive Care Unit
Hospital Infantil La Paz
Madrid, Spain

Suzanne Delport, M.D.
Department of Paediatrics
Kalafong Hospital
Pretoria, Republic of South Africa

Joseph D. DiCarlo, M.D.
Assistant Professor
Department of Pediatrics
Georgetown University Children's
    Medical Center
Washington, DC, USA

Svetozar Dluholucky, M.D., Ph.D.
Associate Professor
Head, Pediatric Clinic
F. D. Roosevelt Hospital
Banska Bystrica, Slovakia

Paloma Dorao, M.D.
Pediatric Intensive Care Unit
Hospital Infantil La Paz
Madrid, Spain

Paulo Roberto Einloft, M.D.
Assistant Professor
Department of Pediatrics
Clinical Chief, Pediatric Intensive Care
    Unit
Hospital São Lucas da PUC and
    Faculdade de Medicina PUC-RS
Porto Alegre RS, Brazil

James C. Fackler, M.D.
Instructor in Pediatrics (Anesthesia)
Harvard Medical School
Director, Multidisciplinary ICU
The Children's Hospital
Boston, Massachusetts, USA

Randall P. Flick, M.D.
Fellow, Pediatric Critical Care
Department of Anesthesiology/Critical
    Care Medicine
The Johns Hopkins University School of
    Medicine
Baltimore, Maryland, USA

Pedro Celiny Ramos Garcia, M.D.
Adjunct Professor
Department of Pediatrics
Chief of In-Patient Service and Pediatric
    Intensive Care Unit
Hospital São Lucas de PUC and
    Faculdade de Medicina PUC-RS
Porto Alegre RS, Brazil

Peter Gasparec, M.D.
Department of Anesthesiology and
    Resuscitation
Children's University Hospital
Bratislava, Slovakia

Barry Gelman, M.D.
Fellow, Pediatric Critical Care Medicine
Department of Pediatrics
University of Miami School of Medicine
Miami, Florida, USA

Eli Gilad, M.D.
Tel-Aviv University
Sackler School of Medicine
Pediatric Intensive Care Unit
Chaim Sheba Medical Center
Tel Hashomer, Israel

Salvatore R. Goodwin, M.D.
Associate Professor of Anesthesiology and
    Pediatrics
University of Florida College of Medicine
Medical Director, Pediatric Intensive Care
Shands Hospital at the University of
    Florida
Gainesville, Florida, USA

William J. Greeley, M.D.
Associate Professor of Pediatrics and
    Anesthesiology
Duke University Medical Center
Durham, North Carolina, USA

Robert S. Greenberg, M.D.
Fellow, Pediatric Critical Care Medicine
Department of Anesthesiology/Critical
    Care Medicine
The Johns Hopkins University School of
    Medicine
Baltimore, Maryland, USA

Eric L. Gunnoe, M.D.
Fellow, Pediatric Critical Care
Department of Anesthesiology/Critical
    Care Medicine
The Johns Hopkins University School of
    Medicine
Baltimore, Maryland, USA

Darryl R. Gwyn, M.D.
Fellow, Pediatric Critical Care
Department of Anesthesiology/Critical
    Care Medicine
The Johns Hopkins University School of
    Medicine
Baltimore, Maryland, USA

Steven E. Haun, M.D.
Assistant Professor
Division of Critical Care Medicine
Department of Pediatrics
The Ohio State University School of
    Medicine
Columbus, Ohio, USA

Gabriel J. Hauser, M.D.
Associate Professor of Pediatrics and
    Critical Care Medicine
Chief, Pediatric Critical Care Medicine
Director, Pediatric Intensive Care Unit
Georgetown University Children's
    Medical Center
Washington, DC, USA

William R. Hayden, M.D.
Associate Professor
Rush Medical College
Director, Rush-Cook County Hospital
    Pediatric Critical Care Program
Chicago, Illinois, USA

Jan A. Hazelzet, M.D.
Division of Pediatric Intensive Care
Department of Pediatrics
Sophia Children's Hospital
University Hospital/Erasmus University
Rotterdam, The Netherlands

Mark A. Helfaer, M.D.
Assistant Professor
Departments of Anesthesiology/Critical
*   Care Medicine, and Pediatrics*
The Johns Hopkins University School of
*   Medicine*
Baltimore, Maryland, USA

Robert Henning, F.R.C.A.
Staff Specialist in Intensive Care
Royal Children's Hospital
Melbourne, Victoria, Australia

Peter Hudec, M.D.
Pediatric Clinic, PICU
F. D. Roosevelt Hospital
Banska Bystrica, Slovakia

Zeev Kain, M.D.
Assistant Professor
Department of Anesthesiology
Yale University School of Medicine
New Haven, Connecticut, USA

Elizabeth W. Kelley, M.D.
Assistant Professor
Department of Anesthesiology
Bowman Gray School of Medicine
Wake Forest University
Winston-Salem, North Carolina, USA

Frank H. Kern, M.D.
Assistant Professor of Pediatrics and
*   Anesthesiology*
Duke University Medical Center
Durham, North Carolina, USA

Delio J. Kipper, M.D.
Assistant Professor
Department of Pediatrics
Attending Physician, Pediatric Intensive
*   Care Unit*
Hospital São Lucas da PUC and
*   Faculdade de Medicina PUC-RS*
Porto Alegre RS, Brazil

Alan S. Klein, M.D.
Associate Professor of Anesthesiology and
*   Pediatrics*
University of Florida College of Medicine

Attending Physician, Pediatric Intensive
*   Care*
Shands Hospital at the University of
*   Florida*
Gainesville, Florida, USA

Patrick M. Kochanek, M.D.
Associate Professor
Departments of Anesthesiology/Critical
*   Care Medicine and Pediatrics*
University of Pittsburgh School of
*   Medicine*
Children's Hospital of Pittsburgh
Pittsburgh, Pennsylvania, USA

Fernando Konrad, M.D.
Fellow, Pediatric Critical Care
Hospital São Lucas da PUC and
*   Faculdade de Medicina PUC-RS*
Porto Alegre RS, Brazil

Brian R. Krafte-Jacobs, M.D.
Fellow, Critical Care Medicine
Department of Critical Care Medicine
George Washington University School of
*   Medicine*
Children's National Medical Center
Washington, DC, USA

Karol Kralinsky, M.D.
Pediatric Clinic, PICU
F. D. Roosevelt Hospital
Banska Bystrica, Slovakia

Ladislav Laho, M.D.
Pediatric Clinic, PICU
F. D. Roosevelt Hospital
Banska Bystrica, Slovakia

Mauri Leijala, M.D.
Cardiothoracic Surgery
University Children's Hospital
Helsinki, Finland

W. Casey Lenox, M.D.
Assistant Professor
Department of Anesthesiology/Critical
*   Care Medicine*
The Johns Hopkins University School of
*   Medicine*
Baltimore, Maryland, USA

Daniel L. Levin, M.D.
Medical Director, Pediatric Intensive
   Care Unit
Department of Pediatrics
University of Texas Southwestern
   Medical Center at Dallas
Children's Medical Center of Dallas
Dallas, Texas, USA

Ann Marie LeVine, M.D.
Fellow, Critical Care Medicine
Department of Critical Care Medicine
George Washington University School of
   Medicine
Children's National Medical Center
Washington, DC, USA

George Lister, M.D.
Professor of Pediatrics and
   Anesthesiology
Department of Pediatrics
Yale University School of Medicine
New Haven, Connecticut, USA

Paul H. Liu, M.D.
Associate Director, Pediatric Critical Care
Phoenix Children's Hospital
Phoenix, Arizona, USA

Robert T. Mansfield, M.D.
Fellow, Pediatric Critical Care Medicine
Departments of Anesthesiology/Critical
   Care Medicine and Pediatrics
University of Pittsburgh School of
   Medicine
Children's Hospital of Pittsburgh
Pittsburgh, Pennsylvania, USA

Linda R. Margraf, M.D.
Assistant Professor
Department of Pathology
University of Texas Southwestern
   Medical Center at Dallas
Children's Medical Center of Dallas
Dallas, Texas, USA

Lynn D. Martin, M.D.
Director, Pediatric Critical Care
Swedish Medical Center/Seattle
Seattle, Washington, USA

Markus Mauderli, M.D.
University of Ear, Nose, and Throat
   Surgery
Inselspital
Bern, Switzerland

Lynne G. Maxwell, M.D.
Assistant Professor
Department of Anesthesiology/Critical
   Care Medicine
The Johns Hopkins University School of
   Medicine
Baltimore, Maryland, USA

Francis X. McGowan, Jr., M.D.
Assistant Professor of Anesthesiology,
   Pediatrics, and Critical Care Medicine
University of Pittsburgh School of
   Medicine
Staff Anesthesiologist
Children's Hospital of Pittsburgh
Pittsburgh, Pennsylvania, USA

Jon N. Meliones, M.D.
Assistant Professor of Pediatrics and
   Anesthesiology
Duke University Medical Center
Durham, North Carolina, USA

Katsuyuki Miyasaka, M.D.
Department of Anesthesia and Intensive
   Care Unit
National Children's Hospital
Tokyo, Japan

Sheila Momberger, M.D.
Fellow, Pediatric Critical Care
Hospital São Lucas da PUC and
   Faculdade de Medicina PUC-RS
Porto Alegre RS, Brazil

Jorge E. Montes, M.D.
Director, Pediatric Critical Care Medicine
Presbyterian Hospital
Albuquerque, New Mexico, USA

Mohan R. Mysore, M.B.B.S.
Fellow, Pediatric Critical Care
Department of Pediatrics
University of Texas Southwestern
    Medical Center at Dallas
Children's Medical Center of Dallas
Dallas, Texas, USA

Vinay M. Nadkarni, M.D.
Assistant Professor of Pediatrics
Thomas Jefferson University School of
    Medicine
Philadelphia, Pennsylvania
Director, Pediatric Critical Care
Medical Center of Delaware, Christiana
    Hospital
Newark, Delaware, USA

Satoshi Nakagawa, M.D.
Clinical Fellow
Department of Critical Care
The Hospital for Sick Children
Toronto, Ontario, Canada

David G. Nichols, M.D.
Assistant Professor
Departments of Anesthesiology/Critical
    Care Medicine and Pediatrics
Director, Pediatric Intensive Care Unit
The Johns Hopkins University School of
    Medicine
Baltimore, Maryland, USA

Edward J. Novotny, Jr., M.D.
Assistant Professor of Pediatrics and
    Neurology
Department of Pediatrics
Yale University School of Medicine
New Haven, Connecticut, USA

**D. Roddy O'Donnell, M.B.B.S.,
M.R.C.P.**
Hospital for Sick Children
London, United Kingdom

Olubunmi A Okanlami, M.D.
Fellow, Pediatric Intensive Care
Department of Anesthesiology/Critical
    Care Medicine

The Johns Hopkins University School of
    Medicine
Baltimore, Maryland, USA

Andrew C. Oken, M.D.
Assistant Professor
Department of Anesthesiology/Critical
    Care Medicine
The Johns Hopkins University School of
    Medicine
Baltimore, Maryland, USA

Anthony L. Palomba, M.D.
Assistant Professor of Pediatrics, Critical
    Care Medicine, and Anesthesiology
Associate Director
Division of Pediatric Critical Care
The Children's Medical Center at
    Montefiore
Bronx, New York, USA

Gideon Paret, M.D.
Instructor
Tel-Aviv University
Sackler School of Medicine
Pediatric Intensive Care Unit
Chaim Sheba Medical Center
Tel Hashomer, Israel

Antonio R. Perez-Atayde, M.D.
Associate Professor of Pathology
Harvard Medical School
Director of Surgical Pathology
The Children's Hospital
Boston, Massachusetts, USA

William H. Perloff, M.D., Ph.D.
Professor of Pediatrics and
    Anesthesiology
University of Wisconsin–Madison
    Medical School
Head, Pediatric Emergency and Critical
    Care
Children's Hospital
Madison, Wisconsin, USA

Juerg Pfenninger, M.D.
University Children's Hospital
Bern, Switzerland

Aroonwan Preutthipan, M.D.
Instructor, Division of Pediatric
*   Pulmonology and Critical Care*
Department of Pediatrics
Faculty of Medicine
Ramathibodi Hospital
Mahidol University
Bangkok, Thailand

Rudolf Riedel, M.D.
Department of Anesthesiology and
*   Resuscitation*
Children's University Hospital
Bratislava, Slovakia

Thomas V. Ringer, M.D.
Fellow, Pediatric Critical Care
University of Wisconsin–Madison
*   Medical School*
Children's Hospital
Madison, Wisconsin, USA

Peter Rock, M.D.
Acting Director, Division of Critical Care
*   Anesthesia*
The Johns Hopkins University School of
*   Medicine*
Baltimore, Maryland, USA

Francisco Ruza, M.D.
Director, Pediatric Intensive Care Unit
Professor of Pediatrics, Universidad
*   Autonóma de Madrid*
Hospital Infantil La Paz
Madrid, Spain

Hirokazu Sakai, M.D.
Department of Anesthesia and Intensive
*   Care Unit*
National Children's Hospital
Tokyo, Japan

Charles L. Schleien, M.D.
Director, Pediatric Critical Care Medicine
Associate Professor
Department of Pediatrics and
*   Anesthesiology*
University of Miami School of Medicine
Director, Pediatric Intensive Care Unit
Jackson Memorial Medical Center
Miami, Florida, USA

Eduardo Julio Schnitzler, M.D.
Chief, Pediatric Intensive Care Unit
Hospital Italiano
Buenos Aires, Argentina

Scott R. Schulman, M.D.
Assistant Professor of Pediatrics and
*   Anesthesiology*
Duke University Medical Center
Durham, North Carolina, USA

Linda L. Sell, M.D.
Associate Professor Clinical Surgery
Department of Surgery
Medical College of Wisconsin
Milwaukee, Wisconsin, USA

Nancy Setzer, M.D.
Associate Professor of Clinical
*   Anesthesiology and Pediatrics*
Department of Anesthesiology
University of Miami School of Medicine
Miami, Florida, USA

Donald H. Shaffner, M.D.
Assistant Professor
Department of Anesthesiology/Critical
*   Care Medicine*
The Johns Hopkins University School of
*   Medicine*
Baltimore, Maryland, USA

Anthony J. Slater, B.Med.Sc.,
M.B.B.S., F.R.A.C.P.
Honorable Senior Lecturer
University of London
Hospital for Sick Children
London, United Kingdom

Linda K. Snelling, M.D.
Assistant Professor of Pediatrics and
*   Anesthesiology*
Brown University School of Medicine
Director, Pediatric Critical Care
Rhode Island Hospital
Providence, Rhode Island, USA

Curt M. Steinhart, M.D.
Associate Professor of Pediatrics, Surgery,
  and Anesthesiology
Medical Director, Pediatric Intensive
  Care Unit
Medical College of Georgia
Augusta, Georgia, USA

Jana A. Stockwell, M.D.
Associate Professor of Pediatrics and
  Anesthesiology
Duke University Medical Center
Durham, North Carolina, USA

Herwig P. Stopfkuchen, M.D.
University Professor
Universitaetskinderklinik
Mainz, Germany

Waldemar Storm, M.D.
Fellow, Pediatric Critical Care Medicine
Department of Pediatrics
University of Wisconsin–Madison
  Medical School
Children's Hospital
Madison, Wisconsin, USA

Subharee Suwanjutha, M.D., F.C.C.P.
Professor of Pediatrics
Division of Pediatric Respiratory Disease
  and Intensive Care
Department of Pediatrics
Faculty of Medicine
Ramathibodi Hospital
Mahidol University
Bangkok, Thailand

**Robert C. Tasker, M.A., M.B., B.S.,
  M.R.C.P.**
Honorable Senior Lecturer
University of London
Pediatric Intensive Care Unit
Hospital for Sick Children
London, United Kingdom

David W. Tellez, M.D.
Associate Director, Pediatric Critical Care
Phoenix Children's Hospital
Phoenix, Arizona, USA

Joseph R. Tobin, M.D.
Assistant Professor
Departments of Anesthesiology/Critical
  Care Medicine and Pediatrics
The Johns Hopkins University School of
  Medicine
Baltimore, Maryland, USA

Edward J. Truemper, M.D.
Assistant Professor of Pediatrics
Medical College of Georgia
Augusta, Georgia, USA

H. Michael Ushay, M.D.
Fellow, Division of Critical Care
  Medicine
Department of Pediatrics
New York Hospital
Cornell University Medical Center
New York, New York, USA

Edwin van der Voort, M.D.
Division of Pediatric Intensive Care
Department of Pediatrics
Sophia Children's Hospital
University Hospital/Erasmus University
Rotterdam, The Netherlands

L. Kyle Walker, M.D.
Assistant Professor
Department of Anesthesiology and
  Critical Care Medicine
The Johns Hopkins University School of
  Medicine
Baltimore, Maryland, USA

**Randall C. Wetzel, M.B., B.S.,
  F.C.C.M.**
Associate Professor
Chief, Division of Pediatric Anesthesia
Department of Anesthesiology/Critical
  Care Medicine
The Johns Hopkins University School of
  Medicine
Baltimore, Maryland, USA

Lauren R. Widner, M.D.
Fellow, Pediatric Critical Care Medicine
Departments of Anesthesiology and
  Pediatrics
University of Florida College of Medicine
Gainesville, Flordia, USA

James D. Wilkinson, M.D.
Assistant Professor of Anesthesiology and
  Pediatrics
Department of Critical Care Medicine
George Washington University School of
  Medicine
Children's National Medical Center
Washington, DC, USA

Kathy Wilkinson, M.B.B.S., M.R.C.P.,
F.R.C.Anes.
Honorable Senior Lecturer
Hospital for Sick Children
London, United Kingdom

Eyal Winkler, M.D.
Tel-Aviv University
Sackler School of Medicine
Pediatric Intensive Care Unit
Chaim Sheba Medical Center
Tel Hashomer, Israel

Arno L. Zaritsky, M.D.
Associate Professor of Pediatrics
Eastern Virginia Medical School
Co-Director, Pediatric Critical Care
  Medicine
Children's Hospital of The King's
  Daughters
Norfolk, Virginia, USA

Juraj Zbojan, M.D.
Head, Department of Neonatology
F. D. Roosevelt Hospital
Banska Bystrica, Slovakia

Jerry J. Zimmerman, M.D., Ph.D.
Associate Professor of Pediatrics
Director of Critical Care Fellowship and
  Research Programs
University of Wisconsin–Madison
  Medical School
Children's Hospital
Madison, Wisconsin, USA

Howard A. Zucker, M.D.
Assistant Professor of Pediatrics
  (Cardiology) and Anesthesiology
Columbia University College of
  Physicians and Surgeons
Pediatric Director, Intensive Care Unit
Babies Hospital
New York, New York, USA

Aaron L. Zuckerberg, M.D.
Assistant Professor
Department of Anesthesiology/Critical
  Care Medicine
The Johns Hopkins University School of
  Medicine
Baltimore, Maryland, USA

Contents

Case 1

Paloma Dorao, Juan C. De Carlos, and Francisco Ruza
Hospital Infantil La Paz
Madrid, Spain

HISTORY

A 10-year-old, 35-kg boy was admitted to the PICU because of acute dizziness, speech disturbances, and weakness in both legs. He had been well until 24 hours prior
to admission, at which time he complained of headache,
paresthesias, and pain in the lower extremities.

There was no history of drug or toxic ingestion, and no
history of recent infectious illness or vaccination. Family
background revealed an uncle who died of miliary tuberculosis 6 years previously. The child's father was treated for
rheumatoid arthritis.

PHYSICAL EXAMINATION

When examined, the child was conscious and in good
condition. His temperature was 36°C. The patient's heart
rate was 75 beats/min with a regular rate, respiratory rate
was 20 breaths/min, and blood pressure was 120/80 mm
Hg. He had good bilateral ventilation and his abdomen
showed no abnormality.

Neurologic examination revealed symmetric weakness
in upper and lower extremities with more proximal muscle
weakness compared with distal musculature. His senses
appeared intact and his reflexes were markedly diminished. Motor and sensory function on the chest and abdomen was preserved. He had positive Kernig and Brudzinski signs. Papilledema was not observed. He had bilateral
facial paralysis, which was more prominent on the right

1

side. All other cranial nerves were preserved. There was no cerebellar ataxia.

LABORATORY DATA

Laboratory values were as follows: hemoglobin 15 g%; white blood cell count 12,050/mm^3 (78% polymorphonuclear leukocytes, 8% lymphocytes); platelet count 118,000/mm^3; lactate dehydrogenase 225 U/l; creatine phosphokinase 82 U/l; aldolase 7 U/l. There was normal hepatic and renal function.

Lumbar puncture results showed cerebrospinal fluid (CSF) containing 2 white blood cells/mm^3, 42 mg% protein, and 64 mg% glucose. The boy's electroencephalographic findings were normal for his age.

Electrophysiologic study revealed delayed motor conduction with signs of demyelination without axonal involvement (Fig. 1.1).

Microbiologic screening results showed no bacteria.

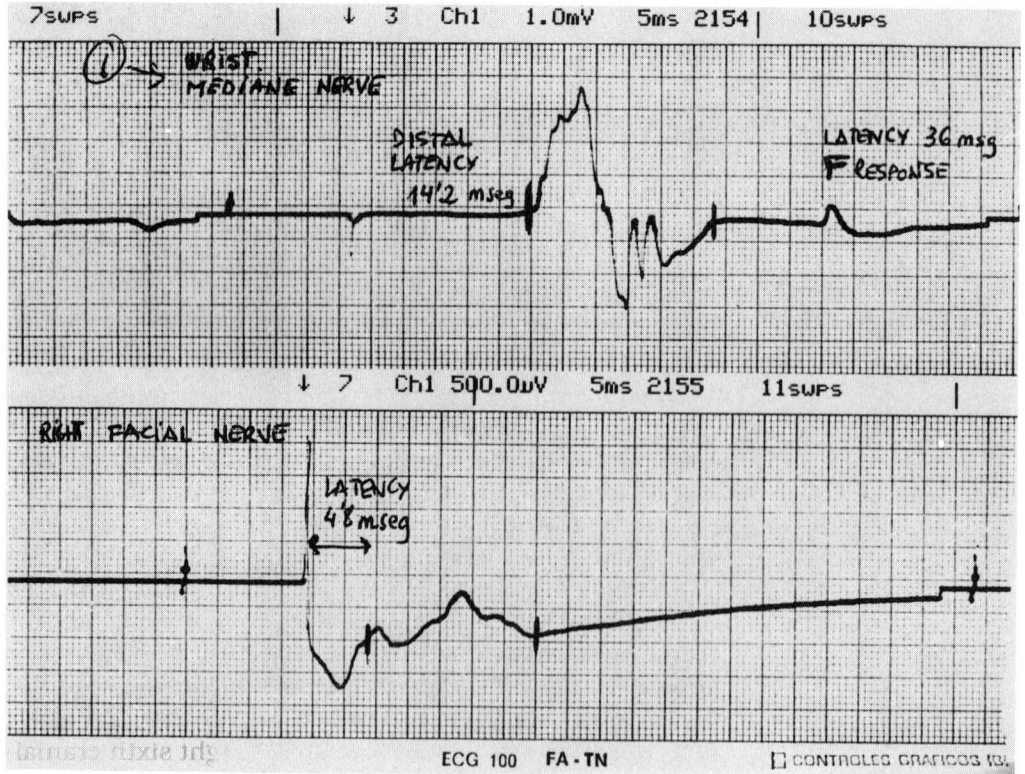

Figure 1.1. Electrophysiologic study at the time of admission.

Serum and CSF were collected for virus isolation and serologic studies.

MANAGEMENT

Twenty-four hours after admission, the child had severe ascending paralysis affecting his respiratory muscles, and loss of airway and swallow reflexes. He was intubated and mechanically ventilated. He had evidence of a sixth cranial nerve involvement with disconjugate gaze.

With the diagnosis of Guillain-Barré syndrome most likely, treatment with polyvalent γ-globulin (Endobulin), 400 mg/kg/d, and plasmapheresis, five sessions-cycle, was started. Through a jugular vein, a Vas-Cath 4000 (Gambro) was inserted, utilizing a Plasmafilter PF 2000 (Gambro). Exchange volume was 1.5 l (50% blood volume) with plasma or seroalbumin. Mean blood flow was 70 ml/min and heparin infusion was set at 20 U/kg/hr. After the first two sessions, paralysis of the sixth and seventh cranial nerves improved, and the child recovered movements in his arms and shoulders. He was weaned from the respirator after the third session.

Mild autonomic dysfunctions with hypertension and urinary retention developed in the child.

Three days after admission, the boy's liver and spleen appeared enlarged, with normal hepatic function. Serologic tests for Epstein-Barr virus, cytomegalovirus, and hepatitis A, B, and C viruses were negative.

Because of family background and the clinical presentation, a tuberculin skin test with 5 U of purified protein derivative was performed, which resulted in 9 mm of induration. Bacilloscopy and mycobacterial culture in bronchial aspirates, gastric content, and CSF were negative. Chest X-ray film appeared normal and CSF adenosine deaminase was 0.3 U/l. The family referred a negative Mantoux test 6 years before. Prophylaxis with isoniazid 5 mg/kg/d was started.

The patient was discharged from the PICU after 11 days with mild residual weakness and absent motor reflexes in both legs. He was sent home 1 week later.

Fifteen days after the initial admission, the child was readmitted because of gait disturbances and blurred vision. Physically, severe weakness affecting both legs, complete areflexia, and bilateral facial and right sixth cranial nerve paralysis were observed. The clinical course was considered a relapse of the Guillain-Barré syndrome; so γ-globulin and plasmapheresis were initiated again for 4 and 5 days, respectively.

Antinuclear antibodies, cryoglobulins, and rheumatoid factor were negative. IgG, IgM, and IgA were slightly decreased for his age (584 mg%, 38.4 mg%, and 31.1 mg%, respectively). Circulating immunocomplexes (57 μg/ml) and decreased C_3 (19.2 mg%) and C_4 (2.5 mg%) were detected. Circulating immunocomplexes measured in plasma and from the plasmapheresis decreased progressively from 67 μg/ml to 15 μg/ml during the 5-day cycle of plasmapheresis.

At that time, the results of the serologic tests for *Borrelia burgdorferi* and viruses that had been taken on the first admission were received. Negative titers for influenza A and B, parainfluenza 1, 2, and 3 adenoviruses, rhinovirus, Epstein-Barr virus, cytomegalovirus, and *Mycoplasma pneumonae* were obtained. IgG, IgA, and IgM titers in CSF and serum against *B. burgdorferi* were detected by enzyme-linked immunosorbent assay (ELISA) (1:500 dilution) and confirmed by immunoblot technique. Cross-reactivity to *Treponema* was ruled out by negative VDRL and fluorescent treponemal antibody.

With the diagnosis of Lyme neuroborreliosis, treatment with ceftriaxone 100 mg/kg/d for 14 days was initiated.

Titers of IgG, IgA, and IgM to *B. burgdorferi* assessed by ELISA and immunoblot techniques remained positive in blood and CSF on the 30th day of the disease. The CSF showed proteins of 320 mg% without pleocytosis (1 white blood cell/mm^3).

The sixth cranial nerve paralysis disappeared after the first session of plasmapheresis and facial palsy progressively improved. The child showed slow remission of weakness in both legs and partial recovery in motor reflexes when he was sent to the general ward. He complained of weakness in his legs and showed mild facial paresis when he was finally discharged in an improving condition.

DISCUSSION

Lyme disease is a multisystem illness that is caused by the tick-borne spirochete, *B. burgdorferi*. Although the disease has a worldwide distribution, only a few sporadic cases have been reported in Spain and those have been mostly in adults.

After the tick bite, early manifestations (weeks or months later) include the characteristic skin lesion: erythema migrans, accompanied by flu-like or meningitis-like symptoms, carditis, and some neurologic disturbances such as lymphocytic meningitis or meningoradiculoneuritis (Bannwarth syndrome in Europe). Late manifestations (usually more than a year after the tick bite) may be oligoarthritis, acrodermatitis chronica atrophicans, and some neurologic disorders such as encephalitis.

Neurologic manifestations are pleomorphic, with lymphocytic meningitis, with or without cranial nerve involvement, and peripheral neuropathy being the most frequent. Other neurologic disturbances such as transverse myelitis, acute encephalitis, chorea, cerebellar ataxia, chronic encephalomyelitis, pseudotumor cerebri, or polyradiculoneuritis are very unusual.

Polyradiculoneuritis or Guillain-Barré-like syndromes caused by *B. burgdorferi* have occasionally been reported. Unlike true Guillain-Barré syndrome, in these cases the neurologic involvement is asymmetric and usually not ascending, pleocytosis may be found in CSF, and the electrophysiologic study shows predominant axonal involvement.

A small number of cases of true Guillain-Barré syndrome have been described in patients with evidence of Lyme disease. There are no descriptions of such severe manifestations with respiratory compromise and need of mechanical ventilation, however. Such severe clinical features are occasionally found in *B. burgdorferi* meningoencephalitis, but not in the peripheral nervous system.

This patient fulfills the diagnostic criteria for Guillain-Barré syndrome. He had a symmetric ascending motor paralysis with areflexia and absence of sensory loss. He also had cranial nerve involvement, which has been described in 50% of the patients, with bilateral facial paralysis the most frequent finding. The disease had an acute onset with a rapid progression of the disease (less than 4 weeks). Involvement of the autonomic nervous system was mild in this case, with mild hypertension and bladder dysfunction. Besides the clinical criteria, the child had albumincytologic dissociation, with high protein content in the CSF and no pleocytosis. Electrophysiologic study confirmed the diagnosis of demyelinating polyneuropathy.

The diagnosis of Lyme disease depends on serologic findings. Although *B. burgdorferi* has been cultured from the CSF and skin of affected patients, isolation and culture of *B. burgdorferi* is not a sufficiently specific technique and not suitable for routine diagnosis. The laboratory diagnosis of Lyme disease is difficult. Indirect immunofluorescent assay techniques (IFA) were initially used, but currently ELISA techniques are preferred, because they can be automated and are easy to standardize. *B. burgdorferi* shares antigenic determinants with other bacteria, so false positive results with ELISA or IFA can be obtained. Therefore, a confirmatory procedure is needed. In this child, positive IgM, IgA, and IgG were confirmed by immunoblot in serum and CSF, and false positive results in relation to connective tissue disorders were ruled out (negative antinuclear antibody and rheumatoid factor). There was no evidence of cross-reaction with spirochete (negative VDRL and fluorescent titer antibody).

Advances in molecular genetics have provided other diagnostic tools such as polymerase chain reaction (PCR) technique. The possibility of detecting genetic material in different body tissues would help to define the pathogenesis of Lyme disease in the future.

A diagnosis of mycobacterial meningitis was initially considered because of the cranial nerve involvement, the positive tuberculin skin test, neck stiffness, and the family history. It was ruled out by the child's normal adenosine deaminase, chloride, cellularity in the CSF, and negative bacilloscopy and cultures. Normal lactate dehydrogenase, creatine phosphokinase, and aldolase, with no myopathic pattern on the electromyelogram, ruled out the possibility of metabolic myopathy. There are different causes of polyneuropathy (Table 1.1). Clinical presentation excluded the

Table 1.1. Differential Diagnosis of Polyneuropathy

Systemic Illness
  Uremia
  Diabetes mellitus
  Porphyria
  Chronic hepatopathy
  Amyloidosis
  Lymphoma, myeloma
  Paraneoplasic syndrome
Drugs
  Vincristine, nitrofurantoin, isoniazid, hydralazine
  Metronidazole, hydantoins, amiodarone
Toxins
  Heavy metals, organophosphorates
Heredity
Infectious
  Acute poliomyelitis
  Botulism
  Diphtheria
  Epstein-Barr virus
  Hepatitis B virus
  Lyme disease
Idiopathic
  Guillain-Barré syndrome
Vitamin Deficiency
  Thiamine, B_6, B_{12}

possibility of chronic polyneuropathy and polyneuropathy associated with systemic illness. There was no history of exposure to drugs or toxic substances, and the clinical presentation in either of those cases would have been different, so polyneuropathy associated with them was ruled out.

Among the possible infectious causes, no clinical signs suggesting botulism, poliomyelitis, or diphtheria were present, and the child had an adequate immunization status. There was no evidence of infectious mononucleosis or hepatitis B infection, with negative serology.

Lyme polyradiculoneuritis is probably best treated with ceftriaxone or cefotaxime, although there may be persistent radicular signs for as many as 24 months with the possibility of relapse.

Plasmapheresis has been reported to be effective in the treatment of severe Guillain-Barré syndrome and other immunocomplex-mediated diseases, mainly because of antibody clearance against neuronal antigens. Immunologic mechanisms have been involved in the pathogenesis of Lyme polyradiculoneuritis, although direct *B. burgdorferi* infection has been suggested.

The immunologic pathogenesis of Guillain-Barré syndrome and the favorable clinical course after plasmapheresis correlated with clearance of circulating immune complexes in this child. The relapse was, in our opinion, due to the transitory clearance of immunocomplexes and antibodies against neuronal antigens achieved by the plasmapheresis. Only after specific antibiotic treatment did the child finally improve.

We suggest the consideration of Lyme polyradiculoneuritis among the etiologic differential diagnosis of Guillain-Barré syndrome because of the possibility of specific antibiotic treatment. If immunologic pathogenesis is considered, severe neurologic disturbances with respiratory compromise might be best treated with plasmapheresis as well as with specific antibiotics.

COMMENTARY

Lyme disease is either becoming more prevalent or clinicians are becoming more aware of it. Despite this, confirmatory laboratory techniques have lagged behind our clinical acumen measured by the lack of specificity and sensitivity of these assays. The type of pathophysiology shown in the case of this patient demonstrates the principle of "the more we look, the more we see." We suggest a potentially broader role for plasmapheresis in any disease with immune complexes as part of the pathophysiology.

Suggested Readings

1. Asbury AK, Cornblath DR. Assessment of current diagnostic criteria for Guillain-Barré syndrome. Ann Neurol 1990;27s:s21–s24.
2. Halperin JJ. Nervous system manifestations of Lyme disease. Rheum Dis Clin North Am 1989;15:635–647.
3. Huppertz HI. Childhood Lyme borreliosis in Europe. Pediatrics 1990; 149:814–821.
4. Steere AC. Lyme disease. N Engl J Med 1989;321:586–596.

Case 2

Aroonwan Preutthipan, Subharee Suwanjutha, and Teerachai Chantarojanasiri

Ramathibodi Hospital
Bangkok, Thailand

HISTORY

A 50-day-old infant boy appeared at the PICU who had difficulty in breathing of 2 weeks' duration and difficulty in swallowing of 1 week's duration (Fig. 2.1).

The infant had an uneventful perinatal course and weighed 3100 g at birth. He was well until 2 weeks prior to admission when the mother noticed xiphisternal and subcostal retraction of the chest wall when the baby inspired. He did not have a cough, nasal discharge, or fever. One week prior to admission, he had further difficulty breathing, and snoring developed. At that time he could no longer tolerate oral feedings. One day prior to admission, the infant became hoarse. His mild respiratory distress was relieved somewhat when he was placed face down or on his side. The mother referred him to a local hospital where they diagnosed "an unusually long soft palate and uvula." The infant was then referred to Ramathibodi Hospital in Bangkok.

Past medical history was unremarkable, and the infant had a bacillus Calmette-Guerrin vaccination at birth.

PHYSICAL EXAMINATION

Vital signs were as follows: temperature 37.8°C (rectal), pulse rate 140 beats/min, respiratory rate 44 breaths/min, weight 3.7 kg, length 56 cm, and head circumference 37.5 cm.

The infant was fully conscious and alert without pallor, cyanosis, jaundice, or lymphadenopathy. The anterior fontanel measured 3×3 cm and was soft. The soft palate and uvula were nearly touching the posterior wall of the oropharynx and the baby was drooling. Cervical lymph nodes were not palpable. The infant had mild inspiratory stridor and a moderate degree of xiphisternal and subcostal retraction. His trachea was in the midline and his breath sounds were equal bilaterally.

No abnormalities were found in examination of the infant's heart and abdomen.

LABORATORY DATA

Laboratory values were as follows: a complete blood count: hemoglobin 12.4 g%, hematocrit 49%, white blood cell count 19,800 (polymorphonuclear leucocytes 59%, lymphocytes 36%, monocytes 4%, basophils 1%), platelet count 512,000, no toxic granulation, and normal red blood cell morphology. Urinalysis and chest X-ray results were normal.

MANAGEMENT

Because of the possibility of upper airway obstruction, an otolaryngologist was consulted. A nasopharyngeal tube was placed, which excluded the diagnosis of choanal atresia. A lateral neck X-ray demonstrated thickening of retropharyngeal soft tissue measuring three times the width of cervical vertebrae 4 (Fig. 2.2). The patient was then given general anesthesia for placement of an endotracheal tube. Through laryngoscopy, we observed a bulging fluctuating mass in the posterior pharyngeal wall. The retropharyngeal abscess was drained and we obtained cultures that grew *Staphylococcus aureus*. Intravenous administration of cloxacillin was presumptuously started and continued for 10 days. The endotracheal tube was removed 2 days after the operation. The infant's general condition improved dramatically during the next few days.

DISCUSSION

The infant was first seen with signs and symptoms of inspiratory airway obstruction with dysphagia and drooling, which suggested that the upper airway was the site

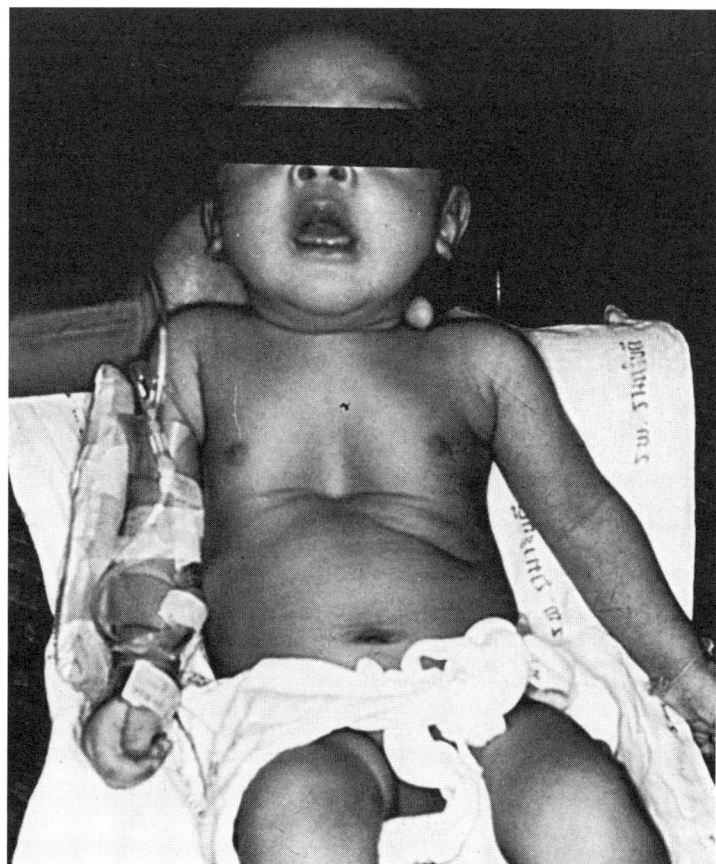

Figure 2.1. The patient: a 50-day-old infant boy.

of lesion. An inflammatory process was not initially considered because of the absence of fever or signs of infection. In addition, the differential white blood cell count was within normal limits. Although the lateral neck X-ray showed thickening of prevertebral soft tissue, making retropharyngeal abscess a possible diagnosis, there was no other clinical evidence to support this. There was no history of local trauma, so hematoma was unlikely. Moreover, adenoid hypertrophy would be an unlikely cause of airway obstruction at this age. The pediatric house officer's initial differential diagnosis included tumor, such as teratoma, angiofibroma, cystic hygroma, or other congenital abnormalities of the nasopharynx.

The diagnosis of retropharyngeal abscess was only made when direct laryngoscopy revealed a fluctuating mass from which aspiration obtained a purulent fluid. The retropharyngeal space is a midline area formed by cervical fascia extending from the base of the skull to the level of

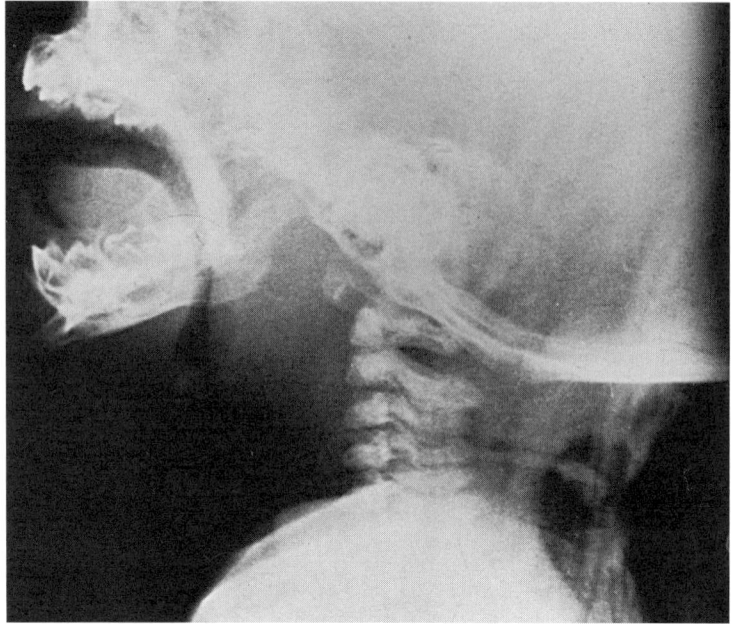

Figure 2.2. Lateral neck X-ray revealing thickening of the retropharyngeal soft tissue measuring three times the width of the C-4 vertebrae.

thoracic vertebrae 2. This area contains two paramedial chains of lymph nodes that receive drainage from the nasopharynx, adenoids, and posterior paranasal sinuses. These structures are prominent in early childhood and atrophy at puberty (1). The diagnosis of retropharyngeal abscess may be difficult in very young children (2). In this infant there was no history of a recent upper respiratory infection. No fever or other signs of bacterial infection were observed. However, he had dysphagia, was drooling, and had symptoms of inspiratory stridor and respiratory distress. A physical examination of his retropharyngeal abscess classically showed an erythematous oropharynx with unilateral fullness in the posterior pharynx. In this patient, the soft palate and uvula were unusually long and nearly touched the posterior pharynx, which misled us into making an incorrect initial diagnosis. A lateral neck roentgenogram is noninvasive, rapid, and provides useful information in the diagnosis of a retropharyngeal abscess. Wholy et al (3) have established norms for the width of the retropharyngeal space by roentgenography. In general, the retropharyngeal space is no wider than the width of the adjacent vertebral body of cervical vertebrae 4 (4). In addition to widening on lateral roentgenography, gas or a gas-fluid level may be present in the retropharyngeal space. If the findings from physical examination and lateral neck roentgenography are equivocal, a CT scan of the neck, examination of the oropharynx under general anesthesia, or an ultrasonographic examination is indicated.

When an abscess is present, surgical treatment is mandatory. Preferably, incision and drainage are performed intraorally under general anesthesia but they may be performed through an external lateral cervical approach (5). Initial management must be directed at securing the airway either by endotracheal intubation or tracheostomy if necessary. Antimicrobial therapy must be directed at the most common organisms including both aerobic and anaerobic bacteria. The common aerobic species were *S. aureus*, *Streptococcus pyogenes*, and *Streptococcus viridans* (6). Bacteroides species were more frequently isolated among anaerobic bacteria (6).

Possible complications of neglected abscess are profound and include rupture with pulmonary aspiration, mediastinal extension, airway obstruction with respiratory arrest, and erosion into the large cervical vessels with massive hemorrhage (7).

Retropharyngeal abscess should be included in the differential diagnosis in any young child with a history of swallowing or upper airway respiratory difficulties. The complications of this disease are significant, and an accurate diagnosis and appropriate treatment for this condition will lower the associated morbidity and mortality.

COMMENTARY

Retropharyngeal abscess represents a great challenge to the pediatric intensive care physician. It requires cooperation among many physicians to secure the airway safely and surgically drain the abscess. There must be consultation with the otolaryngologist, the pediatric intensivist, and the pediatric anesthesiologist. We hesitate to obtain a lateral neck X-ray for acute airway obstruction due to epiglottitis because it may postpone definitive therapy. This case of this infant demonstrates the appropriate use of lateral neck X-rays in airway obstructions that are not immediately life threatening.

References

1. Hammerschlag PE, Hammerschlag MR. Retropharyngeal abscess. In: Feigin RD, Cherry JD, eds. Textbook of pediatric infectious disease. 2nd ed. Philadelphia: WB Saunders, 1987:192–193.
2. Barratt GE, Koopmann CF Jr, Coulthard SW. Retropharyngeal abscess: a ten year experience. Laryngosceope 1984;94:455–463.

3. Wholey MH, Bruwer AJ, Baker HL. The lateral roentgenogram of the neck. Radiology 1958;71:350–356.
4. Seid AB, Dunbar JS, Cotton RT. Retropharyngeal abscesses in children revisited. Laryngoscope 1979;89:1717–1724.
5. Dean LW. The proper procedure for external drainage of retropharyngeal abscess secondary to caries of the vertebrae. Ann Otol Rhinol Laryngol 1919;28:566–572.
6. Asmar BI. Bacteriology of retropharyngeal abscess in children. Pediatr Infect Dis J 1990;9(8):595–596.
7. Schlossberg D, Fugate JS. Retropharyngeal cellulitis. Laryngoscope 1981;91:1738–1742.

Case 3

David W. Bernard, Steven D. Barnes, and David G. Nichols

The Johns Hopkins Hospital
Baltimore, Maryland, USA

HISTORY

An 8-year-old boy was seen following a 1-day prodrome of nonproductive cough, sore throat, rhinorrhea, and low-grade fever. Early on the morning of admission, he awakened his mother complaining of difficulty in breathing and feeling as if he might die. His mother noted that he had a temperature of 104°F and he was making high-pitched noises on inspiration with an associated bark-like cough. His mother placed him next to a steamy shower, but no improvement resulted. His past medical history showed no abnormalities. Review of systems revealed that he could swallow without difficulty and he could lie supine without worsening his respiratory status. His voice was hoarse and muffled but he had not been drooling.

PHYSICAL EXAMINATION

His vital signs when he was examined included temperature of 39.5°C, heart rate of 72 beats/min, respiratory rate of 36 breaths/min, and blood pressure of 135/80 mm Hg. He appeared anxious but was alert and talkative. He had clear rhinorrhea with boggy, erythematous nasal mucosa, but no nasal flaring was apparent. Pharyngeal examination revealed symmetric tonsils with mild enlargement and erythema, but no exudates were present. His neck was supple with bilateral 1-cm anterior cervical nodes that were nontender. Results of cardiovascular examination

15

were normal. Examination of his chest revealed suprasternal retractions with loud inspiratory stridor and symmetric expiratory wheezes, but there was excellent air movement throughout the lung fields. There were no rales or pleural rubs. The abdomen was soft with normal bowel sounds and no masses or organomegaly. His extremities were well perfused with strong pulses. There was no cyanosis or clubbing. Dermatologically, there was a fine macular rash on the boy's chest and back.

LABORATORY DATA

The oxygen saturation determined by pulse oximetry while the child was breathing room air was 97%. Arterial blood gas determination revealed a pH of 7.38, $PaCO_2$ of 39 torr, PaO_2 of 102 torr, and a calculated bicarbonate of 23 mEq/l. Complete blood cell count showed a white blood cell count of 10,700/mm^3 with 90% neutrophils, of which 28% were band forms, 8% lymphocytes, and 2% monocytes. His hemoglobin and platelet counts were normal. The neck radiographs demonstrated subglottic narrowing with a normal epiglottis and normal aryepiglottic folds. There was no evidence of a foreign body. Chest radiographs demonstrated mild hyperexpansion and a right lower lobe density. Cultures of blood and sputum were taken.

MANAGEMENT

The patient received a racemic epinephrine aerosol treatment with subjective improvement of his respiratory status. He was admitted to the hospital with the diagnosis of croup to be managed with humidified oxygen and racemic epinephrine aerosol treatments as needed. Decadron was begun to treat presumptive subglottic edema. Because of the infiltrate on chest radiograph, cefuroxime was started to treat a possible pneumonia. Continuous cardiorespiratory and pulse oximetry monitoring were initiated.

The boy continued on the above therapies for 48 hours with an apparent improvement in his respiratory status. He required no further racemic epinephrine treatments. His fever resolved after 24 hours of antibiotic therapy. His cough became productive of a greenish sputum, Gram stain of which revealed moderate numbers of neutrophils and Gram-positive cocci in clusters.

He awakened early in the morning on the third hospital

day with agitation and obvious apprehension. He developed worsening stridor and respiratory distress that were unresponsive to an aerosolized racemic epinephrine treatment. While being prepared for a portable chest radiograph, the patient became aphonic and suffered a respiratory arrest. Manual self-inflating bag-mask ventilation was unsuccessful. He became bradycardic, necessitating external cardiac compressions. An endotracheal tube was placed under direct laryngoscopy. Thick, purulent tracheal secretions were noted. He was successfully resuscitated following intubation, although he required atropine and epinephrine for cardiovascular instability. Chest radiograph after intubation demonstrated significant obliteration of the tracheal air shadow (Fig. 3.1). The diagnosis

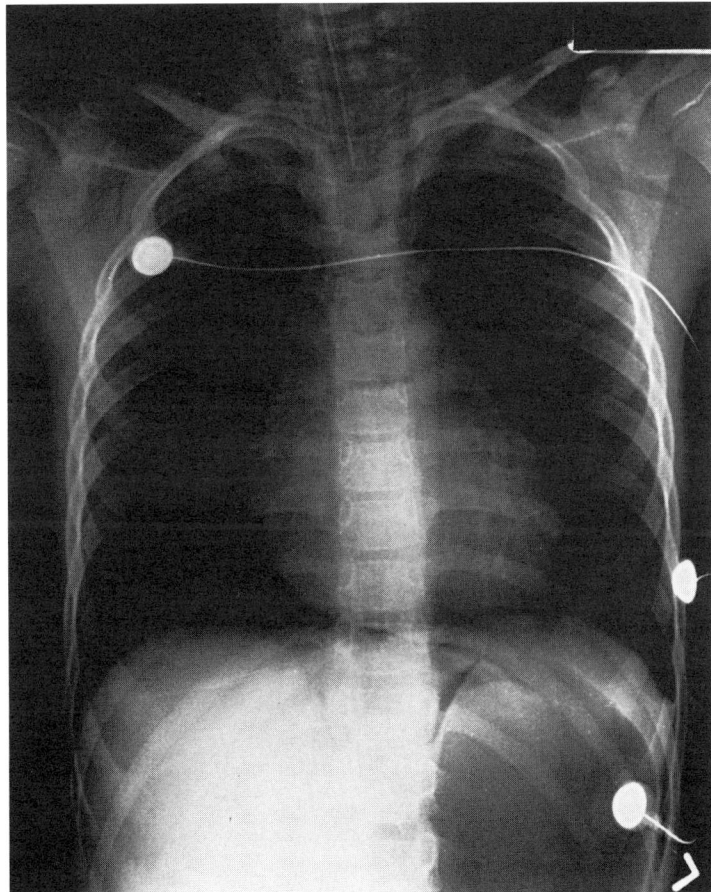

Figure 3.1. The chest radiograph, obtained shortly after intubation and stabilization, demonstrates almost total obliteration of the tracheal air shadow by the intratracheal secretions. Chest hyperexpansion is present secondary to the continued airway obstruction despite establishment of an artificial airway.

of bacterial tracheitis was made, and antibiotics were changed to oxacillin and gentamicin to treat a presumed *Staphylococcus aureus* infection.

His hospital course was complicated by copious, tenacious tracheal secretions that repeatedly obstructed his endotracheal tube. Cultures of these secretions were positive for *S. aureus* and parainfluenza type 2. On the fourth hospital day his clinical condition improved to the point where he could be successfully extubated. Examination after extubation revealed persistent stridor. He was observed to become aphonic and have worsening respiratory distress in the 12 hours following extubation. He was taken to the operating room where fiberoptic laryngoscopy revealed a normal supraglottic area. There were subglottic edema and purulent, inspissated secretions obstructing the subglottic airway (Fig. 3.2). Tracheostomy was performed to provide a patent airway. For several days following tracheostomy copious amounts of secretions were suctioned. Tracheostomy obstruction occurred on one occasion, which necessitated a change of the tracheostomy tube. Subsequently, the boy improved with antibiot-

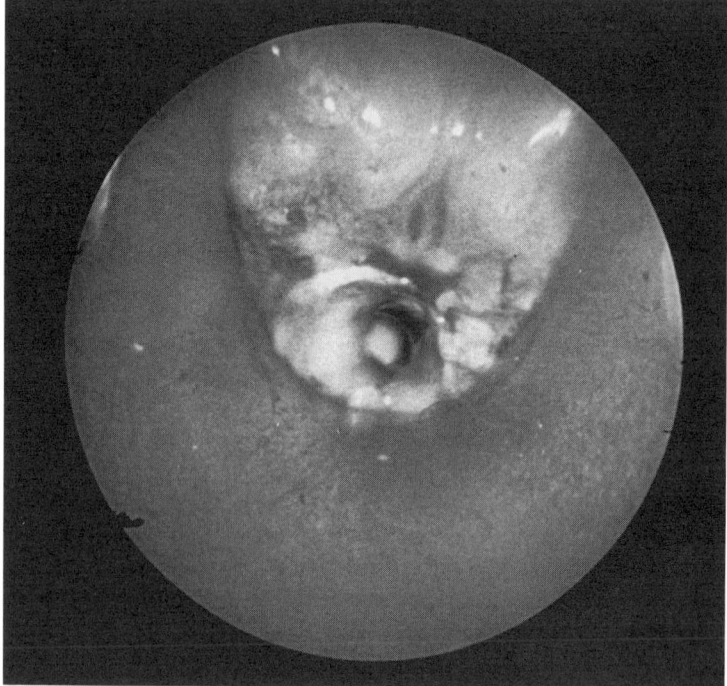

Figure 3.2. Through fiberoptic laryngoscopy, the subglottic inflammation is seen in association with purulent secretions that almost totally obstruct the airway.

ics and meticulous pulmonary toilet. He was discharged home in good condition and the tracheostomy tube was removed 3 weeks after his initial admission.

DISCUSSION

Bacterial tracheitis is an acute upper airway infection consisting of subglottic inflammation and edema, copious purulent secretions, and a normal epiglottis. The nomenclature is controversial but several synonymous terms are used in the literature: membranous laryngotracheobronchitis, nondiphtheric laryngitis, and pseudomembranous croup (1). Bacterial tracheitis should be considered in the differential diagnosis of acute upper airway obstruction.

The clinical differentiation of epiglottitis and croup has been previously well described (2). For bacterial tracheitis the mean age of onset is 4 years and there is a male to female predominance of 2:1 (3). Bacterial tracheitis probably results from bacterial superinfection in the setting of respiratory viral infection, commonly croup (4). Most cases are preceded by a mild illness with rhinorrhea, cough, low-grade fever, and stridor. The classic presentation is with high fever, toxicity, and respiratory distress following a prodromal illness.

Once the diagnosis is suspected, it can be confirmed only by direct tracheobronchoscopy. However, radiographs and laboratory studies can serve as adjuncts. The epiglottis and aryepiglottic folds appear normal on lateral neck radiographs, while there often will be marked subglottic narrowing. Occasionally intratracheal membranes will be interpreted as foreign bodies (1). The white blood cell count can be normal or elevated but will often exhibit a predominance of immature neutrophils. Respiratory viral cultures grow parainfluenza or other respiratory viruses. *S. aureus* is most commonly isolated from tracheal secretions, but *Haemophilus influenza* and *Streptococcus pyogenes* are also pathogens. Blood cultures are usually negative (5). The patient requires an artificial airway in as many as 85% of the cases, but the selection of the appropriate method (intubation versus tracheostomy) is controversial (1). Aggressive pulmonary toilet with frequent suctioning is required. Difficulty arises from obstruction of the airway with the thick secretions. Antibiotics are chosen to treat the common pathogens, but secretions and airway obstruction can remain a problem for some time after appropriate therapy has been instituted (4). Racemic epinephrine aerosols are of no value in relieving the obstruction.

Outcome varies by report but is potentially devastating with respiratory arrest and death. Pneumothorax, toxic shock syndrome, and overwhelming pneumonia have been reported as complications that contribute to the substantial morbidity. Mortality has recently been estimated at 3–5% (1). The diagnosis of bacterial tracheitis should be considered in all children with evidence of upper airway obstruction.

COMMENTARY

The controversy over airway management worldwide has led to widely divergent approaches to the child in respiratory distress. The clearest dichotomy exists in patients with epiglottis. In some centers, patients are immediately taken to the operating room for emergency establishment of an artificial airway, while in other centers the patients are closely observed and treated with antibiotics. Certainly when the airway is compromised to the point of obstruction, no one would argue that an artificial airway needs to be established regardless of the etiology—whether it is epiglottis, croup, or, as in this case, bacterial tracheitis.

References

1. Gallagher PG, Myer CM. An approach to diagnosis and treatment of membranous laryngotracheobronchitis in infants and children. Pediatr Emerg Care 1991;7:337–342.
2. Davis HW, Gartner JC, Galvis AG, Michaels RH, Mestad PH. Acute upper airway obstruction: croup and epiglottitis. Pediatr Clin North Am 1981;28:859–880.
3. Donnelly BW, McMillan JA, Weiner LB. Bacterial tracheitis: report of eight new cases and review. Rev Infect Dis 1990; 12:729–735.
4. Liston SL, Gehrz RC, Leighton GS, Tilelli J. Bacterial tracheitis. Am J Dis Child 1983;137:764–767.
5. Sofer S, Duncan P, Chernick V. Bacterial tracheitis—an old disease rediscovered. Clin Pediatr 1983;22:407–411.

Case 4

Zeev Kain,
Edward J. Novotny, Jr.,
and George Lister
Yale New Haven Hospital
New Haven, Connecticut, USA

HISTORY

A 16-year-old girl was admitted to the PICU because of status asthmaticus following an upper respiratory infection.

The patient had suffered from severe recurrent asthmatic episodes and was treated at home with oral theophylline and prednisone (10 mg/d) as well as albuterol and isoetharine inhalers.

PHYSICAL EXAMINATION

When she was examined at the hospital emergency room (ER), the girl's temperature was 37°C, respiratory rate was 34 breaths/min, heart rate was 170 beats/min, and blood pressure was 107/50 mm Hg. She had mild intercostal and suprasternal retractions with inspiration. By auscultation, she had poor air entry and diffuse inspiratory and expiratory wheezing.

LABORATORY DATA

Her chest radiograph was consistent with acute asthma (Fig. 4.1). Her white blood cell count, hemoglobin concentration, hematocrit, and electrolyte concentrations were normal in her peripheral blood, whereas the theophylline concentration was 47 mg/ml. Treatment with inhaled al-

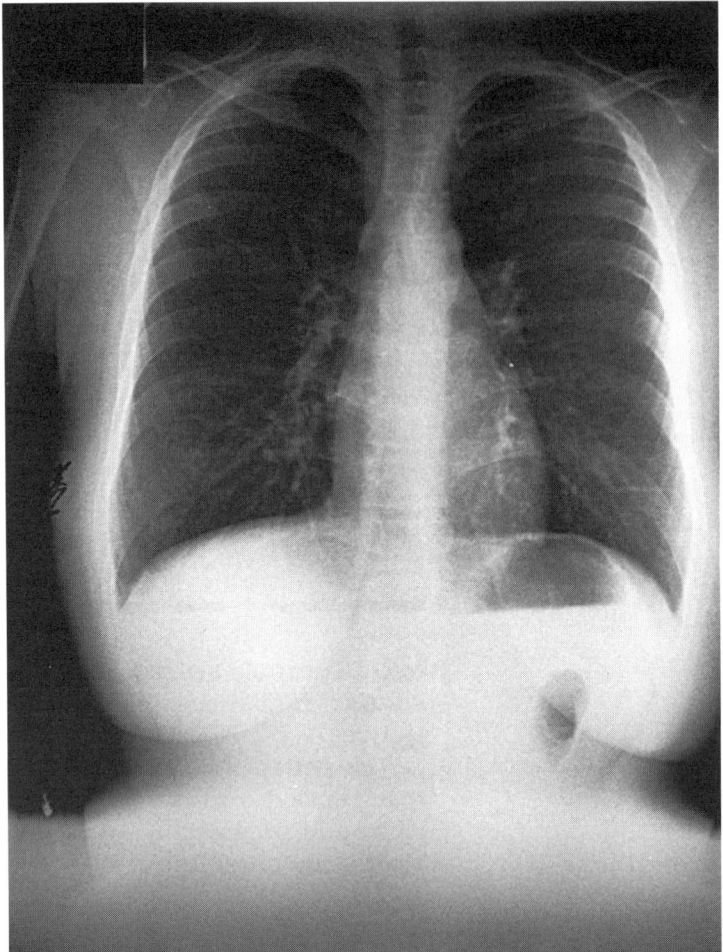

Figure 4.1. Radiograph of the chest obtained in the emergency room. There is marked hyperinflatation but no other specific findings.

buterol did not improve her respiratory function and she was transported to the PICU for further therapy.

MANAGEMENT

Intravenous isoproterenol and methylprednisolone (2 mg/kg/d) as well as frequent inhaled terbutaline, albuterol, and ipratropium were given. Her respiratory condition rapidly deteriorated and she complained of severe shortness of breath. An arterial blood sample had a pH of 7.50, PO_2 of 54 mm Hg, and PCO_2 of 60 mm Hg, while she received 100% O_2 via a non-rebreathing mask. Her trachea was intubated and she had to be sedated and paralyzed (with vecuronium) in order to achieve ventilation with an $FIO_2 < 0.60$ to sustain an arterial saturation greater than 85%. The next day, bilateral tension pneumothoraces developed in the patient and chest tubes were placed. The bronchospasm was refractory to all inhaled medications and the isoproterenol dose was increased gradually. An infusion of theophylline was started (after the blood concentration decreased below 20 mg/ml). On the second hospital day, the patient became febrile to 38.3°C, and a Gram stain of her sputum revealed numerous Gram-positive cocci and polymorphonuclear leukocytes. Bilateral lung infiltrates were seen on chest X-ray and intravenous penicillin G therapy was started.

Four days after starting the isoproterenol infusion (maximum dose 2.2 μg/kg/min), the patient developed hypertension (diastolic pressure 110–120 mm Hg), an intermittent S_3 heart sound, and signs of pulmonary edema (Fig. 4.2). An echocardiogram showed evidence of depressed cardiac contractility and the electrocardiogram

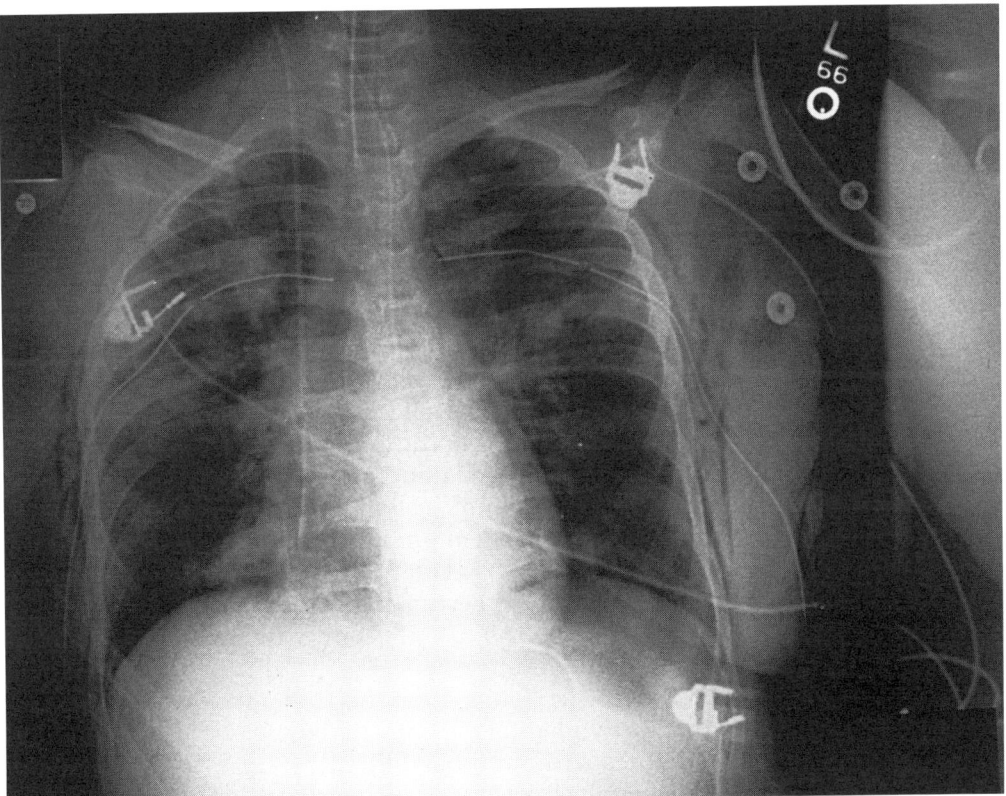

Figure 4.2.   Radiograph of the chest obtained in the ICU. The chest tubes were placed bilaterally for the pneumothoraces, and there is marked pulmonary edema.

(ECG) appeared normal except for the sinus tachycardia. The altered ventricular function was believed to be related to the increased left ventricular afterload and chronic administration of β adrenergic agonists. She had received isoproterenol in high doses on numerous occasions in the hospital and was treated with other β adrenergic agonists at home on a daily basis. The hypertension (which was not responsive to sedation or narcotics) was unexplained. Fluid restriction, furosemide, and hydralazine improved the pulmonary edema and the cardiac dysfunction. The fever did not subside with Penicillin administration and intravenous cefuroxime was started. *Candida albicans* was isolated in the urine and was treated successfully with Amphotericin B bladder irrigation.

On hospital day 9, the patient experienced some ventricular ectopy which was also thought to be related to the isoproterenol. The dose was decreased and intravenous terbutaline was started (0.2 μg/kg/min). After isoproterenol was stopped the ventricular ectopy disappeared and a marked reduction in heart rate was noted. The bronchospasm improved gradually, muscle relaxation was stopped, and sedation was decreased. After 11 days the patient was extubated; however, she remained tachypneic and complained of severe muscle weakness. A peripheral nerve stimulator applied over her left ulnar nerve revealed no adductor pollucis longis muscle movement with electrical stimulation. When electrical stimulation was applied over the orbicularis oculi muscle, however, a sustained tetanus was demonstrated. Eight hours after extubation she had to be reintubated (using no muscle relaxant) because of acute respiratory failure. With mechanical ventilation her air movement was good with only mild expiratory and inspiratory wheezing. A chest X-ray showed left lower lobe atelectasis and right upper lobe infiltrate. A sputum culture grew *Escherichia coli* and the Gram stain showed numerous leukocytes and Gram-negative bacilli. A 7-day course of intravenous clindamycin and ceftazidime was started for presumed pneumonia caused by *E. coli* or anaerobic organisms. One day later, gross myoglobinuria appeared and the serum creatine phosphokinase concentration was 1189 U/l. The myoglobinuria cleared with hydration and diuresis.

Ninety-six hours after the first attempted extubation (her 13th hospital day), the patient was extubated and she breathed with minimal difficulty (Fig. 4.3). She again had severe muscle weakness and complained of myalgia at this time. Neurologic assessment showed quadriparesis and some sensory involvement of all four limbs. Reflexes were

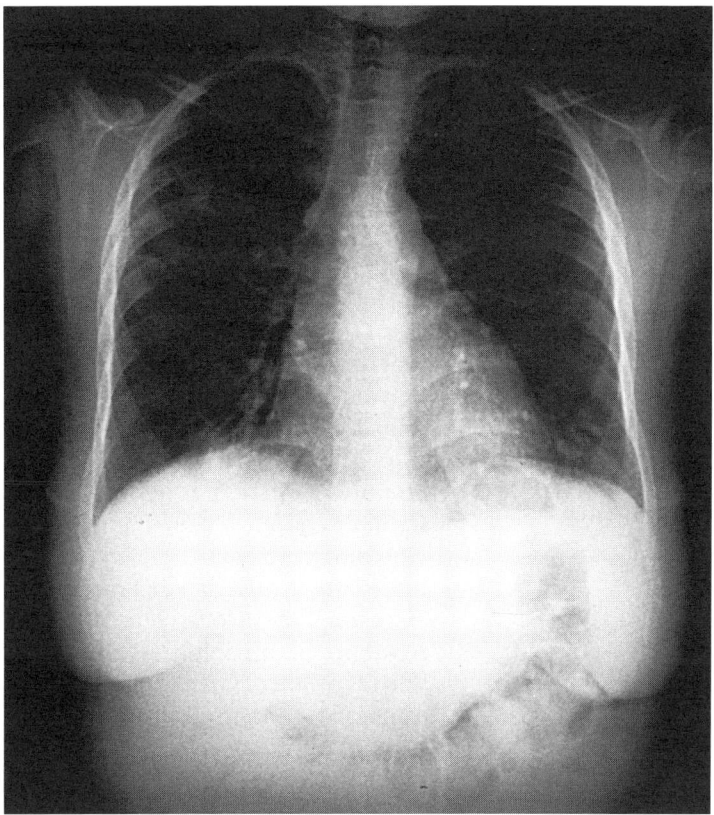

Figure 4.3. Radiograph of the chest obtained after recovery from the respiratory failure.

found to be absent and cortical function was assessed to be normal. Results of examination of the cerebrospinal fluid (CSF) were normal, with protein of 27 mg/dl and no cells. Albumin and IgG concentrations in the CSF were normal; viral and bacterial cultures had no growth. Nerve conduction studies showed evidence of a mixed axonal and demyelinating polyneuropathy. Sensory nerve conduction demonstrated a normal velocity with a low-amplitude response in the upper extremities and absent sural nerve potentials. Electromyography showed a severe diffuse muscle denervation in several muscles in both upper and lower extremities. The denervation was most prominent in the proximal muscles. These findings are most consistent with the clinical diagnosis of Guillain-Barré syndrome. Her respiratory functions continued to improve, intravenous drugs were stopped, and the patient was transferred to a rehabilitation unit. Examination 3 months later revealed marked improvement with minimal neurologic abnormalities.

DISCUSSION

Our patient demonstrated the unusual combination of refractory bronchospasm complicated by Guillain-Barré syndrome. A number of clinical findings were initially unexplained but made more sense once the diagnosis of Guillain-Barré syndrome was made. These include the hypertension (in the presence of depressed myocardial function), the failure to stimulate muscle contraction via a peripheral nerve, and the muscle weakness after the first extubation. Less clear is whether the initial need for mechanical ventilation was related to muscle weakness; however, the patient was able to walk into the ER without assistance, so there may not have been any contribution of Guillain-Barré syndrome to her initial respiratory failure. It is also unclear whether the myoglobinuria was a manifestation of muscle breakdown provoked by Guillain-Barré syndrome alone or in combination with steroids. Although it might be anticipated that rhabdomyolysis could occur with Guillain-Barré syndrome, we could find no report to substantiate this possibility. Of note is the fact that the girl did not have fever nor had she received neuromuscular blockade immediately preceding the myoglobinuria.

The occurrence of a coincident Guillain-Barré syndrome may explain many features of this unusual course. Guillain-Barré syndrome is an inflammatory polyneuropathy causing ascending motor weakness. Individuals with Guillain-Barré syndrome may require ventilatory support, and the disease remits spontaneously after a variable time period. The features that allow diagnosis of Guillain-Barré syndrome include clinical, laboratory, and electrodiagnostic criteria. The occurrence of an antecedent illness, usually a viral infection, is common. Features required for diagnosis include progressive motor weakness of more than one limb and areflexia (1). Other features strongly supportive of the diagnosis include rapid progression and recovery, relatively symmetric involvement, and autonomic dysfunction. Findings in the CSF supportive of Guillain-Barré syndrome include an elevated protein concentration and a white blood cell count of < 10 mononuclear leukocytes/mm^3. However, Guillain-Barré syndrome with normal CSF protein is observed in some patients. Cardiac arrhythmias and hypertension are seen among Guillain-Barré syndrome patients and are thought to be secondary to involvement of the autonomic nervous system (1).

Our patient experienced an upper respiratory infection

and the features required for diagnosis, namely, motor weakness and areflexia. The consistent hypertension, tachycardia, and ventricular ectopy may be the result of drugs administered, but may also represent autonomic dysfunction. We suggest that the initial course and symptoms of Guillain-Barré syndrome were obscured by the necessary treatment for the asthma and respiratory failure. Unfortunately, most of the typical Guillain-Barré syndrome features may be masked in intubated and paralyzed patients.

Critically ill polyneuropathy and an acute myopathy associated with the use of neuromuscular blocking agents should be considered with Guillain-Barré syndrome in the differential diagnosis of this case. Critically ill polyneuropathy is defined as a polyneuropathy found among patients with multiple organ failure and sepsis (2). In contrast, Guillain-Barré syndrome tends to occur in a younger age group and there is usually a history of a predisposing viral illness. Among patients with critically ill polyneuropathy, the polyneuropathy is noted at the peak of the critical illness and involves severe documented sepsis. The severity of the polyneuropathy is similar in both types, but it improves in the majority of patients with Guillain-Barré syndrome, while some of the patients with critically ill polyneuropathy are left with residual neuropathy. Patients with the acute myopathy observed with prolonged use of non-depolarizing neuromuscular blocking drugs usually have normal motor and sensory nerve conduction studies (3). Finally, analysis of electrophysiologic features can distinguish between these three different entities. Since this is the third report of Guillain-Barré syndrome associated with bronchospasm, we suggest that physicians be aware of this syndrome when there is unexplained respiratory failure and muscle weakness in a patient with asthma (4,5).

COMMENTARY

In most disciplines of pediatrics, illnesses are restricted to a single organ system. In the PICU, however, multiple organ systems are often involved in the pathology. The interactions of these pathologies makes critical care challenging as well as interesting. Recognition of two potentially life-threatening illnesses followed by successful treatment and support makes a case such as this gratifying.

References

1. Criteria for diagnosis of Guillain-Barré syndrome. Ann Neurol 1978; 3:565–566.
2. Bolton CF, Laverty DA, Brown JD, Witt NJ, Hahn AF, Sibbald WJ. Critically ill polyneuropathy: electrophysiological studies and differentiation from Guillain-Barré syndrome. J Neurol Neurosurg Psychiatry 1986;49:563–573.
3. Danon MJ, Carpenter S. Myopathy with thick filament (myosin) loss following prolonged paralysis with vecuronium during steroid treatment. Muscle Nerve 1991;14:1131–1139.
4. Hamilton RJ, Puckett R, Bazemore WC. Ventilator dependence in acute severe asthma due to a variant presentation of Guillain-Barré syndrome. Chest 1989;96:1205–1206.
5. Millar AB, Davis SN, Gross MLP. Prolonged ventilation in acute severe asthma caused by the Guillain-Barré-Strohl syndrome. J R Soc Med 1984;77:965–966.

Case 5

Jan A. Hazelzet, Edwin van der Voort, Wim Blom, and Coriene Catsman-Berrevoets
*Sophia Childrens Hospital
Rotterdam, The Netherlands*

HISTORY

A 6-month-old infant boy was transferred from a general hospital to our PICU, with a respiratory insufficiency. Seven weeks prior to admission, he was admitted to the general hospital with diarrhea and vomiting that were not responsive to dietary changes. Finally, he was treated with elemental feeding and given loperamide with reasonable success. On the day of transfer, the infant had hypotonia and apnea, with a slightly impaired level of consciousness.

The boy was the third child of healthy Dutch parents, born after an uneventful pregnancy of 32 weeks, with a birth weight of 2470 g. The neonatal period was uncomplicated.

PHYSICAL EXAMINATION

Physically, this was a premature-appearing, sweating infant. His weight was 6650 g (50th percentile for age), skull circumference was 0.46 m (97th percentile for age), heart rate was 180 beats/min, arterial blood pressure was 100/50 mm Hg, and rectal temperature was 39.8°C. Eye examination results, including funduscopy, were normal, with the exception of ocular bobbing and a slight facial diplegia. There was a general hypotonia and paresis grade 4, a maximal head lag, and a slipping-through phenomenon at vertical suspension. The reflexes were symmetrical (+2). Ear, nose, throat, heart, lungs, and abdomen showed no abnormal findings. Three days following admission, a deterioration in the boy's clinical situation occurred. Hypotonia increased and ptosis of the eyes worsened. His eyes showed myoclonic movements and pinpoint pupils. There was an irregular respiration, sometimes gasping, sometimes tachypneic. The infant seemed awake. The reflexes were diminished (−2). The next day he had areflexia, tachycardia, and a very irregular breathing pattern. The situation was complicated by severe paroxysmal bradycardias. He was then intubated and mechanically ventilated.

LABORATORY DATA

Extensive analysis of hematology, clotting function, liver enzymes, renal and thyroid function, immunoglobulins, vitamins A, B_1, B_6, B_{12}, E, lactate, pyruvate, and cerebrospinal fluid (CSF) showed no abnormalities. Microbiologic investigation revealed no recent bacterial or viral infection.

Electroencephalography, electromyography, and brainstem auditory evoked potentials repeatedly showed no abnormalities. Echoencephalography, CT scan, and magnetic resonance imaging also were normal. There was no gastroesophageal reflux. Urine analysis for metabolic diseases revealed a normal amino acid pattern, with dicarboxylic aciduria consistent with medium-chain triglyceride feeding.

MANAGEMENT

The diagnostic work-up proceeded with a goal to discriminate brainstem encephalitis, parainfectious disease, metabolic encephalopathy, neuromuscular disease, neurodegenerative disorder, and malignancies.

During the diagnostic work-up, the infant was treated with antibiotics, acyclovir, atropine, and immunoglogulins. Immunoglobulins were administered on the suspicion of Guillain-Barré disease. After 3 days of mechanical ventilation there was such an improvement that he could be extubated. One day later, however, he became irritable, tachypneic, pale, and hypotonic. The infant was sweating profusely and he had pinpoint pupils. Once again, there were periods of extreme bradycardias and respiratory distress necessitating endotracheal intubation. During the next several days, episodes of more or less severe autonomic dysfunction consisting of sweating, priapism, bradycardias, fluctuations in blood pressure, pinpoint pupils, and paresis of muscles including bulbar muscles were observed. These periods lasted for 2–4 days.

Because of the fact that the urine screening for metabolic diseases had already been performed, we did not immediately repeat this investigation. For this reason, it took some time to discover that there were metabolites of propyleneglycol derivatives as well as some unknown comounds in the urine. Propylene glycol is used as a solvent in many drugs, but not in those we used in this patient. The clinical picture was one of hypoadrenergic or a hypercholinergic. Therefore, we analyzed the patient's serum for known drugs with an adrenergic-blocking action and we estimated the plasma enzyme cholinesterase. This enzyme could not be demonstrated in plasma and was clearly decreased in erythrocytes. This information, together with the clinical picture, was very suggestive of the presence of a cholinesterase blocker in the plasma of the patient. For this reason we started with an antidote, obidoxim 5 mg/kg intravenously. In the course of 2 days, there was an evident improvement: the respiratory insufficiency disappeared, the infant was extubated, there were no bradycardias, the diarrhea and other autonomic symptoms vanished, and his neurologic condition improved.

After extensive analysis of several samples of urine of different days using gas chromatography mass spectrometry, we could identify the unknown compounds as fenthion and bayoxon as well as their metabolites. These substances are organic phosphate compounds often used in domestic animals as insecticides. The family of the patient had two dogs and was also in the possession of these drugs. We told the parents of the probability of an exogenous cause of the disease of their child. Considering the possibility of a so-called Munchausen syndrome by proxy, we asked the parents to talk with a confidential doctor to find an explanation for this matter. Because of the medical and psychologic problems the family had been through the previous year, the parents were referred to intensive psychiatric treatment. Two years after the admission, the boy and his family are in a stable situation, but still under psychiatric treatment.

DISCUSSION

This case can be divided into two separate problems: organophosphate intoxication and possible Munchausen by proxy. Diagnosis of poisoning is based on history of exposure, characteristics, and severity of symptoms. Clinical signs of poisoning with most insecticides and herbicides occur within minutes to a few hours. Organophosphates can be absorbed through the skin; they act by phosphorylating the active site of acetylcholinesterase. This inactive complex is so stable that organophosphates are referred to as irreversible inhibitors of acetylcholinesterase. Cholinesterase activity returns only after new enzyme is generated or following administration of a cholinesterase reactivator. If a patient is not treated with a cholinesterase reactivator, red blood cell cholinesterase may require several months to return to preexposure levels. Signs and symptoms of organophosphate toxicity result from accumulation of acetylcholine at the receptor sites and consist of excessive salivation, diarrhea, pupillary constriction, wheezing, bradycardia, muscle fasciculations, confusion, loss of reflexes, and respiratory and cardiovascular depression.

Serious, acute organophosphate poisonings are diagnosed by history, the presence of cholinergic signs, and the response to antidote administration (3). Death can occur within minutes following a large acute exposure. It may be useful to obtain a blood sample for red blood cell cholinesterase, but treatment should not be delayed until the results are available. Sensitive methods are available to measure urinary metabolites of several organophosphates such as malathion and parathion. The identification of urinary metabolites may be clinically useful to confirm or identify the agent in a poisoning; however, the test requires special technology and results are not likely to be quickly available.

Anticholinergic treatment must be initiated immediately if a severe organophosphate poisoning is suspected (2). Atropine antagonizes the central and muscarinic cholinergic signs. It will not reverse respiratory impairment caused by muscle weakness. For a child younger than 12 years of age, an initial intravenous atropine dose of 0.05 mg/kg is followed by a maintenance dose of 0.02–0.05 mg/kg, repeated every 10–30 minutes until cholinergic signs are reversed. A cholinesterase reactivator such as pralidoxime is the antidote for organophosphate poisoning. Enzyme reactivation occurs most markedly at the neuromuscular junction, with rapid restoration of normal skeletal response: normalization of diaphragm excursion and respiratory effort. Central effects do not respond to pralidoxime, because the drug is unable to penetrate the blood-brain barrier. A child is given 25–50 mg/kg infused over a 15- to 30-minute period.

Children afflicted with Munchausen by proxy have parents who consistently give fraudulent clinical histories, fabricated signs, and even intoxicate them, causing harmful medical investigations, hospital admissions, and treatment. Meadow published a list of warning signs, which should warn us and make us suspicious of the possibility of this syndrome. There is extensive literature on this subject (1).

COMMENTARY

It is often easier to diagnose what a problem is rather than what it is not. Munchausen syndrome by proxy illustrates this point. Identifying that a set of signs and symptoms can only be explained by an exogenous toxin administered in the hospital requires a great deal of fortitude and expertise. In the United States, medical staff are obligated to report even slightly suspicious cases to the authorities. This obligation does not exist worldwide, and this case illustrates that the system works well even in the absence of this law. As always, the medical and psychiatric needs of the child are the first priority.

Suggested Readings

1. Meadow RJ. Munchausen syndrome by proxy. Arch Dis Child 1982; 57:92–98.
2. Mortensen ML. Management of acute childhood poisonings caused by selected insecticides and herbicides. Pediatr Clin North Am 1986; 33(2):421–445.
3. Zwiener RJ, Ginsburg CM. Organophosphate and carbamate poisoning in infants and children. Pediatrics 1988;81:121–126.

Case 6

Nancy Setzer
Jackson Memorial Hospital
Miami, Florida, USA

HISTORY

A 2-year-old, 10-kg girl was admitted to the PICU directly from the operating room following complete repair of her tetralogy of Fallot.

The child was born at full term, and was diagnosed with both tetralogy of Fallot and esophageal atresia. The esophageal atresia was repaired at 9 days of age through a right thoracotomy. Postoperatively, she developed episodic cyanosis and had a left Blalock-Taussig shunt placed at 17 days of age. Following these surgeries, she recovered uneventfully except for a persistent barking cough and mild hoarseness. Prior to this admission for complete cardiac repair, she was receiving digoxin and had been in good health, with no history of pulmonary infections, and only mild cyanosis with exuberant crying.

The patient's intraoperative course was unremarkable. General anesthesia was induced with intramuscular ketamine (5 mg/kg) and maintained with fentanyl (150 µg/kg), pancuronium, and isoflurane. The anesthesiologist noted that there appeared to be narrowing of the glottis during intubation and that a size 4.5 endotracheal tube would only pass with difficulty; there was a small audible leak around the tube with a sustained inspiratory pressure of 20 cm H_2O.

The tetralogy repair consisted of a pericardial patch to enlarge the pulmonary outflow tract and annulus, a right ventricular infundibular resection, and a Dacron patch closure of the ventricular septal defect. The Blalock-Taussig shunt was ligated at the initiation of cardiopulmonary bypass at which time coronary anatomy was noted as normal. Surgical repair was completed through atrial and pulmonary artery incisions, without the need for ventriculotomy. Total aortic cross-clamp time was 48 minutes with a cardiopulmonary bypass time of 108 minutes. She was weaned from bypass using dobutamine 10 μg/kg/min and nitroprusside 1 μg/kg/min. Following chest closure, the patient was transferred to the PICU.

PHYSICAL EXAMINATION

The vital signs at the time of admission were as follows: blood pressure 107/55 mm Hg; central venous pressure 10 mm Hg; left atrial pressure 12 mm Hg; respiratory rate 16 breaths/min; rectal temperature, 102°F.

Physically, the child was unresponsive, with pupils equal and reactive to light. She was intubated and mechanically ventilated with bilateral breath sounds and an inspiratory tidal volume of 150 ml; oxygen saturation was 100% with an F_1O_2 of 100%. The remainder of her physical examination demonstrated diminished pulses in her left arm, chest wall scars from previous surgeries, and a fresh surgical mediastinal incision. Capillary refill time was 4 seconds. Monitors on admission included a right radial arterial line, right internal jugular central venous line, left atrial line, Foley catheter, and mediastinal drainage tubes.

MANAGEMENT

One hour after admission, as the child began to emerge from anesthesia and cough, she had acute hemodynamic deterioration with hypotension to a systolic pressure of 66 mm Hg, elevation of the central venous pressure to 17 mm Hg, with diminished peripheral perfusion and decreased urine output. There was moderate drainage of blood from her mediastinal and chest tubes (10 ml/kg) and an audible leak around her endotracheal tube with each mechanical ventilation. Oxygen saturation remained at 100% with an F_1O_2 of 70% and good bilateral chest expansion.

Several therapeutic maneuvers were instituted concomitantly. The nitroprusside was discontinued, and blood was given to replace that lost through the chest tubes. The dobutamine infusion was increased to 15 μg/kg/min and two doses of $CaCl_2$ (10 mg/kg) were administered. Analysis of blood gas taken during this episode was as follows: pH 7.18, pCO_2 77 mm Hg, pO_2 221 mm Hg, and HCO_3^- 28 mEq/l. In view of the increasing leak around the endotracheal tube and hypercarbia, the endotracheal tube was changed under direct visualization to a 5.0-uncuffed tube by the original anesthesiologist. It was noted that the glottic opening appeared to be larger than during the initial laryngoscopy several hours previously. This tube had a small leak; exhaled tidal volume as measured by spirometry increased from 100–200 ml. Over the next 10 minutes, there was a dramatic increase in systolic blood pressure to 88 mm Hg, with a decrease in central venous pressure to 11 mm Hg. Follow-up analysis of blood gases demonstrated resolution of the hypercarbia. The child was weaned from mechanical ventilation and extubated the morning after surgery. The remainder of her ICU course was unremarkable. Postoperatively, there was no clinical evidence of recurrent laryngeal or phrenic nerve injury.

DISCUSSION

Although the hemodynamic compromise in this child was easily treated, hypotension in infants following open heart surgery requires rapid careful consideration of all the physiologic and anatomic perturbations that may be present. Hemodynamic deterioration may be precipitous, and therapy instituted without all of the data needed to accurately diagnose the cause of the instability.

Postoperatively, the child with tetralogy of Fallot is likely to develop right and left ventricular failure for a number of reasons. Frequently, the pulmonary outflow tract is reconstructed using a pericardial patch across the pulmonary valve annulus. Unusually (<1% of patients), the child is left with marked pulmonary valvular insufficiency. Acute elevations of pulmonary vascular resistance with resultant right ventricular afterload can increase the amount of regurgitation and potentially precipitate acute right-sided heart failure (1). The patient described above developed hypercarbia upon awakening from anesthesia, coughing and "fighting the ventilator," which increased the leak around the endotracheal tube and decreased effective ventilation. Carbon dioxide is a potent pulmonary vasoconstrictor. This elevation of pulmonary vascular resistance results in acute right ventricular dilatation and failure. It is recognized that a similar phenomenon occurs in intubated children with a patent foramen ovale who exhibit transient cyanosis and arterial oxygen desaturation during coughing and straining while emerging from general anesthesia. Transthoracic echocardiography has demonstrated acute intraatrial right to left shunting during such episodes in these normal children (2).

It is probable that some of the hypotension was a consequence of acute right ventricular failure, which led to diminished left ventricular preload. With right ventricular failure and dilatation, there was probably a shift of the interventricular septum (comprised of the very compliant Dacron patch) into the left ventricular cavity, creating diminished left ventricular volume.

There are other reasons for decreased myocardial function following open heart surgery and cardiopulmonary bypass. During aortic cross-clamping, the heart is not perfused; the myocardium is preserved by a cardioplegia solution that uses cold temperatures and high levels of potassium to arrest the heart in diastole. Although myocardial metabolism is minimized by these maneuvers, invariably there is a small amount of metabolism occurring, as evidenced by decreased myocardial cellular pH and elevated coronary sinus lactic acid levels. As with any organ that has sustained an ischemic injury, some degree of dysfunction may be anticipated following reperfusion.

Other intraoperative factors that are linked to myocardial injury include intraoperative coronary damage (direct or through embolism) and the need for a ventriculotomy resulting in direct muscle damage.

In our patient, other major diagnoses that needed to be considered and rapidly excluded during the period of acute instability were hypovolemia related to blood loss and pericardial tamponade. Excessive blood loss as a solitary cause was considered unlikely because of the elevated right heart filling pressure. Pericardial tamponade is an ever present possibility in the fresh postoperative patient, particularly when there has been copious bleeding from the surgical drains that abruptly ceases, suggesting occlusion of the drainage tube. This is most likely in the clinical setting of progressively elevating cardiac filling pressures with hypotension and poor cardiac output. As such, it may be difficult to clinically differentiate tamponade from isolated myocardial failure following cardiac surgery. Although the diagnosis may be made by transthoracic echocardiagraphy, the amount of time needed to order and obtain the study may preclude its usefulness in the hemodynamically unstable patient.

Continuous transesophageal echocardiography is an exciting, relatively new modality that is used intraoperatively to monitor cardiac function, filling volumes, and anatomical structural abnormalities in adults and larger children. It is anticipated that with development of smaller probes and less expensive hardware, the usefulness of this monitoring modality may be extended to the intubated child in the ICU.

The significance of a leak around the endotracheal tube during mechanical ventilation needs to be considered. It has been demonstrated in animal models that capillary perfusion of the tracheal mucosa ceases and histologic damage occurs when the pressure on the trachea exceeds 25 mm Hg; this correlates with an audible leak around the endotracheal tube at a similar inspiratory pressure (3). To date, there has been no prospective data linking leak pressure with subglottic stenosis in the intubated child in the ICU.

COMMENTARY

This case represents the complicated challenges of managing a child who has just undergone cardiac surgery. With all of the perturbations in preload, afterload, and inotropy, the first priority once again is the airway and breathing. An underappreciated process is the fact that positive pressure ventilation provides afterload reduction to the left ventricle by increasing intrathoracic pressure, thus reducing the work the left ventricle has to expend to push blood into the abdominal aorta. This afterload reduction with positive pressure ventilation is of course lost when ventilation becomes ineffective. With an optimally sized endotracheal tube and optimal ventilatory parameters, not only are the blood gases normalized (thus decreasing pulmonary pressures and septal shifts) but the myocardial oxygen supply/demand ratio is improved.

References

1. Fuster V, McGoon DC, Kennedy MA, et al. Long-term evaluation (12 to 20 years) of open heart surgery for tetralogy of Fallot. Am J Cardiol 1980;46:635–642.
2. Moorthy SS, Haselby KA, Caldwell RL, et al. Transient right-left interatrial shunt during emergence from anesthesia: demonstration by color flow doppler mapping. Anesth Analg 1989;68:820–822.
3. Finholt DA, Audenaert SM, Stirt JA, et al. Endotracheal tube leak pressure and tracheal lumen size in swine. Anesth Analg 1986;65: 667–671.

Case 7

Gideon Paret, Eli Gilad, Eyal Winkler, and Zohar Barzilay

Chiam Sheba Medical Center
Tel Hashomer, Israel

HISTORY

A 3-year-old boy was referred to a local emergency room (ER) with nausea 3 hours after he was bitten by a *Vipera palaestinae* snake on his right foot. Past medical history documented a post-traumatic removal of his spleen when he was 18 months old.

Physical examination results were normal except for a blue discoloration and a single fang mark visible on the boy's foot. During the following day the foot became swollen, and the child was transferred to the Sheba Medical Center.

PHYSICAL EXAMINATION

On arrival 30 hours after envenomation, the child was somnolent, with the following vital signs: blood pressure 95/45 mm Hg, pulse rate 125 beats/min, and respiratory rate 20 breaths/min. The child had edema and discoloration extending up to his groin (Fig. 7.1). Subcutaneous hemorrhages were noted at the lateral aspect of the foot. Dorsalis pedis and tibialis posterior pulses were easily palpable. No abnormalities of the heart or lung were noted.

LABORATORY DATA

Laboratory studies at the time of admission revealed the following results: hemoglobin 6.5 g/100 ml, white blood cell count 11,700/mm^3, platelets 16,000/mm^3. Prothrom-

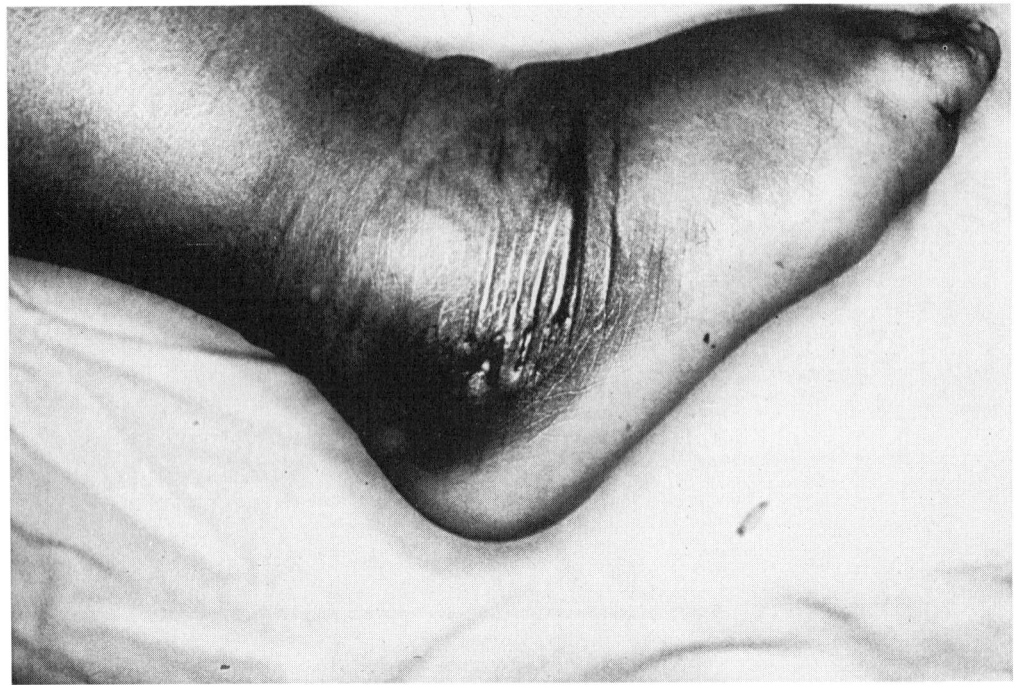

Figure 7.1. Right foot showing envenomation site 30 hours postinjury.

bin time (PT) was 14.7 seconds (62% of normal) and activated thromboplastin time was 33.7 seconds (normal 30–36 seconds). Fibrin degradation products were normal. Total protein was 6.5 g/100 ml (albumin 3.2 mg%). Arterial blood gas analysis showed a compensated metabolic acidosis: pH 7.34, PCO_2 28 mm Hg, PO_2 60 mm Hg, and bicarbonate 14.2 mm/l (F_IO_2 0.3). Chest X-ray, ECG, cardiac enzymes, and results of liver and kidney function tests were normal.

MANAGEMENT

Fluid resuscitation was begun with intravenous 5% albumin (100 ml), packed red blood cells (150 ml), crystalloids (300 ml), and sodium bicarbonate. Six hours after admission (36 hours after the bite), local progression of the hematoma and swellings, as well as nausea and vomiting, were noted. Five vials (10 ml/vial) of *V. palaestinae*-specific antivenin (Rogoff Institute, Petah Tikva, Israel) were given, followed by gradual relief of signs and symptoms. No immediate adverse effects were noted. Within 12 hours after admission, the boy had a swollen right leg, but was in good general condition, hemodynamically stable, and all laboratory results were normalized.

On the following day, 72 hours after envenomation, he became dyspneic and tachypneic. His temperature was 38°C. Moist rales were heard over both lung fields. Mean central venous pressure was 8 mm Hg. Arterial blood gas samples showed severe hypoxemia: pH 7.32, pCO_2 49 mm Hg, pO_2 58 mm Hg (on F_IO_2 1.0). Repeat chest X-ray showed severe pulmonary congestion consistent with adult respiratory distress syndrome (Fig. 7.2). Shortly thereafter, despite therapy with oxygen and intravenous furosemide, respiratory insufficiency necessitated tracheal intubation and mechanical ventilation.

Following intubation, the child had the following arterial blood gas values: pH 7.38, PCO_2 42 mm Hg, PO_2 126 mm Hg (F_IO_2 0.4 positive end-expiratory pressure 10 cm H_2O).

Within 72 hours after intubation, clinical and respiratory improvement was noted and weaning from mechani-

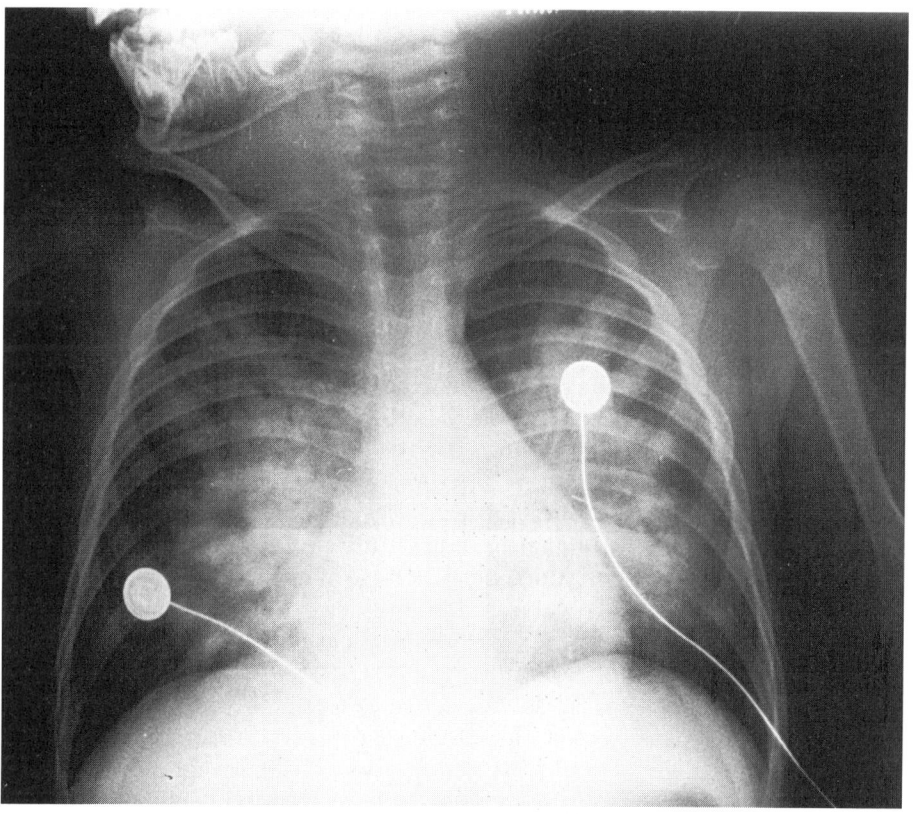

Figure 7.2. Chest roentgenogram: frank pulmonary edema. Heart is not enlarged.

cal ventilation led to extubation on the following day. Swelling of the leg improved and gradually resolved, and the child was discharged on the 10th hospital day. No signs of serum sickness were seen during the hospital course.

DISCUSSION

Snake envenomation is a life-threatening accident that is not uncommon throughout the world. Of the five families of poisonous snakes in the world, *Viperidae* (old world vipers) usually cause primarily local effects and bleeding (1). However, systemic manifestations, including bleeding from the mucous membranes, urinary tract, and into the myocardium and the central nervous system have been described (2, 3). The course of viper bite poisoning is usually more benign in children than in adults, perhaps due to their lesser tendency to develop anaphylaxis (2). Our patient showed all classical features attributed to *V. palaestinae* envenomation, including local skin necrosis, subcutaneous hemorrhage, edema of the affected limb, and thrombocytopenia.

The late respiratory failure is more difficult to explain. Early pulmonary edema is the most severe respiratory feature occurring in scorpion sting (4). Its mechanism remains unclear, and the few studies designed to examine it provide contradictory conclusions. Rahav et al. described two cases of early pulmonary edema due to myocardial failure after scorpion sting (5). Both patients had diffuse ST-T changes, elevation of creatine phosphokinase levels, and reduced left and right ventricular function. Immediate myocardial damage following scorpion sting in two patients was described by Barzilay et al. (6). However, heart failure or respiratory symptoms have not been reported in *V. palaestinae* envenomation (7).

Our patient developed noncardiogenic pulmonary edema and respiratory failure 72 hours after viper envenomation, despite lack of clinical or laboratory evidence of myocardial damage. Two possible explanations are suggested: (1) delayed effect or allergic reaction to the venom or the antivenom (1); (2) alveolar capillary leak secondary to massive release of necrotic tissue factors from the affected limb. Late respiratory failure due to a delayed reaction to the venom has not been reported in the literature. Administration of heterologous serum proteins may precipitate severe early reactions, some of which are due to a hypersensitivity and others to anticomplementary activity of the antivenom (8). However, no immediate reaction or delayed hypersensitivity developed in our patient following antivenom treatment. Furthermore, serum immunoglobulins and complement were within the normal range.

In summary, we described a patient in whom noncardiogenic pulmonary edema developed following *V. palaestinae* envenomation. To our knowledge, late respiratory failure and pulmonary edema have not been reported following *V. palaestinae* envenomation. Further studies are warranted to examine its origin.

COMMENTARY

Snake bite is an unusual case for many PICUs. In caring for snake bite victims, late respiratory failure and pulmonary edema are unusual complications. It is gratifying to apply the technological PICU tools to restore physiologic stability, regardless of the etiology, so that patients will have such a good outcome.

References

1. Jurkovich GJ, Luterman A, McCullar K, Rameonfsky ML, Curreri PW. Complications of Crotalidae antivenin therapy. J Trauma 1988;28(7): 1032–1037.
2. Ben-Ami M, Hagher H, Katzuni E, Arens R. Recovery from multiple bites by Vipera Xanthina Palestinae. Clin Pediatr Phila 1982;21(10): 599.
3. Myint-Lwin, Phillips RE, Tun-Pe, Warrel DA, Tin-Nu-Swe, Maung-Maung-Lay. Bites by Russell's viper (Vipera Russelli Siamensis) in Burma: haemostatic, vascular, and renal disturbances and response to treatment. Lancet 1985;7(12):1259–1264.
4. Abroug F, Boujdaria R, Belghith M, Nouria S, Bouchouch S. Cardiac dysfunction and pulmonary edema following scorpion envenomation. Chest 1991;100(4):1057–1059.
5. Rahav G, Weiss AT. Scorpion sting-induced pulmonary edema. Scintigraphic evidence of cardiac dysfunction. Chest 1990;97:1478–1480.
6. Barzilay Z, Shaher E, Schneeweiss Z, Motro M, ShemTov A, Neufeld HN. Myocardial damage with life-threatening arrhythmia due to a scorpion sting. Eur Heart J 1982;3:191–193.
7. Winkler E, Chovers M, Almog S, Tirosh M, Halkin H, Ezra D. Vipera Palaestinae bites—clinical experience in Israel. In: Proceedings of the 10th World Congress on Animal, Plant and Microbial Toxins. Singapore, Nov. 1991.
8. Sutherland SK. Venom and antivenom research. Med J Aust 1980; 2:246–250.

Case 8

Jaime Cordero and Jose Baeza
Hospital Luis Calvo Mackenna
Santiago, Chile

HISTORY

An 11-year-old girl was admitted to the PICU for orthopnea, epigastric pain, and progressive edema. There were no contributing historical factors in this case, and the child was well prior to the time of her admission with no history of recent illness. Her family and social history were noncontributory.

PHYSICAL EXAMINATION

This was a well-nourished, alert, Tanner 2 child. The vital signs were as follows: blood pressure 105/60 mm Hg, heart rate 112 beats/min, temperature 36.3°C, respiratory rate 16 breaths/min. Cranial examination revealed perioral cyanosis. Her upper airway was normal. She had some expiratory wheezing and muffled heart sounds without any murmur or gallops. She had poor peripheral perfusion. Abdominal examination showed a mild degree of hepatomegaly.

LABORATORY DATA

Analysis of arterial blood gases, hematocrit, blood urea nitrogen, glucose, and electrolytes showed normal values. A chest X-ray revealed a rounded cardiac enlargement and signs of pulmonary congestion. The ECG showed a peaked P wave with diminished voltage in all leads. There were no signs of ischemia.

MANAGEMENT

Because of the suspicion of cardiogenic shock, 40% oxygen was administered by mask, furosemide (3 mg/kg), dopamine (6 μg/kg/min), and dobutamine (4 μg/kg/min) were initiated. A 2D echocardiogram was performed that demonstrated a pericardial effusion, signs of cardiac tamponade, and a mobile echodense image attached to the apex that moved freely inside the pericardial cavity (Fig. 8.1).

The girl continued to demonstrate progressive cardiovascular and respiratory impairment; endotracheal intubation and mechanical ventilation were instituted. dobutamine was increased to 14 μg/kg/min. A pericardiocentesis was performed, draining 900 ml of hemorrhagic fluid with 35.8 g/l albumin content, 330 red cells mm^3, and 8600 white cells mm^3, 70% of them neutrophils. This procedure transiently relieved her symptoms, but she worsened 4 hours later. A pericardial drain was placed, and the patient remained in stable hemodynamic and respiratory condition for 24 hours, draining 300 ml of serous hemorrhagic fluid.

Twenty-four hours after admission, the patient suffered a sudden cardiovascular decompensation with hypotension, and was unresponsive to the administration of inotropic agents and volume. She was placed on mechanical

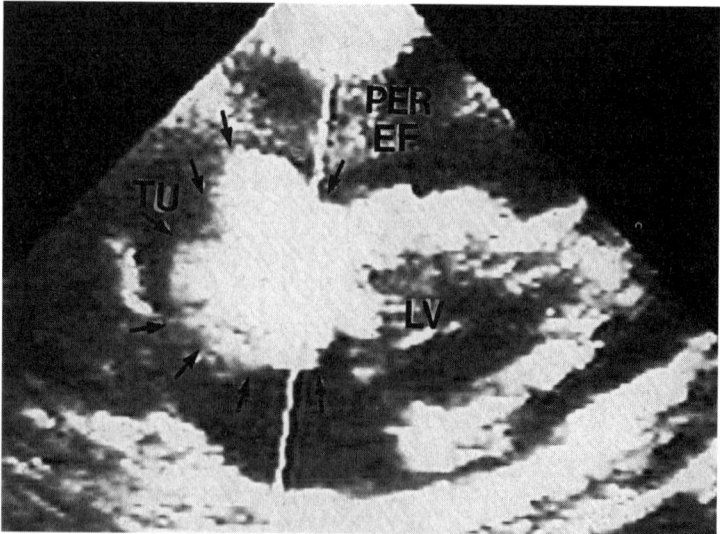

Figure 8.1. Echocardiography. Large pericardial effusion. Echodense image attached to the apex is shown in *white arrows*. *TU*, tumor; *PER EF*, pericardial effusion; *LV*, left ventricle.

ventilation with 100% oxygen concentration, with oxygen saturations around 70%. The pericardial drain was changed, but no fluid was obtained. Ventricular tachycardia was treated with lidocaine, cardioversion, and bretylium. The rhythm deteriorated to ventricular fibrillation, which was treated with electrical defibrillation without success. The patient died after 90 minutes of cardiopulmonary resuscitation.

The necroscopy revealed multiple primary myocardial tumors in both ventricles, the largest being located in the apex of the heart (4 cm × 6.5 cm × 4 cm) (Fig. 8.2). Smaller tumors were found in the aortic arch, main pulmonary vessels, and visceral pericardium.

The cytologic analysis of the pericardial effusion showed anaplastic sarcomatous cells. Histology revealed alveolar rhabdomyosarcoma (Fig. 8.3). Reactive myocarditis and pericarditis were demonstrated and histologic signs of shock were seen in lungs, liver (center lobule necrosis), and kidneys (tubular necrosis).

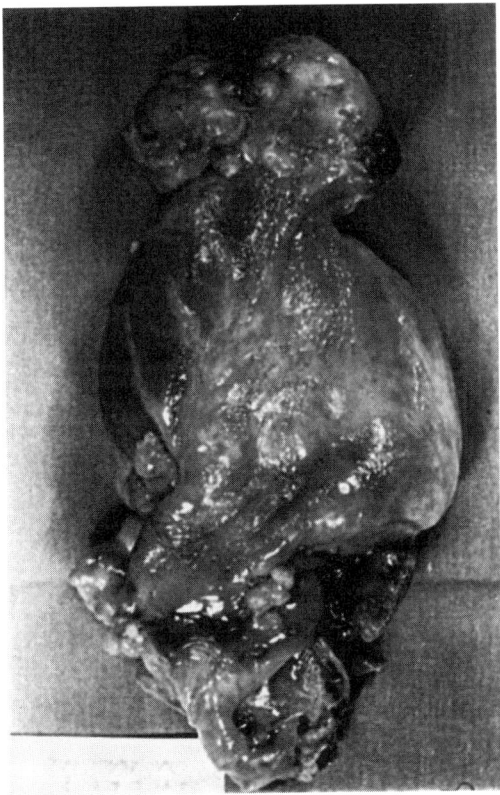

Figure 8.2. Primary rhabdomyosarcoma of the heart. The main tumoral mass involves the apex; smaller tumors appear in between the great vessels, and diffuse fibrinous pericarditis is shown.

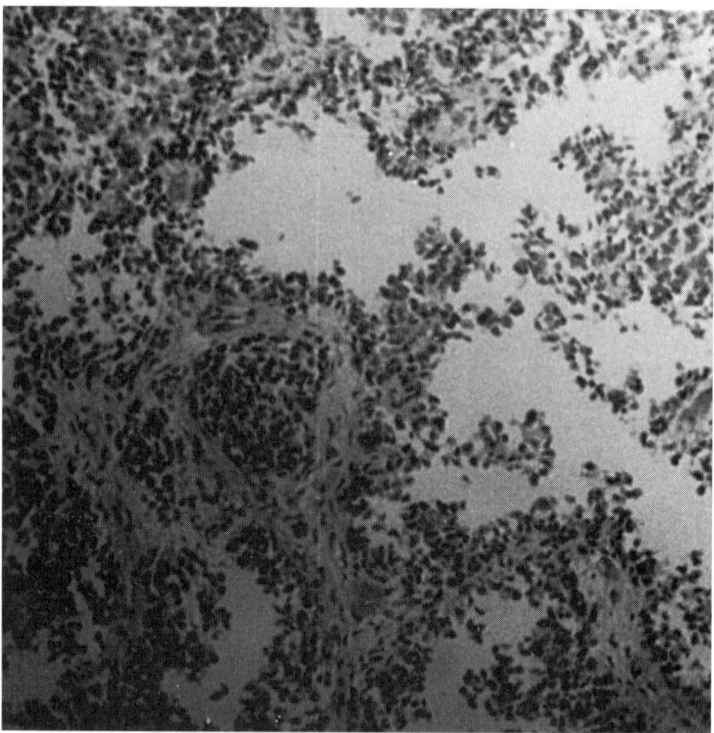

Figure 8.3. Alveolar rhabdomyosarcoma. Undifferentiated round, loosely cohesive tumoral cells separated by fibrous septrum. (hematoxylin & eosin × 210)

DISCUSSION

A case of primary cardiac rhabdomyosarcoma in an 11-year-old girl with pericardial effusion and cardiac tamponade with rapidly progressive heart failure is described. Tumoral invasion of the pericardium may give a clinical picture of acute respiratory distress, chest pain, palpitations, heart failure, and extracardiac symptoms such as fever and myalgia. If the conduction system of the heart is involved, arrhythmias may occur that may become intractable.

Primary cardiac tumors rarely occur (0.001–0.28% incidence), 2% of which are rhabdomyosarcomas. Such tumors are uncommon in our patient's age group. Among females, the highest incidence is between 40 and 50 years of age, whereas among males, the distribution is bimodal, with a frequency in younger children and after 50 years of age. Metastatic heart tumors are 10 to 40 times more frequent than primary ones. Seventy-five percent of primary cardiac tumors are nonmalignant, with rhabdomyomas being more frequent in children. Among malignant tumors, rhabdomyosarcoma has the poorest clinical course. Rhabdomyosarcoma originates in the myocardial fibers and has a positive reaction with myoglobin. The septal origin of this tumor is seen in 35% in children and only 5% in adults, which suggests an embryonic cell origin in the primary rhabdomyosarcoma of the septum. The majority of primary cardiac sarcomas disseminate systemically, mainly to the lungs.

The echocardiographic findings of an echodense image attached to the apex suggest a tumor, but the rapid decompensation did not allow further diagnostic studies. The 2D echocardiography is the main diagnostic noninvasive procedure for cardiac tumors, making it possible to identify their exact nature, depending on the ultrasonographic findings. Magnetic resonance imaging is also useful in the diagnosis and follow-up of treatment. Cardiac catheterization is useful for patients who may be candidates for surgery. Another important diagnostic element is the finding of tumoral cells in the pericardial aspirate, because aspiration is an accessible and rapid test.

Although surgery only offers an actuarial survival rate of 14% after 24 months (compared with a median survival of 11 months for primary cardiac sarcomas), it often permits an improved quality of life. Cardiac transplantation is the treatment for patients with nonresectable, locally aggressive tumors affecting only the heart. Chemotherapy hasn't improved the prognosis either alone or in combination with surgery. Radiotherapy has been used occasionally, but no changes in prognosis have been reported.

Primary cardiac sarcomas have a very low incidence but should be suspected in cases of serohemorrhagic pericardial effusions, rapidly progressive dyspnea, heart failure, or arrhythmias. The evaluation includes an echocardiogram and the search for tumoral cells from pericardiocentesis. A prompt diagnosis might contribute to improving the possibility and quality of survival.

COMMENTARY

When a previously healthy child is admitted to the PICU with signs of cardiac failure, the most likely cause is a virally induced myocarditis. As intensive care physicians, we will provide respiratory and cardiac support, but the outcome often seems independent of our best efforts. This exceptional case provides insight into the profound effects that pericardial disease has upon hemodynamic physiology. This area of cardiac physiology is often unappreciated. Diagnostic tools we have to definitively diagnose entities such as restrictive pericarditis are inexact at best. Pericardial disease as a general category should be considered for any patient with cardiopulmonary dysfunction.

Suggested Readings

1. Aravot D, Banner N, Madden B, et al. Primary cardiac tumors—is there a place for cardiac transplantation. Eur J Cardiothorac Surg 1989;3:521–524.
2. Cooley D. Surgical treatment of cardiac neoplasms: 32 years experience. J Thorac Cardiovasc Surg 1990;38:176–182.
3. Hui K, Green L, Schmidt W. Primary cardiac rhabdomyosarcoma: definition or a rare entity. Am J Cardiovasc Pathol 1988;1:19–29.
4. MacAllister H. Primary tumors of the heart and pericardium. Curr Probl Cardiol 1979;4:1–51.
5. Moriarty A, Nelson W, MacGaley B. Fine needle aspiration of rhabdomyosarcoma of the heart. Light and electron microscopic findings and histologic correlation. Acta Cytol 1990;34:74–78.
6. Poole, Jr. G, Breyer R, Holliday R, et al. Tumors of the heart: surgical considerations. J Cardiovasc Surg 1984;25:5–11.
7. Putnam J, Sweeney M, Colon R, Lanza L, Frazier O, Cooley D. Primary cardiac sarcomas. Ann Thorac Surg 1991;51:906–910.
8. Reece J, Cooley D, Frazier O, Hallman G, Powers P, Montero C. Cardiac tumors: clinical spectrum and prognosis of lesions other than classical benign myxoma in 20 patients. J Thorac Cardiovasc Surg 1984;88:439–446.
9. Satoh M, Horimoto M, Sakurai K, Funayama N, Igarashi K, Yamashiro K. Primary cardiac rhabdomyosarcoma exhibiting transient and pronounced regression with chemotherapy. Am Heart J 1990;120:1458–1460.
10. Szucs R, Rehr R, Yanovich S, Tatum J. Magnetic resonance imaging of cardiac rhabdomyosarcoma, quantifying the response to chemotherapy. Cancer 1991;67:2066–2070.
11. Watanabe A, Teitelbaum G, Henderson R, Bradley W. Magnetic resonance imaging of cardiac sarcomas. J Thorac Imaging 1989;4:90–92.

Case 9

**Pedro Celiny Ramos Garcia,
Paulo Roberto Einloft,
Delio J. Kipper,
Fernando Konrad,
Francisco Bruno, and
Sheila Momberger**
*São Lucas Hospital
Porto Alegre RS, Brazil*

HISTORY

A 3-month-old malnourished infant girl was admitted to the PICU with severe respiratory distress.

The baby was well up until 1 month of age when she was admitted for diarrhea and septicemia. She was discharged to home and presented on this admission with tachypnea, retractions, and perioral cyanosis. Four days after admission, it was discovered that the parents had a history of drug addiction.

PHYSICAL EXAMINATION

The infant's vital signs at the time of admission were as follows: temperature 37.5°C; respiratory rate 90 breaths/min; heart rate 110 beats/min; and blood pressure normal.

The patient was dyspneic, utilizing accessory muscles, with perioral cyanosis and diffuse rales on chest auscultation. The baby had significant retractions. The remainder of the physical examination showed no abnormalities.

LABORATORY ANALYSIS

On an F_IO_2 of 40% by face mask, laboratory values were as follows: pH 7.36; pCO_2 42 mm Hg; pO_2 36 mm Hg, with an oxygen saturation of 66%. White blood count was 12,000 (13% bands, 56% segmented neutrophils, 28% lymphocytes, platelet count 528,000). Chest X-ray showed a diffuse infiltrate. Cultures for bacteria and fungi were negative.

MANAGEMENT

As the infant's respiratory condition worsened, mechanical ventilation (Sechrist IV 100 B-model) was initiated via endotracheal tube with treatments of β-2 adrenergic agonists. The ventilatory status worsened dramatically shortly after mechanical ventilation was initiated. A chest X-ray showed a right-sided pneumothorax and a thoracocentesis was performed. The radiographic picture progressed to one of adult respiratory distress syndrome. Inotropic agents (dopamine and dobutamine) and antibiotics (cefoxitin plus amikacin) along with intravenous sulfamethoxazole plus trimethoprim and dexamethasone were administered. Laboratory test results were as follows: immunofluorescence tests for influenzae 1:40; adenovirus not reactive, respiratory syncytial virus 1:10; parainfluenzae 1:40; enzyme-linked immunosorbent assay (ELISA) for human immunodeficiency virus (HIV) was negative for the child and positive for both parents. The infant's general clinical status worsened daily with arterial hypoxemia and hypertension. On day 16, the nasotracheal tube was changed from nostril to orotracheal because the nose showed signs of necrosis. At this time the presence of candidiasis in the retropharynx was observed. The arterial blood gases over the next days showed the same pattern of hypoxemia, with no response to modifications of the parameters of the ventilator. The chest radiograph worsened and by day 24 the infant died. On the day prior to her death, the western blot analysis for HIV was positive.

DISCUSSION

The first case of acquired immunodeficiency syndrome (AIDS) in children was reported in 1982 and since then the number of new cases is growing throughout the world. AIDS is caused by the human lymphotropic T virus (HTLV-III) and the diagnosis is made by direct evidence of the viral antibody in the main viral proteins. ELISA is one of the diagnostic tests. When a positive result is seen by ELISA, confirmation with a more specific test, like the western blot is necessary. In underdeveloped countries diagnosis is very difficult. The "stigma" of the diagnosis, the costs of the test, as well as the incubation period all make AIDS a challenge to diagnose. Another problem is the time course of exposure, symptom development, and the time at which the assays turn positive (i.e., the so-called immunologic window). In the present case, the child had a history that was typical of an immunodeficient patient, but the parental history of drug addiction was not discovered until after the child showed no improvement with the first treatment. All the complications related to this case are found in other cases of AIDS: that is, protracted or repeated episodes of diarrhea, pulmonary interstitial disease, repeated fungal infections, and failure to thrive. Death occurs in 81% of these children when the disease progresses to pulmonary disease with hypoxemia and respiratory insufficiency.

Better diagnostic techniques to identify children at risk as well as new therapeutic modalities are required for these patients. Use of immunoglobulins in children with AIDS is not well established and there are few protocols with antiviral medications. Finally, we describe the case of this infant to demonstrate that these cases are increasingly common in Brazilian PICUs, and we need a "high suspicion index" to make the diagnosis. Prevention of the disease through education via the media seems to provide the most immediate hope until more definitive approaches are developed.

COMMENTARY

The case of this patient demonstrates the microcosm of the ICU reflecting the AIDS epidemic. As health care deliverers, it is our obligation to educate the population about the mode of transmission and the means of prevention of this viral illness. Undoubtedly, this approach will have the greatest immediate impact upon the disease. As ICU workers, we have learned to initiate therapy directed against *Pneumocystis carinii* as a matter of course when we see patients such as these even if a definitive diagnosis has yet to be made. The prospects for these children seem to be getting slightly better with improved ICU care and antimicrobial therapy. Other therapeutic maneuvers such as newer antiviral agents should also prove helpful for these patients. Earlier identification of the infection is on the horizon. An improved, rapid, simple serologic test for diagnosing HIV infection in neonates has already been described (5).

Suggested Readings

1. Burroughs HM, Edelson PJ. Tratamento medico da crianca infectada pelo HIV. Clin Pediatr Amer Norte 1991;1:47–72.
2. Husson RN, Comeau AM, Hoff R. Diagnosis of human virus infection in infants and children. Pediatrics 1990;86:1–10.
3. Notterman DA, Greenwald BM, Maio-Hunter AD, Wilkinson JD, Krasinski K, Borkowsky W. Outcome after assisted ventilation with acquired immunodeficiency syndrome. Crit Care Med 1990;18:18–20.
4. Sanders-Laufer D, DeBruin W, Edelson PJ. Infeccoes pelo "Pnemocystis carinii" na crianca infectada pelo HIV. Clin Pediatr Amer Norte 1991;01:73–93.
5. Miles SA, Bolden E, Magpantay L, et al. Rapid serologic testing with immune complex-dissociated HIV p 24 antigen for early detection of HIV infection in neonates. New Engl J Med 1993;328:279–302.

Case 10

Ladislav Laho,
Svetozar Dluholucky,
Juraj Zbojan, Karol Kralinsky,
and Peter Hudec

F. D. Roosevelt Hospital, Banska
Banska Bystrica, Slovakia

HISTORY

A 3-month-old infant girl was admitted to the PICU after abdominal surgery. The child was in good health until her admission to the hospital with an incarcerated inguinal hernia. She was immediately brought to the operating room where it was discovered that she had a necrotic ascending colon that required resection.

PHYSICAL EXAMINATION

The child was conscious, with regular breathing and a good state of hydration. Her heart rate was 130 beats/min and she had good capillary refill with a blood pressure of 85/55 mm Hg. Her respiratory rate was 22 breaths/min. She had a tense and tender abdomen with markedly diminished bowel sounds. Her lungs and heart appeared normal.

MANAGEMENT

Because of the prospect of the need for long-term parenteral nutrition, an 18-gauge left subclavian catheter was placed. A chest X-ray showed that the tip of the catheter was located in the right atrium and there was no evidence

57

Table 10.1. Composition of Infused and Pericardial Fluids

Parameter	Infused	Pericardial Fluids
Na (mmol/l)	16	120
K (mmol/l)	20	9.5
Glucose (mmol/l)	444	55.2
Proteins (g/l)	0	6.3
Amino acids (g/l)	8.0	
Osmolality (mmol/kg)	575.0	320.0
Amount (ml)	60	80

of air or fluid in the chest. Parenteral nutrition was initiated. Two hours after the initiation of the infusion, circulatory failure abruptly developed in the child. Cardiopulmonary resuscitation and cardiac life support was initiated. Pericardiocentesis was performed that resulted in withdrawal of 80 ml of translucent fluid. The intravenous catheter was removed. The child continued her cardiovascular decompensation and died shortly thereafter.

An autopsy revealed the same translucent fluid in the pericardial sac and a small amount of similar fluid in both right and left pleural spaces. No perforation was found within the right atrium. The composition of the parenteral nutrition and the pericardial fluid is shown in Table 10.1.

DISCUSSION

This complication occurred during the first month of the initiation of central parenteral nutrition in our hospital in 1982. Since that time, other authors have described similar complications (1,2). The mechanisms of such complication are not completely clear, for there are differences in the ages of patients, catheter material, composition of parenteral nutrition, and composition of pericardial and pleural fluids. Common to all the cases, however, is the placement of the catheter tip in the right atrium. Since 1982, we have not placed our catheter tips in the right atrium. Instead, we have placed them in the superior vena cava. In more than 500 subsequent cases, there have been no similar complications.

COMMENTARY

This case illustrates one of the many iatrogenic complications that are the consequence of invasive monitoring in an intensive care setting. It is always challenging to balance the risk and the benefits of what we do. The indications in the literature strongly suggest that the tips of catheters used to infuse hypertonic fluids should be placed in a great vein and not the right atrium. This is true of percutaneous central venous catheters as well (3). Transudation of fluid into the pericardial sac leading to pericardial tamponade does not require a puncture of the right atrium. In contradistinction, it seems that central venous catheters used only for monitoring pressures can be placed in a number of positions in the thorax.

References

1. Franciosi RA, Ellefson RD, Uden D, et al. Sudden unexpected death during central hyperalimentation. Pediatrics 1982;69:305–307.
2. Giacoia GP. Cardiac tamponade and hydrothorax as complications of central venous parenteral nutrition in infants. JPEN 1990;15:110–113.
3. Mupanemunda RH, Mackanjee HR. A life-threatening complication of percutaneous central venous catheters in neonates. Am J Dis Child 1992;146:1414–1415.

Case 11

Robert S. Greenberg, Mark A. Helfaer, and Lynn D. Martin

The Johns Hopkins Hospital
Baltimore, Maryland, USA

HISTORY

A 5-year-old girl was admitted to the PICU with a closed head injury and right midshaft compound femoral fracture after being struck by an automobile.

PHYSICAL EXAMINATION

Vital signs were stable, but she was noted to have a waxing and waning mental status (Glasgow coma scale = 13/15 [motor 5/6, verbal 4/5, eyes 4/4]). The remainder of her physical examination and CT scan of her head showed no abnormality. After her leg was splinted in the emergency room (ER), the patient was admitted to the PICU for observation and monitoring prior to urgent open debridement and reduction of the fracture.

MANAGEMENT

Upon arrival at the PICU, the girl's vital signs were stable, and while she was still on the transport stretcher, a right femoral nerve (3-in-1) block was performed as previously described (1). A 22-gauge regional block needle was placed using sterile technique, and 2 ml of lidocaine 2% with epinephrine 1:200,000 followed by 20 ml (1 ml/kg) of bupivacaine 0.25% were injected with pressure distal to the injection site. It was noted at that time that her writhing and squirming—which made effective assessment of her mental status difficult—ceased several minutes after placement of the block. She was then transferred to the ICU bed comfortably. She became calm and more lucid. Her Glasgow coma scale improved to 14/15 (eyes 3/4).

Four hours later, still awaiting transfer to the operating room, the patient began to experience a return of pain from the fractured leg. At this point, after we reprepared the groin area, the arterial pulse was located just below the inguinal ligament. A catheter (20-gauge, 2-inch Angiocath, Cat 38-2818-1, Deseret Medical, Sandy, Utah) was placed just lateral to the artery and passed into the nerve sheath. A gentle "give" upon placement without eliciting a paresthesia, an inability to aspirate blood, and easy injection of 3 ml of lidocaine 2% with epinephrine 1:200,000 without a change in heart rate confirmed proper placement of the catheter. This was followed by 3 ml of bupivacaine 0.25% with excellent relief of pain. The catheter was sutured in place and a T-piece connector was attached with a stopcock to allow further injections. The site was covered with a clear semiocclusive dressing to allow observation of the site. Soon thereafter, the patient was transferred to the operating room for her procedure.

DISCUSSION

This case reports the use of a soft intravenous catheter for the delivery of local anesthetic in a child after traumatic compound fracture of the femur. Although there has been reported use of such a technique in adults (2) and use of multiple, single injections in children (3–6), this is the first description of this percutaneous technique in a PICU reported in the American literature.

The 3-in-1 technique described by Winnie (1) blocks the femoral nerve, the lateral femoral cutaneous nerve, and the obturator nerve. In so doing, it provides analgesia to the anterior, medial, and lateral aspects of the leg above the knee. To provide complete analgesia of the leg, however, one must perform a sciatic nerve block as well (7). Femoral nerve blockade can provide prolonged pain relief in the situation where one does not want to obscure mental status changes or peripheral nervous system changes (especially in the contralateral limb and in the ipsilateral limb distal to the knee). It does not require moving the patient to the lateral position as in, for example, placement of a caudal catheter (which would also obscure the examination of the entire lower portion of the body). Because of this patient's head trauma, we did not offer centrally acting analgesics that might cloud the ability to assess mental status changes and cause hypoventilation, resulting in a rise in intracranial pressure.

Potential complications of this technique include hematoma, inadvertent intravascular injection, neuropathy and intraneural injection, and infection. Systemic toxicities including seizures, cardiac depression, and arrhythmias will depend on the anesthetic agent used and the dosage delivered. Careful attention to sterile technique, paresthesias elicited, and gentle advancement of the catheter should reduce the incidence of infection and nerve trauma. Test doses, using small dilute concentrations of epinephrine, will alert the physician to possible intravascular injections by an increasing heart rate and blood pressure. Finally, making sure not to exceed maximum milligram per kilogram dosage of local anesthetic (2.5 mg/kg of bupivacaine, 7 mg/kg of lidocaine with 1:200,000 epinephrine) (8) will minimize the likelihood of toxic reactions.

COMMENTARY

The administration of local anesthetic via a percutaneous femoral nerve sheath catheter is a technique that is relatively simple and effective and deserves more frequent consideration. The role of this technique, especially with respect to the care of critically injured children, holds promise as another element for providing effective analgesia without confounding the examination.

References

1. Winnie AP, Ramamurthy S, Durrani Z. The inguinal paravascular technic of lumbar plexus anesthesia: the "3-in-1 block." Anesth Analg 1973;52:989–996.
2. Tondare AS, Nadkarni AV. Femoral nerve block for fractured shaft of femur. Can Anaesth Soc J 1982;29:270–271.
3. Denton JS, Manning MPRA. Femoral nerve block for femoral shaft fractures on children: brief report. J Bone Joint Surg Br 1988; 70-B:84.
4. Grossbard GD, Love BRT. Femoral nerve block: a simple and safe method of instant analgesia for femoral shaft fractures in children. Aust NZ J Surg 1979;49:592–594.
5. Yaster M, Maxwell LG. Pediatric regional anesthesia. Anesth 1989; 70:320-338.
6. Dahl JB, Daugaard JJ, Dahl J. [Employment of a femoral catheter in fracture of the femur in a child]. Ugeskr Lgæer 1982;149(21):1395.
7. Rosenblatt R. Continuous femoral anesthesia for lower extremity surgery. Anesth Analg 1980;59:631.
8. Sethna NF, Berde CB. Pediatric regional anesthesia. New York: Churchill Livingstone 1989:665.

Case 12

David H. Beyda,
Paul R. Bakerman,
Paul H. Liu, and
David W. Tellez
Phoenix Children's Hospital
Phoenix, Arizona, USA

HISTORY

A 12-day-old full-term infant boy born to a gravida 3 para 0 mother was admitted with status epilepticus.

The infant's birth weight was 7.5 pounds and the baby had Apgar scores of 5 at 1 minute and 8 at 5 minutes. Prenatal history was noncontributory with a delivery via vacuum extraction. The baby received ampicillin and gentamicin immediately after birth for foul-smelling amniotic fluid, and the culture grew *Gardnerella* species. The baby was discharged on day 3 of life on oral ampicillin in apparently good health. On the day prior to admission, the mother stated that the baby was fussy and irritable, nipple feeding with difficulty. On the day of admission, the mother stated that the baby refused to eat and began to have extensor posturing 1 hour prior to being seen in the emergency department at an outlying hospital.

At the outlying hospital, the baby had a temperature of 101°F rectally. Generalized tonic-clonic seizures were noted that persisted for more than an hour despite administration of 20 mg/kg of phenobarbital to the infant. The baby eventually stopped seizing and was transferred to the Pediatric Critical Care Unit at Phoenix Children's Hospital.

PHYSICAL EXAMINATION

Vital signs upon arrival at Phoenix Children's Hospital were stable and the child was lethargic. The anterior fontanel was full but soft. The baby's ears and nose appeared normal and his lungs were clear to auscultation. His heartbeat was regular and his abdomen was soft without organomegaly. Femoral pulses were 1 + bilaterally. Capillary refill time was 3–4 seconds. Skin turgor was decreased. Neurologically, there was intermittent extensor posturing, arching back, and extremities with some jerkiness. Pupils were 2 mm, sluggish, and reactive. Funduscopy did not reveal papilledema or retinal hemorrhages. Cranial nerves II–XII were grossly intact.

LABORATORY DATA

Laboratory values were as follows: white blood cell count 14,000/mm^3, hemoglobin 13.7 g/dl, hematocrit 37.6%, 64% polymorphoneuclear leukocytes, 1% band forms, 21% lymphocytes, 14% mononuclears. Chemistry values were: glucose 66 mg/dl, blood urea nitrogen 35 mg/dl, creatinine 1 mg/dl, sodium 133 mmol/l, potassium 2.6 mmol/l, chloride 120 mmol/l, and CO_2 13 mmol/l. Prothrombin time

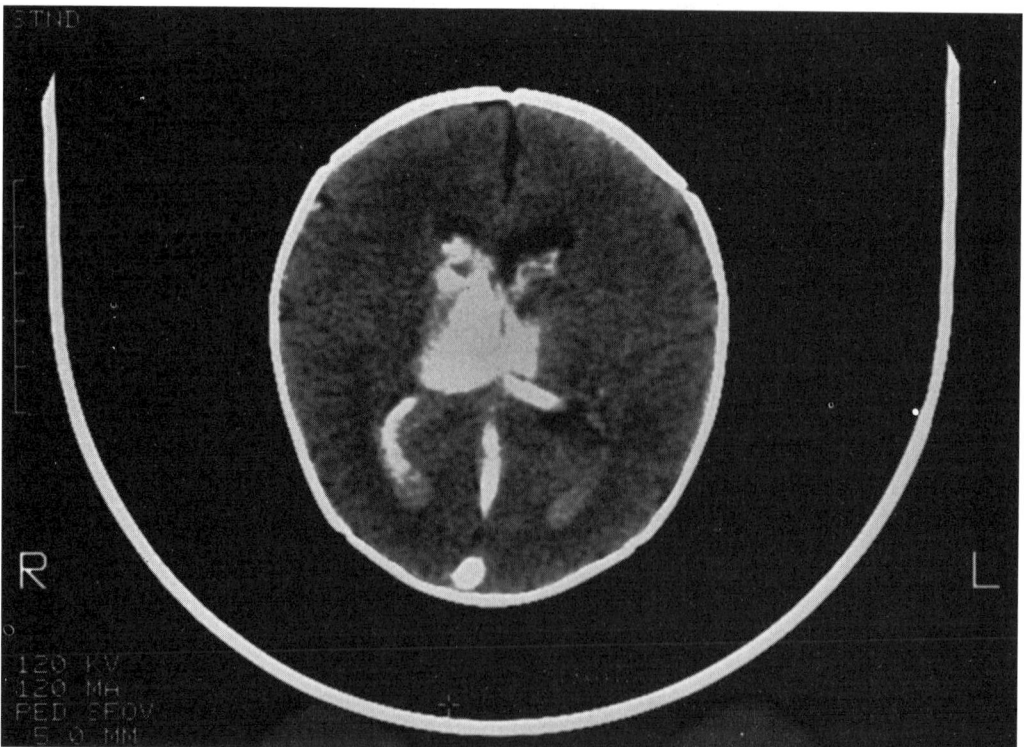

Figure 12.1. Computed tomography (CT) scan of the head.

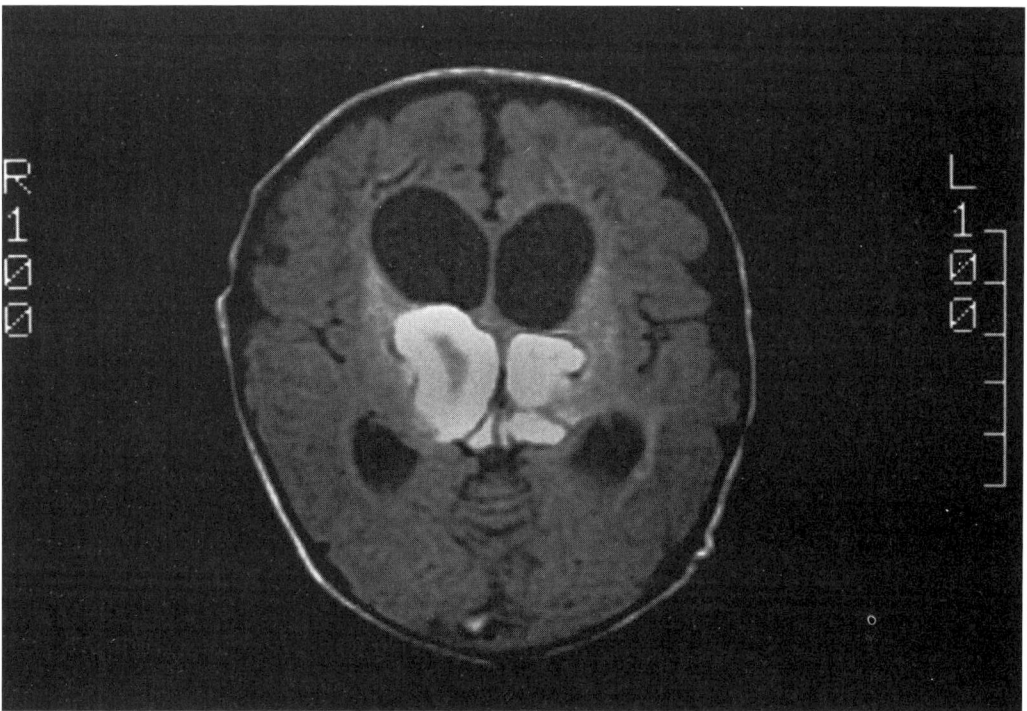

Figure 12.2. Magnetic resonance imaging (MRI) of the head.

was 11.4 seconds, partial thromboplastin time was 30.5 seconds, and results of urinalysis were normal. Phenobarbital 48 μg/ml was measured. Cerebrospinal fluid (CSF) showed moderate red blood cells with no organisms.

CT scan of the head revealed a large amount of ventricular blood in the right thalamus with a small amount of left thalamic blood (Fig. 12.1) as well as hydrocephalus. The findings were consistent with a grade 4 intracranial hemorrhage. Ultrasonagraph of the head revealed extensive intracerebral hemorrhage involving both thalami, choroid plexus, and white matter tracts superolaterally to both ventricles, with intraventricular hemorrhages. Magnetic resonance imaging (MRI) of the head revealed extensive bilateral hemorrhage in the thalamus with intraventricular blood and moderate hydrocephalus (Fig. 12.2).

HOSPITAL MANAGEMENT

Because of initial presentation of posturing and sundowning of both eyes (decorticate), the infant was electively intubated and ventilated. He was started on phenobarbital and phenytoin to control the seizures. The patient was extubated 2 days after admission without any problems and phenytoin was discontinued. Phenobarbital levels remained at approximately 48 μg/ml and the infant gradually improved neurologically. The posturing and jittering decreased. He did not feed well and required nasogastric infusions. Head circumferences were followed and did not change significantly.

Following unsuccessful attempts to place a left femoral venous line, a right femoral venous line was placed with a 3-French 5-cm Cook catheter without problems on the second day after admission. This line was discontinued after 5 days. Approximately 10 days after placement, the right leg became swollen, with poor perfusion. There was a good femoral pulse, but no posterior tibial or dorsalis pedis pulses in the right leg. A color Doppler evaluation of the venous system of the lower extremities was performed, which showed complete occlusion of the external iliac vein, common femoral veins, superficial femoral vein, and popliteal vein on the right leg. In addition, proximal portions of the deep femoral vein and greater saphenous veins showed thrombotic material as well. There was incomplete occlusion in the lower segments of the popliteal vein and proximal portions of the peroneal vein. The deep veins of the left lower extremity were examined to the level of the knee and all were found to be patent with an antegrade flow. The left external iliac vein was also patent. The boy received only conservative therapy. Four days later, a repeat venous ultrasound study demonstrated patency of the right deep vein system, indicating resolution of the thrombus, but there was a newly developed noncompressable thrombus in the deep venous system of the left leg. This lesion also resolved without specific therapy approximately 4 days later.

ECGs were obtained which revealed poorly organized background activity in the presence of multifocal sharpwave activity. Prior to discharge, these improved to normal activity. The infant also had normal visual evoked responses and bilateral brainstem auditory evoked responses. A developmental psychologic consult was obtained. This revealed a potential for significant risk for neurodevelopmental sequelae with some degree of intellectual impairment and neuromuscular involvement on a permanent basis.

Hematology consultation was obtained because of the thrombus and intraventricular hemorrhage. Protein C, protein S, and antithrombin III were obtained from the child, mother, and maternal grandmother. Antithrombin

Table 12.1.   Protein S Levels

	Patient	Mother	Maternal Grandmother	Normal Values
Protein S	59	66	72	57–150
Function	41	47	43	65–150

III and protein C were normal. In all three, protein S-free antigen levels were normal, but protein S functional activity was decreased (Table 12.1).

DISCUSSION

This patient presented with extensor posturing and status epilepticus 12 days after birth. Although the differential diagnosis of seizures in this age group is extensive, common problems include sepsis, metabolic and electrolyte disorders, and trauma. Evaluation in this case included cultures, electrolytes, bleeding studies, and CT scan of the head. CT scan revealed extensive thalamic and intraventricular hemorrhage. Intraventricular hemorrhage is an uncommon problem in full-term newborns; this condition is much more common in premature infants. In premature infants, the germinal matrix is often the source of hemorrhage. Thalamic hemorrhage is a common source of intraventricular hemorrhage in full-term infants, particularly in infants whose clinical symptoms appear after the first week of life. Typical clinical presentation is with sudden dramatic neurologic abnormalities, including altered level of consciousness, vomiting, seizures, apnea, bulging fontanel, irritability, lethargy, jitteriness, posturing, and increased intracranial pressure. In most, but not all cases, predisposing factors for cerebral venous thrombosis were identified, including sepsis, congenital heart disease, coagulopathy, and electrolyte disturbances (1).

Venous stasis or thrombosis occurs commonly with femoral venous cannulation in infants. Most cases of venous thrombosis are self-limiting and do not cause vascular compromise. In this case, this patient had venous thrombosis 2 days after removal of the femoral line. The thrombosis was extensive, with massive swelling, decreased pulses, cyanosis, and coolness of the involved leg. Thrombolysis and heparinization were considered, but in the presence of significant intracranial hemorrhage, this patient was managed without those agents with good results. Patients with significant venous thrombosis should be evaluated for hypercoagulability. As in this case, family history may provide invaluable information since primary hypercoagulability states are inherited.

Primary hypercoagulable states include the following: antithrombin III deficiency, protein C deficiency, protein S deficiency, dysfibrinogenemia, factor XII deficiency, lupus anticoagulant, and disorders of the fibrinolytic system including hypoplasminogenemia, abnormal plasminogen, and plasminogen activator deficiency (2). In the case of this infant, a maternal aunt had a history of recurrent deep vein thrombosis and had documented protein S deficiency. The maternal grandmother also had a history of recurrent deep vein thrombosis; both she and this patient's mother and this child had protein S-free antigen in the normal range but had protein S deficiency by functional assay. Confirmatory testing is often not possible in the acute setting, since these tests may be unreliable during acute thrombosis. Normal levels are reassuring, but low levels may occur due to the acute process. In this patient and his relatives, protein S-free antigen was normal, but the functional activity of this protein was decreased. The inheritance was consistent with an autosomal dominant pattern. Protein S is a vitamin K-dependent cofactor for activated protein C. This complex inactivates factors Va and VIIIa and initiates fibrinolysis. Homozygous protein S deficiency may result in neonatal purpura fulminans, and heterozygous children may present with deep vein thrombosis, stroke, sagittal sinus thrombosis, or thrombosis of other veins (portal vein, renal vein, iliofemoral vein, or inferior vena cava) (3).

COMMENTARY

As our sophistication increases with our understanding of the coagulation cascade, we will find more cases of previously unexplained thrombosis or bleeding. Identification of these disorders not only has implications for the patient but, as in this case, also offers important information for family members as well as important information for genetic counseling for the parents.

References

1. Roland EH, Flodmark O, Hill A. Thalamic hemorrhage with intraventricular hemorrhage in the full-term newborn. Pediatrics 1990;85: 737–742.
2. Schafer AI. The hypercoagulable states. Ann Intern Med 1985;102: 814–828.
3. Pegelow CH, Ledford M, Young J, Zilleruelo G. Severe protein S deficiency in a newborn. Pediatrics 1992;87:674–676.

Case 13

Andrew M. Atz and
Steven D. Barnes
The Children's Hospital
Boston, Massachusetts, USA

HISTORY

A 6-day-old infant girl was admitted to the PICU because of severe dehydration. She was born at home after a reportedly uncomplicated pregnancy at 41 weeks' gestation to a 31-year-old para 2012 mother. The baby was born as a planned home delivery. The mother had taken prenatal vitamins but had no prenatal ultrasound. The infant was delivered by her father after 3 hours of labor. The parents reported the child was immediately vigorous and weighed 7 pounds (3.18 kg) according to a home scale. The parents have two older healthy children, both of whom obtained standard obstetrical care in a hospital setting. On day 2 of life, the parents called their pediatrician, told him of the birth, and were told to bring the infant in for examination. At this time the child appeared healthy and weighed 2.93 kg. The mother reported adequate breast-feeding and passage of meconium stools daily. A phenylketonuria screen was performed, but no further therapy and no routine follow-up was arranged.

The parents called the pediatrician back on day 6 of life reporting that the baby had been awake the previous evening with seeming abdominal pain and was "vomiting everything." The infant was brought to the office immediately and was alert but weighed 2.52 kg and appeared grossly dehydrated. The parents reported that she had been spitting up an increasingly larger amount of nonbilious material every day since birth. It was not projectile in nature and she continued to breast feed aggressively. The baby was noted in the last day to tolerate sterile water feedings better than breast milk, and this had been offered

71

increasingly more often. Initially the parents had not been concerned because the baby was behaving similarly to her older sister who had been diagnosed with infantile colic. Furthermore, the parents reported that although she had passed a small amount of stool daily, she had had no urine output in the previous 4 days. The parents believed that this was to be expected secondary to the persistent vomiting. The baby had been afebrile throughout this course and only in the last 12 hours prior to being seen had become alternately more irritable and lethargic. She was taken immediately to a local hospital.

PHYSICAL EXAMINATION

When we saw her, the baby was lethargic but arousable. Her temperature was 96.7°F and her pulse was 124 beats/min and regular. Respirations were 40–50 breaths/min without retractions. Her blood pressure was 73/37 mm Hg and equal in all extremities. The baby's height was 48 cm; her weight was 2.52 kg; and her head circumference was 34.5 cm. Head examination revealed an open and sunken anterior fontanel. No eye or ear abnormalities were seen. Her mouth had tacky mucosa, and her neck was supple. Examination of the infant's chest revealed clear and equal breath sounds. Cardiovascularly, she had a regular heart rate and rhythm without murmur, rub, or gallop. Pulses were easily palpable and symmetric in all extremities. The abdomen was visibly scaphoid with poorly heard bowel sounds. There was no palpable spleen and the liver was felt 1 cm below the right costal margin. Kidneys were palpable bilaterally and were considered to be of normal size, configuration, and location. Genitourinary examination revealed normal female features and a patent anus. Rectal tone was normal but absent of stool. The infant's skin was remarkable for discrete tenting over the abdomen and thighs. There were no rashes but there was extensive bruising bilaterally at the antecubital fossae and overlying the radial arteries. There was also bruising at the suprapubic area. All bruises corresponded to puncture sites. Neurologic review showed brisk, reactive pupils with gag reflex present. The girl would move all extremities to painful stimuli, and deep tendon reflexes were present and symmetric. Intermittently, the infant would begin rhythmic jerking of the right hand progressing to all the other extremities. There was no change in respiratory or heart rate during this seizure activity.

LABORATORY DATA

Laboratory values were as follows: hemoglobin 21.0 g%, hematocrit 63.0%, platelets 333,000/mm^3, white count 9000/mm^3 (13% band forms, 40% polymorphonuclears, 43% lymphocytes, 3% mononuclears, 1% eosinophils). Electrolytes were: sodium 139 mEq/l, potassium 4.5 mEq/l, chloride 77 mEq/l, and bicarbonate 23 mEq/l. Blood urea nitrogen (BUN) was 145 mg/dl, creatinine 8.3 mg/dl, total bilirubin 3.8 mg/dl, direct bilirubin 0.7 mg/dl, calcium 7.7 mg/dl, ionized calcium 0.77 mg/dl, phosphorus 10.7 mg/dl, and uric acid 39.0 mg/dl. Total protein was 6.5 g/dl and albumin 4.2 g/dl. Enzyme values were as follows: aspartate transaminase (AST) 55 U/l, alanine transaminase (ALT) 21 U/l, and alkaline phosphatase 178 U/l. Anion gap was 44. Prothrombin time (PT) and partial thromboplastin time (PTT) were each more than 150 seconds. Lumbar puncture showed 9 white blood cells (70% lymphocytes, 30% polymorphonucears) with normal cerebrospinal fluid (CSF), glucose, and protein. Arterial blood gas on room air showed pH 7.41, PaCO$_2$ 44 torr, and PaO$_2$ 137 torr. Blood and CSF fluid cultures were taken. It was not possible to obtain a urine culture despite numerous catheterizations and suprapubic taps.

MANAGEMENT

Immediate management of this patient included placement of an intraosseous line in the left tibia with fluid resuscitation with crystalloid. Valium and phenobarbital were administered to control seizures. Ampicillin, cefotaxime, and clindamycin were given for possible sepsis. The coagulopathy was corrected with one dose of vitamin K and 10 ml/kg of fresh frozen plasma. Within the first 6 hours, PT and PTT had returned to normal levels, and no further bleeding occurred. Antibiotics were continued until blood and CSF cultures were negative at 72 hours.

Plain radiographs of the abdomen revealed a large distended stomach and a classic "double bubble" sign consistent with duodenal obstruction (Fig. 13.1). A contrast study through a nasogastric tube confirmed these findings, with no penetration of contrast past the first portion of the duodenum. Once we ruled out a surgical emergency, repair was delayed until resolution of the other problems.

Abdominal ultrasound showed normal-sized kidneys

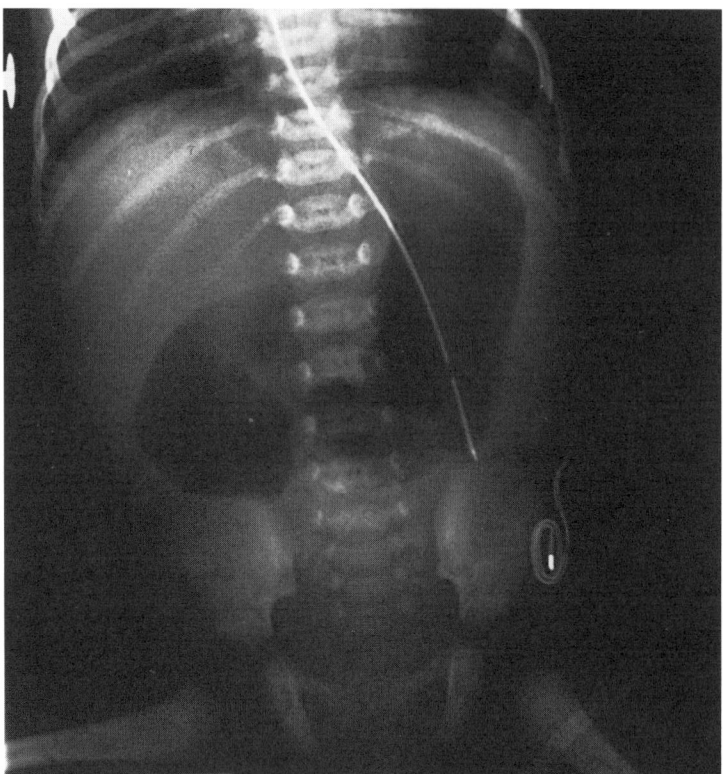

Figure 13.1. Plain radiograph of the abdomen showing distended stomach and first portion of the duodenum, the classic "double bubble" sign.

without cystic or dysplastic changes. Doppler studies revealed normal blood flow to each kidney. Despite aggressive resuscitation with fluid and subsequent use of loop diuretics, there was no urine output. Because of the persistent azotemia, anuria, and elevated uric acid level, as well as the seizure activity, a Quinton Curl peritoneal catheter was placed and dialysis begun. After 24 hours, the baby began to make urine and entered a phase of high-output urine failure requiring careful replacement of urinary losses. On hospital day 5, the BUN was 33 mg/dl, creatinine was 2.7 mg/dl, and uric acid 4.3 mg/dl, and peritoneal dialysis was discontinued. By hospital day 7, the baby began to concentrate urine normally, creatinine, BUN, and uric acid levels were normal, and urine replacement was stopped.

After initial seizure control with valium and phenobarbital, phenobarbital was continued at therapeutic levels. The child had three more seizures of the same character over the next 36 hours. Results of cranial ultrasound were normal, and electroencephalogram (EEG) results were normal for age. Phenobarbital was continued for 5 days, then stopped with no further seizures.

On hospital day 6, the dialysis catheter was removed and an exploratory laparotomy performed. At surgery a restrictive duodenal web and intestinal malrotation were found. The web was excised and a duodenoscopy and Ladd's procedure were done without complications. On postoperative day 6, feedings were started and slowly advanced without difficulty. The child was discharged home in good condition on postoperative day 18.

DISCUSSION

This infant illustrates a case of small bowel obstruction complicated by a bleeding coagulopathy, profound dehydration, renal failure, and seizure activity.

With classic hemorrhagic disease of the newborn (HDN) the coagulopathy is due to a deficiency in vitamin K and decreased activity of factors 2, 7, 9, and 10, which require activation by vitamin K. The normal source of vitamin K is intestinal bacterial synthesis with additional dietary intake of vitamin K. It has been shown that cow's milk has much higher content of vitamin K than breast milk. In classic HDN, bleeding is unusual in the first 24 hours and is variable but usually not life threatening. In HDN the PT and PTT are prolonged, platelet count is normal, and the PT and PTT begin to normalize within 4 hours of administration of vitamin K. To prevent HDN it is now common practice to give infants vitamin K in the first 24 hours of life (1). This infant had not been given vitamin K and was exclusively breast fed with poor absorption secondary to the duodenal web. As in classic HDN, she responded quickly to a dose of vitamin K.

The diagnosis of duodenal obstruction is made by plain radiograph showing the classic "double bubble" sign, as seen in this case. This includes a distended stomach along with a markedly distended first portion of the duodenum with an absence of air distally. The emesis with duodenal obstruction is generally bilious, but this is dependent on the relationship of the obstruction with the ampulla of Vater. This diagnosis has been increasingly made on prenatal sonogram showing two large fluid-filled cystic structures in the abdomen (2). The baby in this case had no prenatal sonogram and a duodenal web proximal to the ampulla explaining her nonbilious vomiting.

This infant also presented interesting physiology related to her renal failure. An anion gap of 44 suggests a sizeable metabolic acidosis. In this case it was secondary to uremia and increased circulating phosphate and sulfate. Complicating this situation was the normal pH of 7.4 and serum bicarbonate of 23 mEq/l. Obviously, a compensatory alkalosis existed. The normal PaCO$_2$ ruled out a respiratory origin and implicated a compensatory metabolic alkalosis. This could be accounted for by persistent vomiting and loss of H+ ions. The degree of hypochloremia (77 mEq/l) further substantiated this notion.

Once indications for dialysis were met, the patient had a Quinton Curl catheter placed. Although hemodialysis is possible, it usually requires two separate large-bore access sites, making it technically difficult. Complications with clotting can also be seen if heparin is not used. Peritoneal dialysis has been used frequently in neonates and with good results. The high peritoneal surface to body weight ratio makes it more efficient in infants than in older children. Peritoneal dialysis is also more efficient in the removal of excessive uric acid as seen in this case, and it lacks the potential dangers of large fluid shifts that hemodialysis might cause (3).

Seizure activity in the neonatal period can be caused by structural defects, intracranial hemorrhage, infection, hypoglycemia, hyponatremia, or hypocalcemia, among others. This infant had normal imaging study and EEG results, and normal sodium and glucose levels. She did have an initial ionized calcium level of 0.77 mg/dl. However, after the calcium level was normalized the infant continued to have seizure activity until dialysis was begun. In infants with acute renal failure it may be difficult to observe the usual symptoms of lethargy, nausea, and vomiting seen with uremia, but seizure activity is commonly seen (4). One could hypothesize that a combination of hypocalcemia with a rapid rate of increase in the BUN level could account for this seizure activity. More suggestive of renal involvement is the cessation of seizure activity once dialysis had begun, despite the discontinuation of anticonvulsants.

COMMENTARY

I chose this complicated case because it illustrates the facilities that pediatric critical care physicians must possess. Management of such an infant requires knowledge of well child care and routine vitamin administration. It also requires the challenge of managing acute renal failure in a neonate as well as the surgical urgency of a small bowel obstruction.

References

1. Glader BE, Amylon MD. Hemostatic disorders in the newborn. In: Bralow L, Ballard RA, Avery ME, Taeusch HW. Diseases of the newborn. 6th ed. Philadelphia: WB Saunders, 1991:780–781.
2. Schnaufer L. Duodenal atresia, stenosis and annular pancreas. In: Welch KJ, Randolph JG, Ravitch MM, O'Neill JA Jr, Rowe MI. Pediatric surgery. 4th ed. Chicago: Year Book, 1986:829–837.
3. Guignard J-P. Neonatal nephrology. In: Holliday M, Barratt TM, Vernier RL. Pediatric nephrology. 2nd ed. Baltimore: Williams & Wilkins, 1987:932–934.
4. Anand SK. Acute renal failure. In: In: Bralow L, Ballard RA, Avery ME, Taeusch HW. Diseases of the newborn. 6th ed. Philadelphia: WB Saunders, 1991:892–897.

Case 14

Suzanne Delport
Kalafong Hospital
Pretoria, Republic of South Africa

HISTORY

This patient was admitted to the PICU shortly after birth with respiratory failure. The baby was full-term, delivered via cesarian section for cephalopelvic disproportion and fetal distress to an 18-year-old primigravida.

PHYSICAL EXAMINATION

The neonate weighed 3.5 kg. The Apgar score was 1 at 5 minutes and remained 1 despite active resuscitative measures. Despite a peak inspiratory pressure of 50 cm H_2O, excursion of the chest was hardly noticeable. On abdominal examination, the liver was palpable 3 cm below the costal margin. The rest of the clinical examination revealed no dysmorphic features or abnormalities.

LABORATORY DATA

Mechanical ventilation was initiated with an F_IO_2 of 1.0 and ventilatory rate of 80 breaths/min. The blood gases revealed a severe combined metabolic and respiratory acidosis. The pH was 6.6, PCO_2 was 80 mm Hg, pO_2 was 32 mm Hg, oxygen saturation was 17%, and there was a base excess of -20 mEq/l.

MANAGEMENT

Surgical emphysema started to develop shortly after birth. An intercostal drain was inserted in the left hemi-

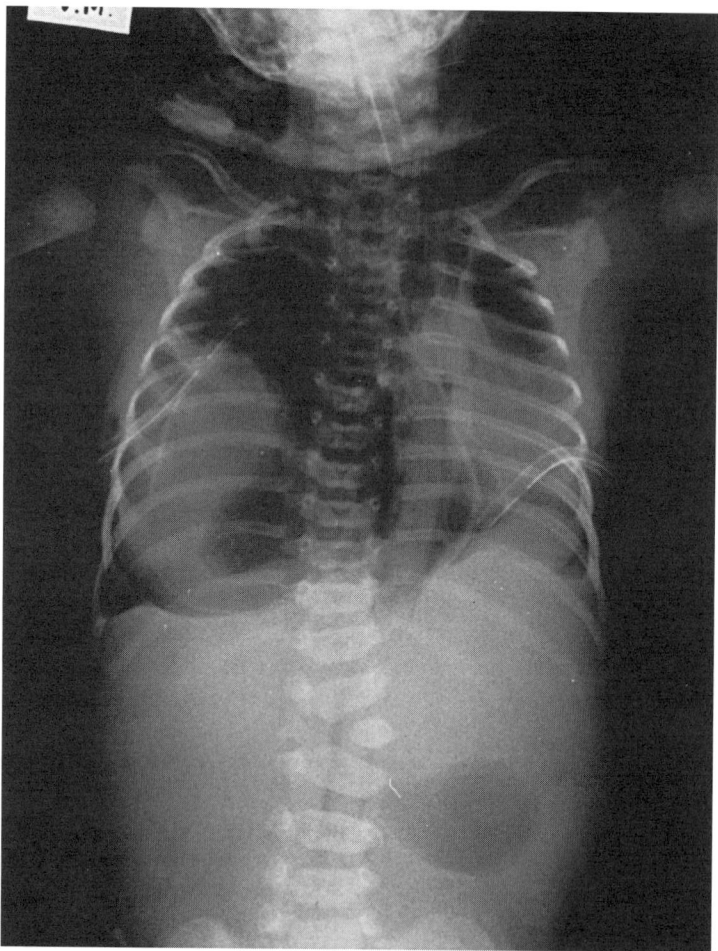

Figure 14.1. Frontal chest X-ray showing surgical emphysema, mediastinal and cardiac displacement to the left, and an opacification in the right hemithorax due to herniation of the right lobe of the liver. Normal lung markings are absent and a lumbar hemivertebra is present.

thorax, followed by a similar drain in the right hemithorax. Air issued from both drains but no clinical improvement was noted. A frontal chest X-ray was obtained (Fig. 14.1). This showed extensive surgical emphysema with displacement of the heart and mediastinum to the left. Normal lung markings were absent and an abnormal opacity was seen in the right hemithorax. The position of the right hemidiaphragm was uncertain. A lumbar hemivertebra was present. No improvement was noted and the patient died 2 hours after birth. An autopsy revealed a large posterolateral defect in the right hemidiaphragm with herniation of the right lobe of the liver into the right hemithorax. Severe bilateral pulmonary hypoplasia was present.

Both lungs were rudimentary and barely visible. The pericardium was adherent to the left lateral chest wall. Both pulmonary arteries were aplastic. A single pulmonary vein was present on each side posterior to the heart and opened into the right atrium. A large patent foramen ovale was present with a small left atrium.

DISCUSSION

Congenital left-sided diaphragmatic hernias are associated with hypoplasia of the ipsilateral lung due to compression by intrathoracic bowel (1). Chronic mediastinal displacement may also lead to hypoplasia of the contralateral lung.

Congenital right-sided diaphragmatic hernias on the other hand rarely present with acute life-threatening respiratory distress after birth (2). The more favorable prognosis in contrast to left-sided hernias is a consequence of the diaphragmatic defect being occluded by the liver, thereby preventing the passage of intestine into the hemithorax with subsequent interference of lung development (2).

Clinically, right-sided hernias may be seen as mild respiratory distress, an asymptomatic intrathoracic mass, progressive liver herniation after birth, or intestinal herniation (2).

The full adult complement of airways is established by the 16th week of gestation. The severity of pulmonary developmental abnormalities depends on the timing and extent of visceral herniation into the chest. Larger diaphragmatic defects are present in nonsurvivors, allowing for more viscera to be displaced into the chest at an earlier stage of development (3).

In this neonate, herniation of the liver probably took place before the 16th gestational week with subsequent arrest of ipsilateral pulmonary development. Contralateral pulmonary hypoplasia occurred because of mediastinal displacement.

A wide variety of anomalies have been reported in association with diaphragmatic hernias. The central nervous system is most frequently involved, followed by the cardiovascular system (4). Cardiac abnormalities are reported to be present in about 23% of these infants and nearly any type has been described (5). The presence and type of cardiac defect must be established prior to surgical intervention for repair of the hernia.

COMMENTARY

The therapeutic approaches to diaphragmatic hernias is incredibly varied. When extracorporeal membrane oxygenation (ECMO) is available, patients are often placed on this support either before, during, or after definitive repair. Candidacy for ECMO in this case would be contraindicated given the degree of pulmonary hypoplasia and the anatomical abnormality of the great vessels. If ECMO is available, some centers operate early and some operate following days of stability. We have not yet been able to prospectively identify which patients would definitely benefit from any one of these various approaches.

References

1. de Lorimier A, Tierney D, Parker H. Hypoplastic lungs in fetal lambs with surgically produced congenital diaphragmatic hernia. Surgery 1967:62:12–17.
2. Campbell DN, Lilly JR. The clinical spectrum of right Bochdalek's hernia. Arch Surg 1982:117:341–344.
3. Harrison MR, Adzick NS, Nahnyama DK, de Lorimier AA. Fetal diaphragmatic hernia: fatal but fixable. Semin Perinat 1985:9:103–112.
4. Caplan MS, MacGregor SN. Perinatal management of congenital diaphragmatic hernia and anterior abdominal wall defects. Clin Perinat 1989:16:917–938.
5. Greenwood RD, Rosenthal A, Nadas AS. Cardiovascular abnormalities associated with congenital diaphragmatic hernia. Pediatrics 1976: 57:92–97.

Case 15

Jeffrey Burns, Antonio R. Perez-Atayde, and James C. Fackler

The Children's Hospital
Boston, Massachusetts, USA

HISTORY

A 5-day-old male infant with profound hypoxemia and hypotension was transferred from a tertiary care center for extracorporeal membrane oxygenation (ECMO). The infant was a 38-week gestational product of a 27-year-old gravida 3, para 2, A-positive, Combs-negative, hepatitis B-negative, gonococcus-negative, RPR-nonreactive mother delivered by cesarean section (after epidural anesthesia) for breech presentation. The birth weight was 3.47 kg and Apgar scores were 7 and 8 at 1 and 5 minutes, respectively. There was no meconium. At 30 minutes of life, the infant developed respiratory distress and was transported to a tertiary care neonatal ICU. There was no alcohol, drug, or tobacco use during the pregnancy. It was complicated only by premature labor at 33 weeks, which was controlled with 24 hours of magnesium sulfate. The mother had a healthy 4-year-old daughter but lost a full-term infant girl who died in the neonatal period. The clinical diagnosis was pulmonary hypoplasia; autopsy permission was refused. The infant's father and mother were not related by blood and were in good health.

PHYSICAL EXAMINATION

At the initial examination, the infant was reported as irritable but vigorous, with a loud cry and in moderate respiratory distress. Vital signs were notable for heart rate

83

of 110–133 beats/min; respiratory rate of 70–90 breaths/min, blood pressure of 65–85/35–67 mm Hg, and temperature of 98.2° F. The baby was normocephalic with a cephalohematoma, and the fontanel was flat and soft, with ears in normal position, nares patent, and palate intact. The clavicles were intact, with moderate intercostal and subcostal retractions with decreased aeration bilaterally by auscultation. The precordium was quiet, with a normal S_1S_2 with S_2 split and a grade II/VI systolic murmur heard at the upper left sternal border, and pulses were diminished throughout with 5-second capillary refill. The abdomen was soft, with a three-vessel cord, without organomegaly. The infant had normal male anatomy, with a patent anus with meconium stool passed. There were no dysmorphic features. He had normal tone and a nonfocal examination.

LABORATORY DATA

An arterial blood gas analysis at 30 minutes of life showed a pH of 7.28, $PaCO_2$ of 40 mm Hg, and a PaO_2 of 40 mm Hg in room air. Repeat arterial blood gas values 30 minutes later in a 90% Oxyhood were as follows: pH 7.30, $PaCO_2$ 42 mm Hg, and PaO_2 150 mm Hg. Complete blood count at that time revealed white blood cell count 15.5, hematocrit 44%, platelets 299,000, with 37% neutrophils, 1% bands, and 50% lymphocytes. Glucose level was 80 by Chemstrip and electrolyte levels were as follows: sodium 139 mEq/l, potassium 4.5 mEq/k, chloride 106 mEq/k, CO_2 21 mEq/l. Chest X-ray was read as well-inflated lung fields with slightly granular appearance to the left lung, streaking atelectasis of the left lower lobe, and fluid in the major and minor fissure. The heart size appeared normal. Blood and urine for culture were obtained, and the infant was given one dose of ampicillin at 100 mg/kg and one dose of gentamicin at 2.5 mg/kg.

MANAGEMENT

Differential diagnosis at that time included respiratory distress syndrome or pneumonia. At 19 hours of life, the patient was intubated in response to arterial blood gas values of pH 7.32, $PaCO_2$ 62 mm Hg, PaO_2 53 mm Hg, HCO_3 31 mm Hg, despite administration of >30 ml/kg colloid and crystalloid and base therapy with tromethamine. For the next 6 hours, a regimen was maintained consisting of packed red blood cell transfusions, alkalinization to keep pH >7.40, dopamine at 10 μg/kg/min to keep mean arterial pressure (MAP) >45 mm Hg, fentanyl, pancuronium, and pressure control ventilation at a rate of 50, peak inspiratory pressure (PIP) at 40, positive end-expiratory pressure (PEEP) at 7, and F_IO_2 at 1.0. The baby remained profoundly hypoxemic with a PaO_2 <40 mm Hg. The patient was eventually stabilized with a PaO_2 >60 mm Hg, then given several doses of surfactant via endotracheal tube. He was maintained on dopamine and dobutamine to keep MAP >50 mm Hg and pressure control ventilation with 80% F_IO_2 and PIP >38 to maintain PaO_2 >60 mm Hg. Laboratory data during this time were notable for negative culture results, normal coagulation parameters and bilirubin level, and serum glucose >60 mg/dl on D20W at 100 ml/kg/d of maintenance fluids. On day 4 of life, the infant again developed a period of profound hypoxemia with PaO_2 <40 mm Hg for more than 8 hours despite maximal support. Echocardiogram showed no structural heart disease or evidence of shunting, and the baby was transferred to receive ECMO.

On arrival, he was stabilized on high frequency oscillatory ventilation with a PaO_2 >150 mm Hg on an F_IO_2 of 1.0, but had a physical examination consistent with profound low output state of unclear etiology. At this time there was no coagulopathy; pyruvate, NH_3, and liver function tests were normal, although the creatinine level was >3.0 mg/dl. Chest X-ray revealed a normal cardiothoracic ratio with bilateral granular opacities. Blood pressure was 35/25 mm Hg with an MAP of 30 mm Hg despite administration of dopamine (20 μg/kg/min), dobutamine (20 μg/kg/min) and epinephrine at 0.6 μg/kg/min. His 12-lead ECG (Fig. 15.1) showed severe global ST-segment elevation

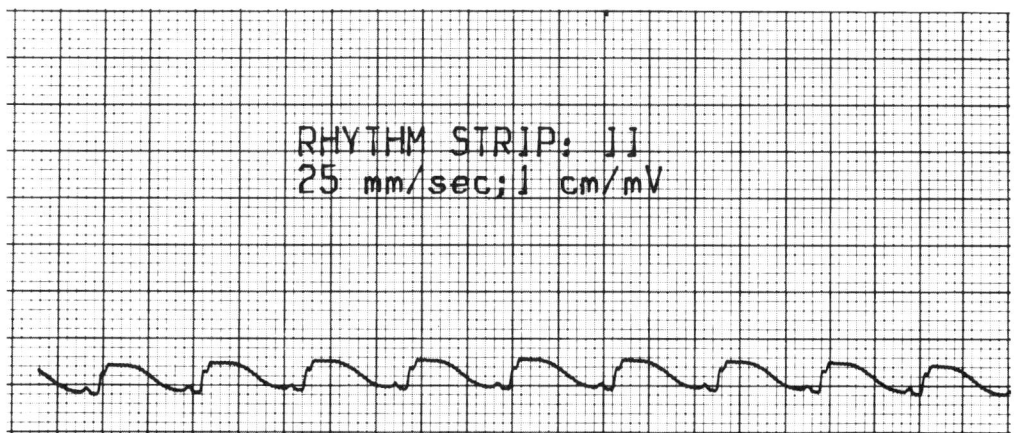

Figure 15.1. Twelve-lead ECG of patient in case report.

consistent with myocardial ischemia. The infant's echo-cardiogram revealed normal cardiac anatomy without evidence of shunt. He had biventricular dysfunction with a normal origin of the coronary arteries and laminar flow pattern in the abdominal aorta consistent with a normal aortic arch.

Given the patient's profound hypotension, which was unresponsive to maximal inotropic support and severe myocardial ischemia, along with progressive metabolic acidosis and decreased urine output, the infant was placed on venoarterial ECMO for both cardiac and pulmonary support. Although hemodynamic parameters were immediately stabilized on ECMO and pressors were able to be withdrawn, the infant showed clinical evidence of seizure activity. Serial head ultrasound revealed no structural abnormalities but serial EEGs demonstrated frequent electroencephalographic seizures along with progressive periods of burst suppression (despite anticonvulsant therapy). Serial ECGs and creatine phospokinase-MB band isoenzyme showed continued severe myocardial ischemia and multiple attempts to decrease venoarterial ECMO flows were impossible because of profound hypotension and desaturation.

The medical team and family agreed on withdrawal of ECMO support by day 8 of life because of profound neurologic devastation and myocardial failure. Autopsy permission was granted for needle biopsy of selected organs.

Autopsy Findings

At autopsy there was evidence of cardiac failure with anasarca, bilateral serous pleural effusions, and serous ascites. The heart appeared enlarged and flabby. The autopsy was limited to small tissue samples of skeletal muscle, heart, liver, kidney, and lungs. With the exception of the heart, histologic examination of these organs was unremarkable. The myocardium, however, had the microscopic characteristics of glycogenesis with marked enlargement of myocytes having clear sarcoplasm and the appearance of plant cells (Fig. 15.2). Ultrastructural studies confirmed a glycogen storage disease restricted to the heart muscle. Subsequent analysis revealed that the activity of phosphorylase kinase was markedly diminished in the heart (15% of standard controls) but normal in other tissues (100% in skeletal muscle). All other enzyme activity (e.g., debranching enzyme and other glycolytic enzymes) was normal in the samples tested.

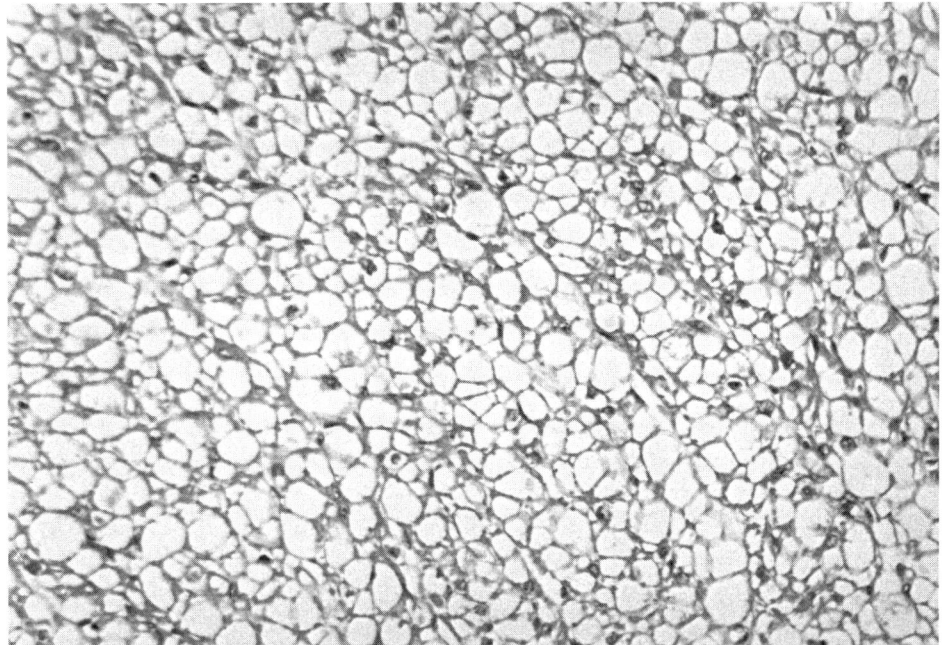

Figure 15.2. Autopsy specimen of heart muscle.

DISCUSSION

All inborn errors of metabolism are single gene disorders, almost all being inherited in an autosomal or X-linked recessive manner. Thus parents, as carriers of a recessive autosomal gene, will have a risk of 1:4 for recurrence in each future pregnancy. For the X-linked recessive disorders, if the mother is a carrier then the risk is 1:2 that a son will be affected and 1:2 that a daughter will be a carrier. All inborn errors of metabolism result in the genetic inability to produce the full complement of a particular protein, almost all of which function as enzymes. The phenotypic expression depends on whether the affected individual lacks production of a necessary end product, accumulates precursors that may be toxic, or has an increased activity of normal alternate pathways with an increase in normal metabolites.

Most states in the United States screen for phenylketonuria, hypothyroidism, and galactosemia. Several screen for other inborn errors of metabolism such as hemoglobinopathies, congenital adrenal hyperplasia, maple syrup urine disease, homocystinuria, galactosemia, adenosine deaminase deficiency, and biotinidase deficiency. However, the limitations of newborn screening are that results may not be available until after the onset of clinical symptoms. This is especially important for some of the more acute inborn errors of metabolism such as congenital adrenal hyperplasia, maple syrup urine disease, and galactosemia. Clinical suspicion is essential for diagnosis. The features of inborn errors of metabolism include a wide variety of clinical expression that usually changes with age. Neonatal onset often has a life-threatening presentation. The infant will more typically have a subacute presentation such as hypotonia, decompensation with intercurrent illnesses, liver disease or seizure disorder, or progressive coarsening of features. The child or adolescent will have either a behavioral-psychiatric presentation or neurologic manifestations such as ataxia, progressive weakness, seizures or, again, symptoms exaggerated only during physiologic stress. Certain clinical features are common to inborn errors of metabolism, such as vomiting, jaundice, diarrhea, seizures, coma, and dysmorphic features such as abnormal hair or eyes. Diagnostic categories useful for developing a differential diagnosis include metabolic acidosis, hyperammonemia, hypoglycemia with or without ketosis, as well as neurologic symptoms and liver dysfunction.

After supportive measures have been undertaken, evaluation should proceed systematically. The earliest preintervention samples of body fluids provide the greatest basis for making a successful diagnosis. However, the precise diagnosis may often require specific biochemical analysis of tissues. Also useful are quantitative serum and urine amino acid analysis, quantitative urine organic acid screen, blood lactate, pyruvate and ammonia, urinary reducing substances and ketone bodies, and quantitative urine carnitive analysis. A full-thickness skin biopsy for fibroblast culture should be obtained and refrigerated.

The inborn error of metabolism identified at necropsy in this case is quite rare. In all types of glycogenesis reported to date, abnormal deposition of glycogen in the heart parallels systemic glycogen deposition (e.g., Pompe's disease). The finding of markedly increased glycogen concentration in the heart but not in muscle or liver implies a defect of a cardiac isozyme of glycogen metabolism of glycolysis. There are only a few case reports in the literature of phosphorylase kinase deficiency confined to the heart with pathologic features identical to those of this patient. Phosphorylase kinase is a complex enzyme composed of four subunits—one is a catalytic subunit and three are regulatory subunits. It is postulated and this case supports the fact that the known different functional properties of phosphorylase kinase in different tissues suggest the existence of tissue-specific isoenzyme. The function of the phosphorylase kinase isozyme in the heart has yet to be fully elucidated.

The recognition of specific inborn errors of metabolism will always be difficult. For the pediatric intensive care physician who is often the first to evaluate an acutely ill infant or child, the presentation and diagnostic criteria for inborn errors of metabolism must be part of a systematic approach to differential diagnoses. Fortunately, there exists a wide spectrum of successful treatments for these disorders if they are recognized. Therapeutic modalities include vitamin supplementation (pyridoxine, homocystinuria), supplement of deficient product (biotinidase deficiency), dietary adjustment to prevent substrate accumulation phenylketonuria, and drug therapies to limit accumulation of toxic metabolites (penicillamine in Wilson's disease) or encourage nitrogenous waste excretion (sodium benzoate and phenylacetate in urea cycle disorders). Finally, organ transplantation is available for storage disorders (bone marrow) or urea cycle defects (liver).

COMMENTARY

With the human genome project in progress, it is likely that many of these genetic disorders (especially the single-gene disorders) will have "gene addresses" accurately identified. The hope is that once the address is located gene replacement therapy will be a future possibility. As is always the case, astute clinicians will be necessary for the accurate identification and diagnosis of these patients early in their illnesses before irreversible damage has taken place. When very ill neonates are admitted to the PICU, the results of neonatal screening may be unavailable. We must maintain the standards for well-child care in the PICU whenever possible.

Suggested Readings

1. Burton BK. Inborn errors of metabolism: the clinical diagnosis in early infancy. Pediatrics 1987;79:359–369.
2. Servidei S, Metley LA, Chodosh J, Dimauro S. Fatal infantile cardiopathy caused by phosphorylase kinase. J Pediatr 1988;113:82–85.
3. Ward JC. Inborn errors of metabolism of acute onset in infancy. Pediatr Rev 1990;11:205–216.
4. Eishi Y, Takemura T, Sone R, Yamamura H, Naruaawa K, Ichinohowama R, Tanaka M, Hatakyama S. Glycogen storage disease confined to the heart with deficient activity of cardiac phosphorylase kinase: a new type of glycogen storage disease. Hum Pathol 1985;16:193–197.

Case 16

Eduardo Julio Schnitzler
Hospital Italiano
Buenos Aires, Argentina

HISTORY

A 12-month-old boy, previously in good health, was hospitalized for status epilepticus and acute renal failure (ARF). Three days prior to admission, he had developed bloody diarrhea and oral ampicillin was prescribed. Two days prior to admission, he had been admitted to another hospital, where examination was not contributory except for evidence of dehydration and blood-streaked stools. During a 24-hour hospital stay, the patient received intravenous fluids and became progressively more lethargic and oliguric with development of generalized tonic-clonic convulsions. Lorazepan and phenytoin were administrated without control of the seizures, which did respond to phenobarbital (18 mg/kg/d). He was transferred to the PICU in critical condition.

PHYSICAL EXAMINATION

At the time of examination, the child was unconscious, hypotensive, and edematous. His pulse rate was 170 beats/min, his blood pressure was 55/24 mm Hg, his temperature was 37.5°C, and his weight was 8.8 kg (10th percentile). He was mildly cyanotic, with cold extremities and slow capillary refill. During initial evaluation he required crystalloid resuscitation (200 ml 0.9% saline solution), was responsive only to deep pain (Glasgow coma score = 6), and his pupils were small and reactive with normal fundoscopy. The child was intubated and mechanically ventilated. The abdomen appeared normal. Lax anal sphincter tone with rectal mucosal prolapse were noted.

91

LABORATORY DATA

Laboratory data at the time of admission included the following values: hemoglobin 8.5 g/dl, anemia characterized by red cell fragmentation (schistocytes and helmet cells), white blood cell count $26400/mm^3$ ($26.4 \times 10^3/l$) with 75% neutrophils, reticulocyte count 2.2%, platelets $105,000/mm^3$, prothrombin time (PT) 19 seconds (control 12 seconds), partial thromboplastin time (PTT) 60 seconds (control 40 seconds), blood urea nitrogen (BUN) 40 mg/dl (14.3 mmol/L), negative sodium 130 mmol/l, potassium 3.7 mmol/l, blood glucose 200 mg/dl (11.1 mmol/l), PaO_2 230 torr (30.5 kPa, pH 7.18, $PaCO_2$ 30 torr (3.98 kPa), bicarbonate 10 mmol/l, Ca 5.4 mg/dl (1.3 mmol/l), serum glutamic oxaloacetic transaminase (SGOT) 311 U/l, serum glutamic pyruvic transaminase (SGPT) 120 U/l, lactate dehydrogenase 4650 U/l, conjugated bilirubin 0.3 mg/dl, total bilirubin 0.8 mg/dl, and protein 4.4 g/dl (albumin 2.7 g). Chest X-ray and cerebrospinal fluid analysis showed no abnormalities. A catheter inserted into the bladder yielded 5 ml of urine which gave a + + test for protein and a + + test for hemoglobin. The sediment contained 8 white blood cells and 12 red blood cells per high power field.

MANAGEMENT

During the next few hours, 240 ml of human plasma and dobutamine (10 μg/kg/min) were administered to achieve a blood pressure of 90/40 mm Hg. On the first hospital day, the infant was hypocalcemic with metabolic acidosis. Hypocalcemia was corrected by means of cautious use of intravenous calcium gluconate, but the metabolic acidosis persisted (serum bicarbonate ranged between 10 and 15 mmol/l) despite several doses of intravenous sodium bicarbonate (2 mEq/kg). Packed red blood cells (20 ml/kg) were administered. A nasogastric tube was inserted, fluids were restricted, and multiple samples were obtained for culture. Ampicillin, gentamicin, and metronidazole were started. Urine and serum toxicology screens were negative. Cultures of rectal swabs disclosed no pathogenic microorganisms, and blood culture and assay for verotoxin (VT) were negative. On the second hospital day, the boy began to display abdominal tenderness. Abdominal X-ray showed massive colonic dilatation. Films from a barium enema examination revealed diffuse

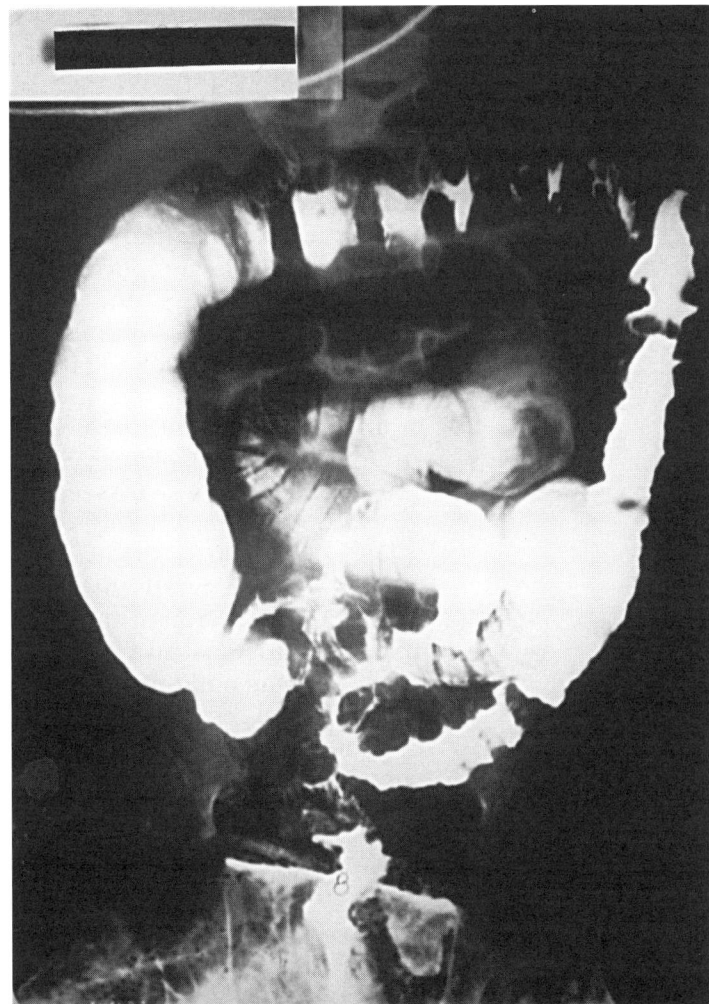

Figure 16.1. Barium enema showing thumb-printing pattern of colonic mucosa.

mucosal irregularity and thumb-printing of the sigmoid and transverse colon (Fig. 16.1). Abdominal signs worsened until the boy demonstrated classical findings of peritonitis. An exploratory laparotomy showed necrosis from the cecal valve to sigmoid. Total colectomy and an end ileostomy were performed. A venous left subclavian double-lumen catheter was inserted by means of the percutaneous Seldinger technique. The infant was anuric, and creatinine was 3 mg/dl (265 μmol/l), BUN 80 mg/dl (28.6 mmol/l), potassium 7.5 mmol/l, and arterial lactate 61 mg/dl (6 mmol/l). Continuous venovenous hemodiafiltration (CVVHDF) was used. Ultrafiltration was performed with partial replacement, allowing a fluid deficit of as much as

50 ml/hr. A balanced, isotonic, potassium-free solution was provided as replacement fluid. At the start of CVVHDF, central venous pressure was 16 mm Hg and decreased to 8 mm Hg. After a negative fluid balance was achieved, BUN was 45 mg/dl (16.1 mmol/l), and creatinine was 2.5 mg/dl (220 µmol/l). The procedure was performed without heparin due to systemic bleeding. The hemodynamic instability prevented continuation of the procedure. The postoperative course was complicated by several hypotensive episodes, hypothermia, and neurologic deterioration (Glasgow coma scale = 3). Pupils were fixed and mydriatic and lactacidemia increased (240 mg/dl). An active hemolytic process continued and the boy required several blood transfusions. His white blood cell count dropped to 5,300/mm^3 (5.3 × 10^3/l), platelet count was 11,300/mm^3, PT was 19 seconds, PTT was 60 seconds, factor II was 30%, factor V was 66%, factor VII/X was 28%, factor VIII was 90%, and factor IX was 30%. The liver profile showed the following: SGOT 645 U/l, SGPT 294 U/l, ammonia 225 µg/dl (159 µmol U/l). Treatment at this time included repeated plasma infusions and adjustment of the catecholamine support. The child died on the second postoperative day as a result of refractory shock. An autopsy was performed.

The pathologic diagnosis of the colectomy demonstrated hemorrhagic necrosis with thrombosis of small vessels, resulting in full-thickness involvement (transmural infarction) and areas of focal mucosal and submucosal injury (Fig. 16.2). Autopsy (central nervous system excluded)

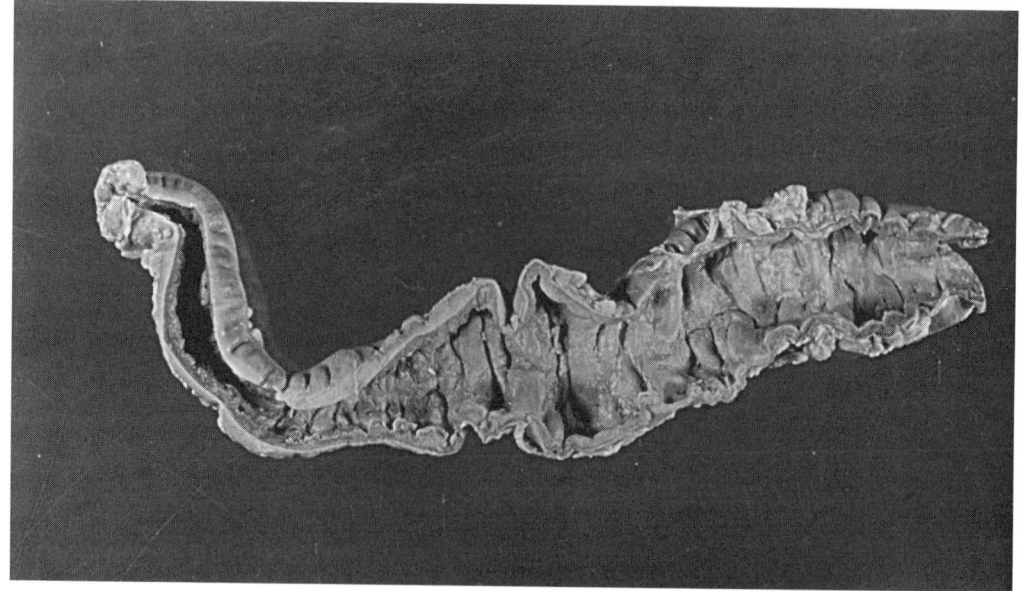

Figure 16.2. Gross specimen of resected colon.

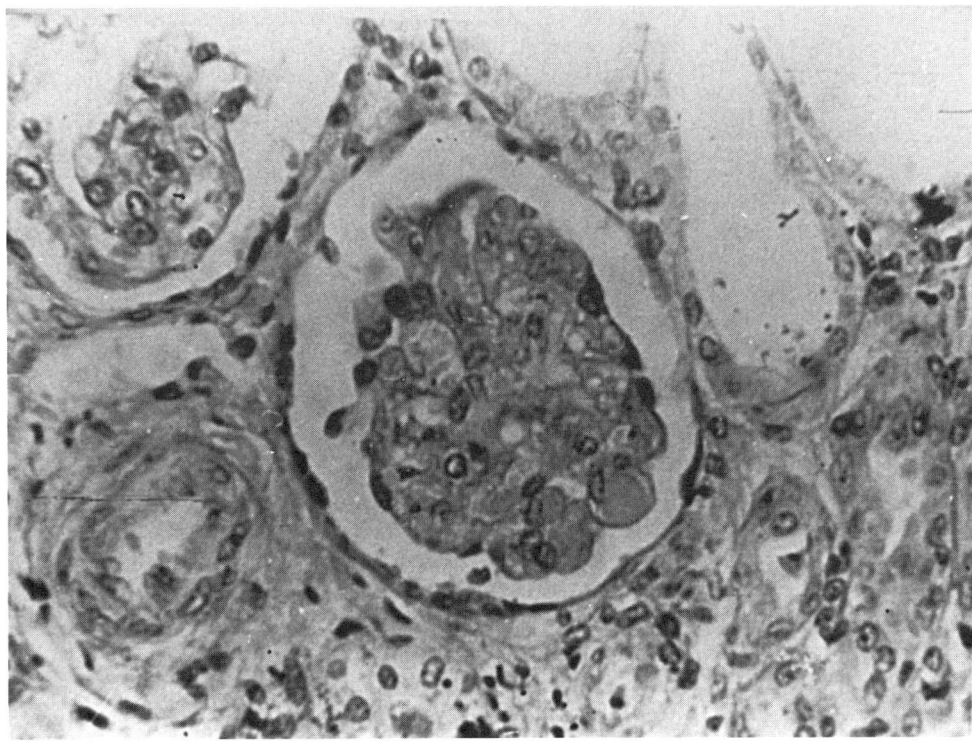

Figure 16.3.   Glomerular capillary thrombosis, subendothelial and mesangial swelling.

demonstrated liquid blood and clots in the abdominal cavity. The lungs showed partial collapsed areas without other lesions. Multiple sections through the heart disclosed recently focal interstitial endomyoepicardial hemorrhages. A few platelet thrombi in small vessels (capillary) and scanty myocytolysis were observed. Hemorrhagic lesions in the mesenteric and juxtapancreatic lymphatic tissue, retroperitoneum, pancreatic connective septum, and lamina propria of the gastric mucosa and small gut were reported. Examination of the liver revealed confluent hemorrhagic necrosis with periportal hepatocyte preservation (50% of liver involvement). Kidney examination showed frequent glomeruli thrombosis with variable capillary collapse, mesangiolisis, thrombus in afferent arteriolar interlobular arteries (with middle wall necrosis) and patchy cortical necrosis (Fig. 16.3).

DISCUSSION

The patient had a sudden onset of renal insufficiency associated with proteinuria, hematuria, and edema. Signs of his illness were bloody diarrhea, anemia, thrombocytopenia, status epilepticus, and shock. This constellation can be caused by a number of infectious etiologies. Hemorrhagic colitis by *Shigella, Yersinia, Escherichia coli, Salmonella,* or *Campylobacter* infections are possibilities. Among the acute vascular problems, intussusception or malrotation with volvulus has to be ruled out. Hemorrhagic shock and encephalopathy syndrome are marked by encephalopathy, shock, and diarrhea with high fevers, which were absent in this patient. The peripheral smears did not support this latter diagnosis.

Hemolytic uremic syndrome is a multisystem disorder characterized by three cardinal features: microangiopathic hemolytic anemia, thrombocytopenia, and acute renal failure. Besides this, gastrointestinal, neurologic, cardiac, hepatic, adrenal gland, and pancreatic involvement have been recognized. Coagulation disorders are frequently present. Shock is an uncommon complication. This syndrome was first described by Gasser in 1955 and Gianantonio reported a significant number of children in Argentina in 1964. A wide variety of agents have been suggested as causative, but until fairly recently the etiology of the classic syndrome has remained unclear. In 1985, Karmali demonstrated an association between classic hemolytic uremic syndrome and intestinal infection with verotoxin-producing *E. coli* (VTEC). VT is almost identical with Shiga-like toxin and a receptor for VT has been recently demonstrated. We did not find *E. coli* 0157:H 7 or VT in coproculture or fecal assay. In classic hemolytic uremic syndrome reported in Argentina, less than 20% of coprocultures and 50% of fecal assays for VT have been positive, and if antibiotics were administrated previously, these positive results were even lower.

Several reports of gastrointestinal tract involvement in hemolytic uremic syndrome have been published. These include colonic stricture, perforation, toxic megacolon, and pseudomembranous colitis. Colonic gangrene is a serious ischemic lesion secondary to vascular thrombosis. The sudden decompensation with hypotension and a bulging and painful abdomen with bloody stools could indicate this complication. The demonstration of colonic mucosal edema, thumb-printing, and scattered filling defects in barium contrast studies is characteristic of ischemia. The initial presentation of hemolytic uremia syndrome may mimic other gastrointestinal diseases: acute appendicitis, intussusception, or ulcerative colitis.

Central nervous system involvement is another problem that contributes to the morbidity and mortality of this syndrome. The most common clinical presentations are seizures. In the last 10 years, 221 patients were admitted to our hospital with a diagnosis of hemolytic uremic syndrome. Of these, 56 (25.3%) had seizures and 8 presented with status epilepticus. Neurologic involvement may be secondary to metabolic alterations (hyponatremia, hypocalcemia, acidosis) or hypertension. Microthrombi in cerebral vessels and vasculitis have been described with ischemic changes and cerebral edema.

Acute renal failure may be oligoanuric with a nephritis sediment. It has been reported that prolonged oliguria is associated with a poor prognosis. Hypertension is present in about 30% of the cases. Our patient had been anuric for 2 days. CAVHF or CVVHDF, either spontaneous or pump-driven, are safe methods for treatment of acute renal failure after abdominal surgery. There is some evidence that they are even useful for clearing detrimental mediators linked to multiorgan failure. In the renal tissue, the typical findings of hemolytic uremic syndrome were observed. Microangiopathic hemolytic anemia is one of the cardinal features of hemolytic uremic syndrome. Coagulation factor abnormalities vary from series to series with no constant abnormalities demonstrable. Elevation of serum transaminases has been noted and appears to reflect minor liver involvement in this syndrome.

Other reports include signs of cardiac dysfunction, myocarditis, and microthrombi in autopsy. In the present case, pathologic heart examination revealed some myocardial lesions.

The recent advances in the knowledge of the pathogenesis were published by Kaplan. First, the causal agent produces a toxin (VT or Shiga-T) and this unites with the cell receptor (GB3). Protein synthesis is inhibited and cell injury or death results. Red blood cell injury provokes the release of Von Willebrand multimers and thrombosis may ensue.

COMMENTARY

Hemolytic uremic syndrome is a difficult diagnosis to make, especially early in the disease process. This is important if one believes the reports that early dialysis may favorably influence the outcome, which would dictate early interventions. In addition, hemolytic uremic syndrome needs to be differentiated from the increasingly common hemorrhagic shock and encephalopathy (1).

Reference

1. Levin M, Pincott JR, Hjelm M, et al. Hemorrhagic shock and encephalopathy: clinical, pathologic, and biochemical features. J Pediatr 1989;114:194–203.

Suggested Readings

1. Gianantonio CA, Vitacco M, Mendilaharzu F, Gallo GE, Sojo ET. The hemolytic-uremic syndrome. Nephron 1973;11:174–192.
2. Kaplan BS, Cleary TG, Obrig TG. Recent advances in understanding the pathogenesis of the hemolytic uremic syndrome. Pediatr Nephrol 1990;4:276–283.
3. Siegler R. Management of hemolytic uremic syndrome. J Pediatrics 1988;112:1014–1020.
4. Whitington PF, Friedman AL, Chesney RW. Gastrointestinal disease in the hemolytic uremic syndrome. Gastroenterology 1979;76: 728–733.

Case 17

Gabriel J. Hauser and Joseph V. DiCarlo

Georgetown University Children's Medical Center
Washington, DC, USA

HISTORY

A 12-day-old infant girl was admitted to our hospital. She was the product of normal spontaneous vaginal delivery at 39 weeks' gestation after an uncomplicated pregnancy. Her birth weight was 2.9 kg. Her nursery course was uneventful except for mild hypothermia that responded to external heating. The baby was discharged from the nursery on her second day of life, and she was fed maternal milk and formula. On the third day of life she became irritable and had decreased oral intake. This continued for over a week with some improvement. She had had no bowel movements for the last 3 days prior to admission. On the day of admission, the baby became lethargic, was reported to have trouble breathing, and refused feeding. There was no history of fever, vomiting, diarrhea, ingestion of toxic substances, maternal perinatal infection, or trauma. The mother denied alcohol or drug abuse, and there was no significant family history.

The baby was examined at a hospital emergency room (ER), where she was found to be limp and unresponsive, with a weak cry and poor sucking ability. Her axillary temperature was 35.4°C, her heart rate was 120 beats/min, and her respiratory rate was 44 breaths/min. Serum glucose concentration was 31 mg/dl. Therefore, a glucose-containing intravenous solution was administered. Serum glucose increased to 88 mg/dl, but no clinical improvement was noted. A lumbar puncture was performed, blood cultures were obtained, and cefotaxime and ampicillin were

99

administered intravenously. She was then transferred to our PICU.

PHYSICAL EXAMINATION

The infant's rectal temperature was 36.2°C, her heart rate was 128 beats/min, her blood pressure was 83/59 mm Hg, her respiratory rate was 36 breaths/min, with occasional 5- to 10-second pauses. Her extremities were warm to the touch, the capillary filling time was 2 to 3 seconds, and full pulses were felt at all four extremities.

The baby was pale, obtunded, and responded only to painful stimuli. Her weight was 2.7 kg. There was slight peeling of the skin, but no external signs of trauma. The neck was supple and ear, nose, and throat appeared normal. A clear discharge was noted from the right eye. The heart sounds were normal and no murmurs were heard. The lungs were clear to auscultation, with good air entry bilaterally. The abdomen was soft, not distended, with no organomegaly, and no masses were palpable. There were good bowel sounds. Rectal examination results were normal, with normal-looking stool, which tested guaiac negative. The genitalia were normal.

Her fontanel was full but soft. No spontaneous movements were noted, except for occasional posturing of the upper extremities. Pupils were equal and small, and reacted sluggishly to light. Corneal reflex and gag reflex were absent. There was increased muscle tone in all extremities, occasional fine tremor, absent Moro and grasp reflexes, and a diminished rooting reflex, but no clonus. Patellar reflexes were diminished bilaterally. Fundoscopic examination revealed clear retinae and normal vessels with no hemorrhages and mild papilledema.

LABORATORY DATA

At the referring ER, the hemoglobin was 18.8 g/dl, hematocrit 52.8%, total white blood cell count 13,100 cells/µl, serum sodium was 140 mEq/l, potassium 4.6 mEq/l, chloride 108 mEq/l, bicarbonate 10 mEq/l, blood urea nitrogen (BUN) 5 mg/dl, magnesium 1.9 mg/dl, glucose 31 mg/dl, and calcium 10.1 mg/dl.

At the time of admission to the PICU, the baby's hemoglobin was 16.6 g/dl, her hematocrit was 50%, her erythrocyte count was 4.77×10^6/µl, and her total white blood cell count was 10,900 cells/µl with 42% segmented neutrophils, 41% lymphocytes, 5% monocytes, 5% atypical lymphocytes, 3% eosinophils, 1% bands, and 3% metamyelocytes. Her platelet count was 557,000. Prothrombin time was 9.4 seconds (with a control of 11.2 seconds), partial thromboplastin time was 33 seconds, and fibrinogen was 265 mg/dl. Serum sodium was 136 mEq/l, potassium 4.6 mEq/l, chloride 115 mEq/l, bicarbonate 10.6 mEq/l, anion gap 10 mEq/l, glucose 46 mg/dl, BUN 5 mg/dl, creatinine 0.7 mg/dl, calcium 9.7 mg/dl, phosphorus 3.2 mg/dl, magnesium 1.7 mg/dl, uric acid 5.5 mg/dl, bilirubin 0.2 mg/dl, alkaline phosphatase, 108 mg/dl, aspartate aminotransferase 24 IU/l, alanine aminotransferase 7 IU/l, lactic dehydrogenase 372 IU/l, total protein 4.1 g/dl, albumin 2.2 g/dl, globulin 1.9 g/dl, and ammonia 69 μmol/l. Arterial blood gases with the baby breathing spontaneously in room air were as follows: pH 7.40, PO_2 102 mm Hg, oxygen saturation 98%, pCO_2 18.4 mm Hg, bicarbonate 11.4 mEq/l, base deficit 10.1.

Urine obtained by catheterization had a specific gravity of 1.016, pH of 6.0, 2+ ketones, and a trace of blood, and was negative for glucose, protein, bilirubin, or nitrites. There were 3 red blood cells and 2 white blood cells per high power field.

Cerebrospinal fluid (CSF) was clear, and had 140 white blood cells per high power field (with 50% segmented neutrophils, 31% lymphocytes, and 19% monocytes), and 3800 red blood cells. Glucose was 53 mg/dl (with concomitant serum glucose of 76 mg/dl), and protein concentration was 43 mg/dl.

ECG results were normal. Chest X-ray showed clear lung fields and a normal cardiac silhouette. A CT scan (Fig. 17.1) showed diffuse, symmetric brain edema, with small ventricles and a small subarachnoid fluid collection. Electroencephalogram results showed intermittent epileptiform disturbance confined to the central regions bilaterally, compatible with a seizure disorder.

MANAGEMENT

The patient was intubated and hyperventilated to a pH of 7.48–7.52. A radial arterial catheter was placed for blood gas monitoring. Vancomycin, cefotaxime, acyclovir, and phenobarbital were administered intravenously. Because of the normal anion gap, treatment with sodium bicarbonate was begun, but resulted in no change in serum bicarbonate concentration. After we considered the differential diagnosis of a newborn infant presenting with

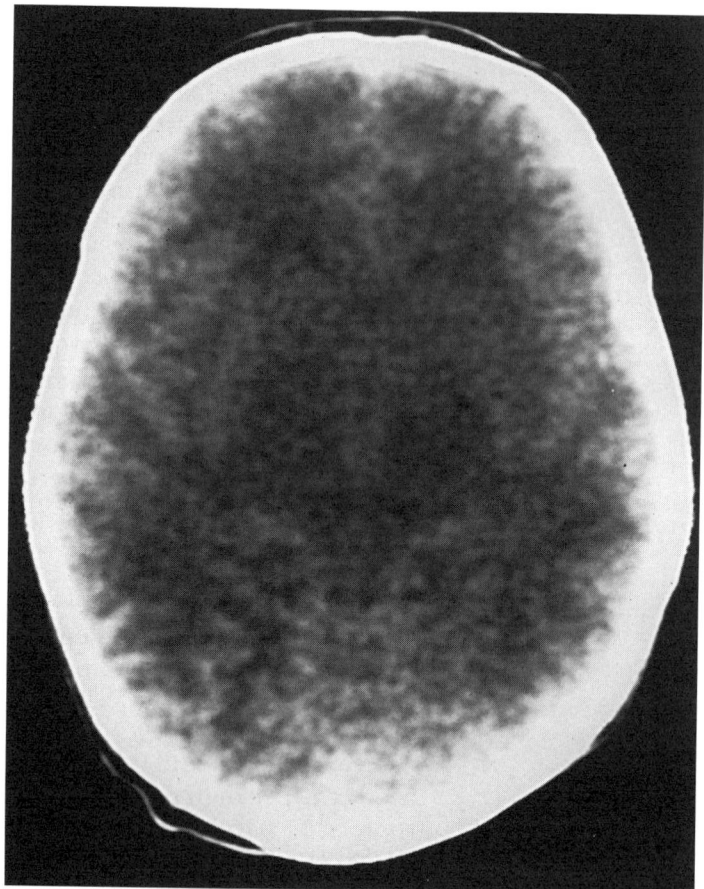

Figure 17.1. CT scan showing diffuse, prominent lucency of the white matter and basal ganglia, with effacement of the cerebral sulci and compression of the frontal horns, compatible with cerebral edema.

cerebral edema, further specific examination revealed that the urine had the odor of maple syrup. Therefore, the 2,4 dinitrophenylhydrazine (DNPH) urine test for the detection of urine ketoacids (derived from high levels of leucine, isoleucine, and valine) was performed at the bedside on the night of admission. A few drops of 0.1% DNPH in 0.1N HCl were added to the patient's urine placed in a test tube and resulted in immediate formation of a yellow precipitate of diphenylhydrazine, while the control urine remained clear. Analysis of the serum amino acid profile showed that the leucine level was 1327 μmol/l (normal 50–100 μmol/l), isoleucine level was 281 μmol/l (normal 20–75 μmol/l), and valine level was 477 μmol/l (normal 80–200 μmol/l).

The diagnosis of the classic form of maple syrup urine disease was made, and the patient was treated with peritoneal dialysis for 3 days until normalization of the DNPH test and of serum amino acid levels were achieved. A special diet devoid of branched-chain amino acids (Analog MSUD Formula, Mead Johnson Laboratories, Evansville, IN) was administered and tolerated well. No improvement in the baby's neurologic status was observed with peritoneal dialysis. Blood, urine, and CSF cultures and serology were negative for bacterial and viral pathogens, and the antibiotic therapy was discontinued. The papilledema had resolved, and head circumference was unchanged. Mechanical ventilation was discontinued. The gag reflex was still absent, and the suck and swallow were abnormal. Therefore, the baby underwent a tracheotomy and a gastrostomy tube was inserted. Her neurologic status gradually improved, and she thrived well on the special formula and was eventually discharged from the hospital. The tracheostomy and gastric tube were subsequently removed, and the baby (today 20 months old) has made progress, although she still has residual neurologic disability.

DISCUSSION

Bacterial sepsis, meningitis, herpes encephalitis, toxic encephalopathy, and extreme hypernatremia should be ruled out in every young infant presenting with lethargy, poor feeding, seizures, metabolic acidosis, and hypoglycemia. However, though less frequently encountered, several metabolic disorders may also cause cerebral edema and have similar clinical appearance. These include aminoacidurias, hyperammonemia syndromes, organic acidemias, disorders of lactate, pyruvate, and carnitine metabolism, as well as galactokinase deficiency and galactosemia. A simple clinical test, smelling the patient's urine, can help in the diagnosis of some of these disorders, such as maple syrup urine disease (maple syrup odor), isovaleric acidemia (sweaty feet-like odor), phenylketonuria (mousy or musty odor), or trimethylaminuria (fishy odor). Ingestion of some spices by the baby or even prenatal ingestion by the mother may sometimes result in peculiar odors and make the diagnosis difficult. After several days of poor oral intake and administration of intravenous fluids, the odors may disappear. Further validation of some of these syndromes at the bedside is possible by simple screening urine tests such as the DNPH test used in our patient. In some cases, early diagnosis may allow the institution of early life-saving therapy (in maple syrup urine disease—peritoneal dialysis). In the era of ever-increasing sophistication of diagnostic and monitoring capabilities in the PICU, the human nose can still be a valuable tool.

COMMENTARY

This case demonstates that the tenets of medicine apply especially in the ICU. A diagnosis is most often made through an accurate history and careful physical examination by an astute clinician. Technology and sophistication are often only helpful adjuvants to what we offer our patients.

Suggested Readings

1. Hauser GJ, Chitayat D, Berns D, Muhlbauer B. Peculiar odours in newborns and maternal prenatal ingestion of spicy food. Eur J Pediatr 1985;144:403.
2. Huttennlocher PR, Hillman RE, Hsia Y. Pseudotumor cerebri in galactosemia. J Pediatr 1970:76:902–905.
3. Lungarotti MS, Calabro A, Signorini E, Garibaldi LR. Cerebral edema in maple syrup urine disease. Am J Dis Child 1982;136:648.
4. Mantovani JF, Naidich TP, Prensky AL, Dodson WE, Williams JC. MSUD presentation with pseudotumor cerebri and CT abnormalities. J Pediatr 1980;96:279–281.
5. Riviello JJ, Jr., Rezvani I, DiGeorge AM, Foley CM. Cerebral edema causing death in children with maple syrup urine disease. J Pediatr 1991;119:42–45.

Case 18

Milan Beier, Rudolf Riedel, Ondrej Benko, Olga Bandzakova, and Peter Gasparec

*Children's University Hospital
Bratislava, Slovakia*

HISTORY

A 3-month-old 3.5-kg girl who was previously healthy was admitted following respiratory arrest. The day prior to admission the child had diarrhea and fever (central temperature 38°C) without aspirin exposure. On the day of admission she had rapid onset of coma and respiratory arrest. Her mother administered mouth-to-mouth ventilation. The infant was vomiting, with possible aspiration, during the resuscitation, and had tonic-clonic seizures. She was still in a coma with restoration of breathing and a regular heart rate. She was immediately taken to the hospital within one-half hour of the arrest.

PHYSICAL EXAMINATION

At the time of admission, the infant was in a coma with poor perfusion. Her mean blood pressure was 45 mm Hg, her heart rate was 150 beats/min, and her respiratory rate was >70 breaths/min, with a rectal temperature of 35°C. Her Glasgow coma scale score was 4, and she was cyanotic and hypothermic, with cool extremities and decreased peripheral perfusion, decreased capillary refill (greater than 5 seconds), mottled skin color, dry mucous membranes, marked decreased skin turgor, and a pulsating anterior fontanel. There was clinical evidence of disseminated intravascular coagulation, with excessive bleeding from venipuncture sites, hematemesis, and melena. A neurologic examination showed sluggish pupillary light reflex, conjugate deviation on doll's eye maneuver, positive corneal reflex, poor response to stimuli, quadruhyperreflexia, repeated generalized tonic-clonic seizures, and no signs of meningeal irritation. Several hours after admission, she developed worsening of the consumptive coagulopathy and hepatomegaly. The infant's status deteriorated despite treatment. Laboratory studies in this hospital showed a red blood cell count of $3.27 \times 10^{12}/1$, hemoglobin content of 8.0 g/dl, white blood cell count of $11.7 \times 10^9/1$, thrombocytopenia with a platelet count of $63 \times 10^9/1$, prolonged bleeding time (Duke) of 13 minutes, prolonged clotting time (Lee-White) of 13 minutes, prolonged prothrombin time, plasma levels of aspartate transaminase (AST) of 43.9 μkat/l (increased 100 times), alanine transaminase (ALT) 16.9 μkat/l, hyponatremia (123 mmol/l), hyperkalemia (6.62 mmol/l), hypoglycemia (1.1 mmol/l), a normal level of plasma urea (5.2 mmol/l), and elevated creatinine level (104 μmol/l). She had severe metabolic acidosis with respiratory alkalosis. With the suspicion of Reye syndrome, the infant was transported to our hospital (Children's University Hospital, Department of Anesthesia and Resuscitation).

MANAGEMENT

Laboratory findings on admission to the PICU showed (Table 18.1) thrombocytopenia, prolonged prothrombin and partial thromboplastin times, very low fibrinogen level, and elevated aminotransferase values while blood ammonia concentration was only mildly elevated (80.4

Table 18.1. Laboratory Values in Infant With Hemorrhagic Shock and Encephalopathy

Day	1	2	3	4	5	8	10	15
PLT × $10^9/1$	51	36	35	49	82	68	117	261
Quick (sec)	105	34	37	25	18	19	19	18
PTT (sec)	116	45	51	44	48	37	34	44
Fbg (g/l)	0	3.0	2.5	2.3	2.0	1.7	2.3	5.6
AST* (μkat/l)	39	65	94	49	21	6.3	1.2	0.9
ALT* (μkat/l)	14	30	36	15	10	4.8	1.6	0.9

* Normal value 0.067–0.400 μkat/l.
Abbreviations: ALT, alanine aminotransferase; AST, aspartate aminotransferase; Fbg, fibrinogen; PLT, platelets; PTT, partial thromboplastin time.

mmol/l). The hemoglobin concentration decreased to 7.1 g/dl, and the white blood cell count was increased to 14.1 $\times$ $10^9/1$, with 70% neutrophils and 25% lymphocytes. We found elevated levels of serum bilirubin, hyponatremia, hyperkalemia, and a normal blood glucose level. Renal function was impaired, with raised plasma urea (8.9 mmol/l) and creatinine levels (158.9 μmol/l). She had severe metabolic acidosis (pH 7.03, pCO_2 21 mm Hg, standard bicarbonate 7.6 mmol/l, and base deficit of 24.8 mmol/l) with a compensatory respiratory alkalosis. Chest X-ray and ECG appeared normal. Hepatitis B surface antigen was negative. Other laboratory studies including toxicologic and metabolic screens, cerebrospinal fluid (CSF) analysis, microbiologic specimens from nasopharyngeal secretions, sputum, urine, stool, and CSF failed to show any abnormality. The respiratory distress and hypotension were treated vigorously with mechanical ventilation and intensive fluid resuscitation. Treatment of the shock required large volumes of blood products. Consumptive coagulopathy was managed aggressively with fresh-frozen plasma, platelet, and fibrinogen infusions. Hyperventilation, mannitol, and dexamethasone were implemented to attempt control of the presumed elevated intracranial pressure. Anticonvulsant drugs were necessary to control seizures. Broad-spectrum antibiotics were administered. The patient survived with serious neurologic sequelae. Electroencephalographic study showed diffuse slowing and epileptiform activity. Ultrasound findings showed cerebral edema, progressing after 1 month to hydrocephalus ex vacuo. Plasma levels of urea cycle amino acids and carnitine were normal. One year later, the girl showed moderate severe neurologic deficits and electroencephalogram with diffuse abnormalities and θ waves.

DISCUSSION

In 1983 Levin et al (1) from the Hospital for Sick Children in London reported a series of 10 children with hemorrhagic shock and encephalopathy who had acute onset of shock, fever, bleeding, seizures, and coma. The recognition of similar patients followed in Great Britain (2), North America, the Netherlands, and Israel. We believe that hemorrhagic shock and encephalopathy represent a distinct clinical entity, but many questions about the disorder remain unanswered. This syndrome presents a challenge to differentiate if from sepsis (3), toxic shock syndrome, infantile Reye syndrome (4), and hemolytic uremic syndrome.

This is a clinical entity now being recognized with increasing frequency. It has rapid onset of shock, fever, seizures, and coma followed by disseminated intravascular coagulation, diarrhea, acidosis, and hepatorenal dysfunction. This syndrome occurs more often between 2 and 10 months of age (5), which represents a vulnerable period for thermoregulatory balance. The failure to identify a bacterial, viral, or toxic cause (6) may indicate that the appearance of hemorrhagic shock and encephalopathy is an unusual response to various insults (7). Despite aggressive medical support, there is a high mortality and survivors have severe neurologic deficits. We describe one similar patient from Czechoslovakia who suddenly developed shock, seizures, coma, consumptive coagulopathy, elevated plasma activity of hepatic enzymes, acidosis, and renal dysfunction.

COMMENTARY

This syndrome is a challenge to diagnose and a disappointment to treat. It is clear that either the incidence of the disease is increasing or our awareness of it is increasing. To me this syndrome bears a similarity to the conditions caused by the Hantaan viruses. It will be interesting to see whether an etiologic agent for hemorrhagic shock and encephalopathy is identified in the near future.

References

1. Lewvin M, Kay JDS, Gould JD, et al. Haemorrhagic shock and encephalopathy: a new syndrome with a high mortality in young children. Lancet 1983;2:64–67.
2. Levin M, Pincott JR, Hjelm M, Taylor F, et al. Hemorrhagic shock and encephalopathy: clinical, pathologic, and biochemical features. J Pediatr 1989;144:194–203.
3. Zimmermann JJ, Dietrich KA. Current perspectives on septic shock. Pediatr Clin North Am 1987;34:131–163.
4. DeLong GR, Glick TH. Encephalopathy of Reye's syndrome: a review of pathogenetic hypotheses. Pediatrics 1982;69:53–63.
5. Joint British Paediatric Association and Communicable Disease Surveillance Centre scheme for haemorrhagic shock encephalopathy syndrome: surveillance report for 1982–4. Br Med J 1985;150:1578–1579.
6. Haemorrhagic shock and encephalopathy [Editorial]. Lancet 1985;2:535–536.
7. Chaves-Carballo E, Montes JE, Nelson WB, Chrenka BA. Hemorrhagic shock and encephalopathy. Am J Dis Child 1990;144:1079–1082.

Case 19

Joseph V. DiCarlo, Gabriel J. Hauser, and Heidi J. Dalton

Georgetown University Children's Medical Center Washington, DC, USA

HISTORY

A 5-year-old girl was admitted to our hospital for failure to thrive and Moebius syndrome (maldevelopment of multiple cranial nerve nuclei, which in her case resulted in ptosis, hemifacial immobility, and vocal cord paralysis). She presented to an emergency department with stridor, respiratory failure, and severe hypotension. Her vocal cord paralysis had been discovered in the perinatal period, and was managed with tracheostomy. She was decannulated uneventfully 10 months prior to this admission. Her growth failure was of unclear etiology; gastroesophageal reflux was eventually treated with a Nissen fundoplication and gastrostomy, but she failed to grow despite supplemental feedings. The gastrostomy tube was removed 1 month prior to admission when she developed a gastrocutaneous fistula. At the age of 5 years she weighed 10.4 kg, below the 5th percentile. Despite these difficulties, she is a functional child who attends school.

Three weeks prior to the present admission, the girl had chicken pox, from which she recovered uneventfully. Four days before this hospitalization, fever, cough, and diarrhea developed, and the child was diagnosed with pharyngitis which was treated with amoxicillin and dexamethasone. She improved, but acutely developed gagging and choking the day of admission. During transport to the emergency department of a community hospital, paramedics suctioned oropharyngeal secretions flecked with blood.

By this time her stridor was severe, her perfusion was poor, and she was hypotensive (blood pressure 70/50 mm Hg). The initial arterial blood gas (100%) oxygen was pH 7.13, $PaCO_2$ 45 torr, PaO_2 73 torr, base deficit -12.9, with an oxygen saturation of 87%. The oxygenation worsened soon after intubation, until the trachea was suctioned for 150 ml of frothy pink secretions. The blood pressure improved with administration of lactated Ringer's solution (450 ml) and infusion of dopamine (5 μg/kg/min). The child was transported to a PICU.

PHYSICAL EXAMINATION

When physically examined, the patient was found to be cachectic, pale, and small for her chronologic age. Her vital signs were as follows: temperature 36.3°C (rectal), pulse rate 160 beats/min, respiratory rate 35 breaths/min (mechanical), and blood pressure 55/48 mm Hg. Her skin was pale, warm, nonicteric, and dry. Her eyes were sunken and her conjunctiva were pale. Her pupils were reactive with a right lateral gaze preference. The mucus membranes were dry. The patient had bilateral axillary and inguinal lymphadenopathy. Her lungs were clear to auscultation. There were no extra heart sounds, murmurs, or rubs. Peripheral pulses were faint. Her abdomen was soft, without organomegaly.

LABORATORY DATA

Her chest X-ray revealed hyperinflation with prominent interstitial lung markings (Figs. 19.1 and 19.2). The left lower lobe was atelectatic, with a small heart size. Her arterial blood gases initially revealed pH 7.13, $PaCO_2$ 45 torr, PaO_2 73 torr, and base deficit -12.9. This was followed by a period of stabilization (pH 7.55, $PaCO_2$ 17 torr, PaO_2 449 torr, and base deficit -7.0). When the patient decompensated subsequently, her arterial blood gas values were as follows: pH 7.33, $PaCO_2$ 38 torr, PaO_2 201 torr, base deficit -6.2. The complete blood count revealed a hemoglobin of 10.1 g/dl, a hematocrit of 31.5%, and a platelet count of 337,000/mm^3, white blood cell count of 5200/mm^3 (19% bands, 63% segments, 16% lymphocytes). Electrolyte assay demonstrated the following values: sodium 142 mEq/l, glucose 266 mg/dl, potassium 3.2 mEq/l, blood

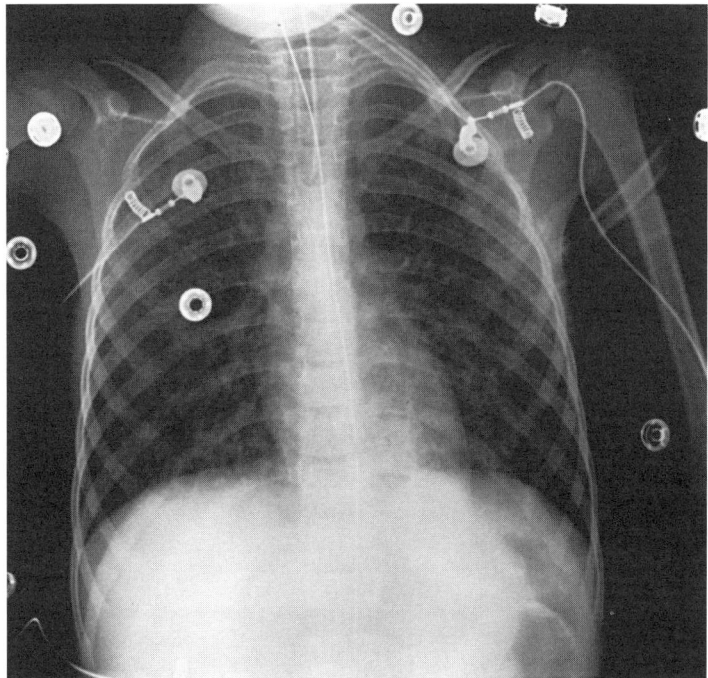

Figure 19.1.   Initial chest X-ray. Interstitial chronic lung disease with hyperinflation; heart size is normal.

urea nitrogen (BUN) 12 mg/dl, chloride 114 mEq/l, creatinine 0.7 mg/dl, bicarbonate 12 mEq/l, and calcium 8.0 mg/dl.

MANAGEMENT

On arrival at the PICU, the child again became hypotensive, with her blood pressure responding to further fluid administration and an increase in the dopamine infusion to 15 μg/kg/min. The central venous pressure after resuscitation was 8 mm Hg. Initial mechanical ventilation resulted in hyperoxia, hypocarbia, and alkalosis. Culture samples were obtained and antibiotics were administered. Mechanical minute ventilation was reduced to normalize the pH and carbon dioxide tension, and the F_IO_2 was gradually reduced, with arterial oxygen tension remaining above normal. She became febrile and flushed, and her blood pressure became unstable. Norepinephrine infusion was begun, with temporary improvement in the blood pressure. She soon became mottled, hypotensive (50/30 mm Hg), and bradycardic (80 beats/min). The central ve-

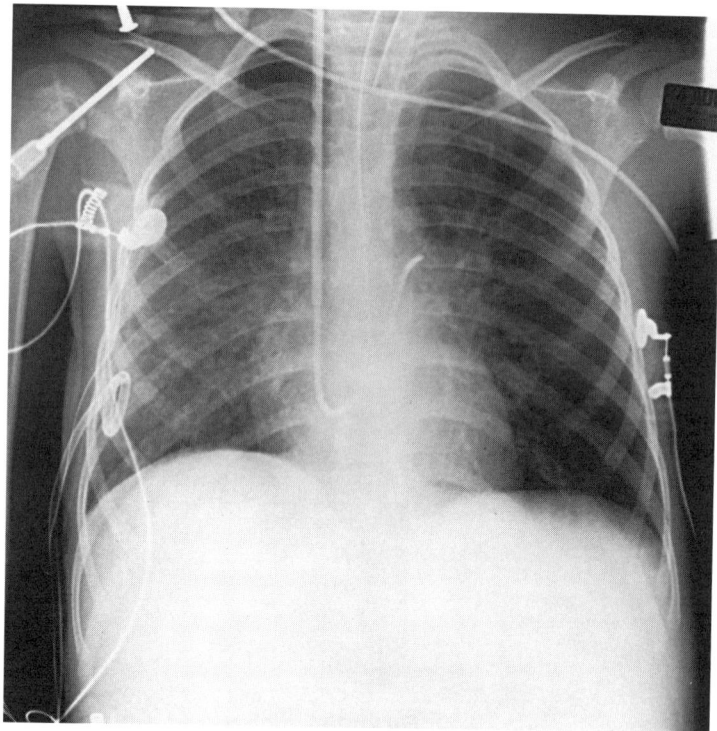

Figure 19.2.   Chest X-ray 5 days later. Heart size is slightly increased; a pulmonary artery catheter is in place.

citation included intravenous administration of epinephrine 0.2 mg, manual hyperventilation, neuromuscular blockade, and dobutamine infusion. An epinephrine infusion resulted in dramatically fluctuating perfusion, pulses, and arterial blood pressure (frequent hypotension in the range of 65–75 mm Hg systolic followed by sustained increases to 135–160 mm Hg systolic). The central venous pressure fluctuated inversely with the arterial blood pressure.

Thus a pattern was established: hemodynamic stability would consistently be achieved with manual hyperventilation, and she would become unstable when the systemic pH decreased to <7.41. Infusion of sodium bicarbonate (1 mEq/kg) would achieve the same stability, as would an intravenous dose of isoproterenol. With rehydration, physical findings suggested right ventricular dysfunction (a heave was notable at the lower left sternal border; the second heart sound was now loudly split; the liver was now palpable 3 cm below the costal margin). An echocardiogram revealed a dilatated right atrium, right ventricle, and pulmonary artery; with moderate tricuspid regurgitation

(3 m/sec); mild pulmonary insufficiency (2.5 m/sec); reasonable left ventricular contractility (shortening fraction 0.34); left ventricular compression by the dilatated right atrium; and estimated pulmonary arterial systolic pressures of 50–60 mm Hg (Fig. 19.3).

The treatment regimen was modified to include hyperventilation to maintain a pH >7.50, oxygenation to maintain the PaO_2 above 100 torr, and infusions of isoproterenol and prostaglandin E_1, to replace the other vasoactive medications. A fiberoptic-tipped pulmonary artery catheter was inserted percutaneously, which measured moderate pulmonary hypertension despite the therapies described above. The data are presented in Table 19.1.

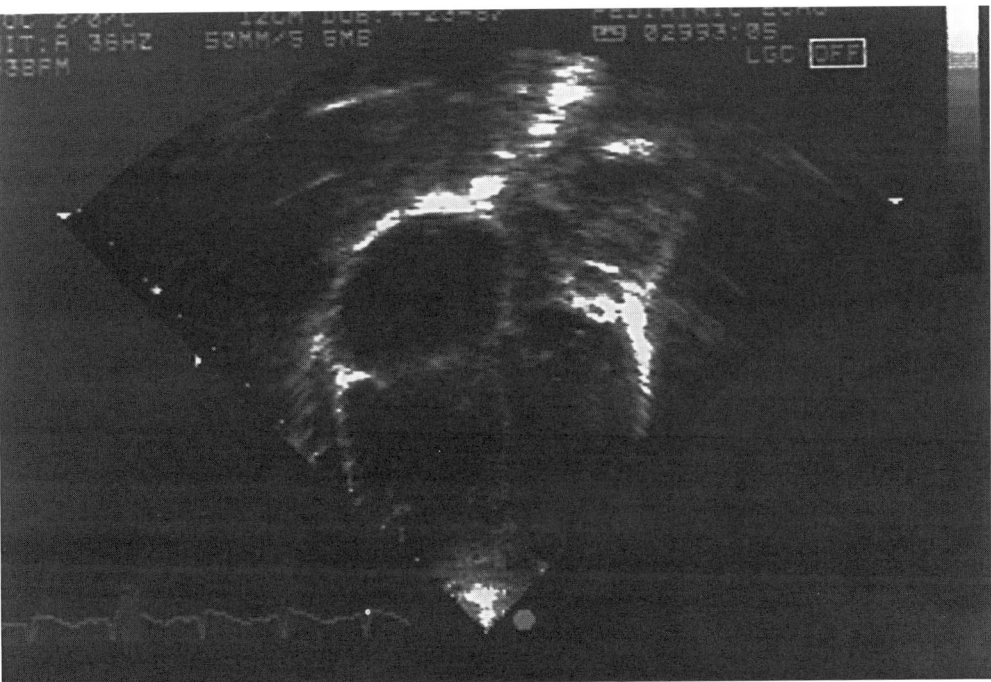

Figure 19.3. Echocardiogram, four-chamber view. The right atrium and ventricle are dilated, to nearly the size of the left ventricle.

Table 19.1.

Measurement	Value
Systemic arterial pressure (mm Hg)	95/65
Pulmonary artery pressure (mm Hg)	45/37 (mean 41)
Pulmonary artery occlusion pressure (mm Hg)	9
Central venous pressure (mm Hg)	11
Pulmonary vascular resistance index (dyne*sec/cm^{5}m^2)	936
Systemic vascular resistance index (dyne*sec/cm^5*m^2)	2080
Cardiac index (l/min/m^2)	2.3

She remained labile for 48 hours, then began a gradual improvement. The pulmonary artery pressures remained elevated, but the cardiac index improved to 3.5 l/min/m². She never developed pulmonary edema, and pulmonary artery occlusion pressure stayed below 10 mm Hg. No bacterial or viral source was found for her illness. After 10 days of supportive therapy, pulmonary function had improved enough to allow extubation. She did well for a day, but then severe coughing and gagging developed during replacement of a nasogastric tube. She did not recover in a reasonable amount of time and was therefore re-intubated. At direct laryngoscopy and bronchoscopy, she was found to have very poor vocal cord function. A tracheostomy was performed. After further recovery, she was again an active child, with good lung function. An echocardiogram 1 month postdischarge was normal, with normal right heart function and pressures and an ejection fraction of 69%.

DISCUSSION

This child had life-threatening pulmonary hypertensive crisis. The diagnosis of pulmonary hypertension was not suspected initially. Its presence, however, was suggested by the success of therapeutic maneuvers that resulted in hyperoxia and alkalosis (and, conversely, the failure of standard therapies for septic shock). The initial chest X-ray should have been helpful. The abnormal lung interstitium may have been the only clue to chronic pulmonary inflammatory changes, and might have pointed to pulmonary hypertension as the culprit in this child who acted "sicker than her X-ray." Secondary pulmonary hypertension occurs almost exclusively in children with chronic lung and/or heart disease; this child is probably not an exception, but had an unusual presentation. With the tracheostomy in place for the first 4 years of her life, she may have been protected from aspiration into the lungs. For the past 10 months she had seemed to do fine without the tracheostomy, but may in fact have been aspirating chronically through dysfunctional vocal cords. Chronic inflammation or hypoxia may have led to pulmonary vascular changes, manifested as life-threatening pulmonary hypertension when she was challenged by an acute infection. A rather high incidence of pulmonary hypertension has been reported in adults with acute respiratory failure. Patients with pulmonary hypertension have a higher mortality rate compared with patients without this risk factor.

Pulmonary hypertension is common in children with adult respiratory distress syndrome, but its presence does not predict mortality. Pulmonary hypertension should be suspected in any child with chronic lung disease who presents with an acute pulmonary or systemic illness. The diagnosis can be supported with echocardiography. The decision to insert a pulmonary artery catheter can be based on its clinical utility in a particular patient.

COMMENTARY

Identifying pulmonary hypertension is often extremely difficult. When suspected, it is often difficult to document but in a situation where it is unexpected, it presents a huge challenge. On the horizon is treatment with inhaled nitric oxide, which seems to be a potent pulmonary vasodilator with a short enough half-life that the systemic effects are minimal. There seems to be no tachyphylaxis to the agent, which will undoubtedly supplant the many nonspecific vasodilators we presently use to treat pulmonary hypertension (1).

Reference

1. Girard C, Lehot J-J, Pannetier J-C, Filley S, French P, Estanove S. Inhaled nitric oxide after mitral valve replacement in patients with chronic pulmonary artery hypertension. Anesthesiology 1992;77: 880–883.

Suggested Readings

1. Goodman G, Perkin RM, Anas NG, Sperling DR, Hicks DA, Rowen M. Pulmonary hypertension in infants with bronchopulmonary dysplasia. J Pediatr 1988;112:67–72.
2. Prielipp RC, McLean R, Rosenthal MH, Pearl RG. Hemodynamic profiles of prostaglandin E_1, isoproterenol, prostacyclin, and nifedipine in experimental porcine pulmonary hypertension. Crit Care Med 1991;19:60–67.
3. Timmons OD, Dean JM, Vernon DD. Mortality rates and prognostic variables in children with adult respiratory distress syndrome. J Pediatr 1991;119:896–899.
4. Villar J, Blazquez MA, Lubillo S, Quintana J, Manzano JL. Pulmonary hypertension in acute respiratory failure. Crit Care Med 1989;17: 523–526.

Case 20

L. Kyle Walker

The Johns Hopkins Hospital
Baltimore, Maryland, USA

HISTORY

A 1-day-old neonate girl was referred to the PICU for extracorporeal membrane oxygenation (ECMO). She was the 2100-g product of a 38 weeks' gestation in a 19-year-old female. The pregnancy was complicated by poor prenatal care and a history of intravenous drug abuse and serology that was positive for the human immunodeficiency virus (HIV). The mother arrived at a hospital emergency room in active labor. With rupture of membranes, thick meconium was noted. As labor progressed, variable decelerations of the fetal heart rate were noted and a scalp pH obtained from the fetus was 7.17. Delivery was by emergent cesarean section and Apgar scores were 6 at 1 minute and 9 at 5 minutes. The infant was intubated in the delivery room and thick meconium was suctioned from below the vocal cords. She was transported to the intensive care nursery, intubated, and ventilated. When the placenta was delivered, it was noted to be small and to have multiple infarcts.

During the first 24 hours of life, arterial blood gases from a umbilical artery line showed hypoxemia refractory to multiple ventilatory maneuvers, with development of increasingly unstable blood pressure requiring boluses of intravenous fluids and initiation of intravenous vasopressor agents. At this time, the PICU was asked to evaluate this patient for ECMO support.

PHYSICAL EXAMINATION

On arrival at the PICU accompanied by the neonatal transport team, the infant was noted to be symmetrically growth retarded with no obvious congenital anomalies. Her vital signs at the time of admission were as follows:

heart rate 178 beats/min, blood pressure 62/38, mean arterial pressure 48 mm Hg, and respiratory rate 60 breaths/min. The skin and general habitus examination revealed an infant who was symmetrically small with weight, length, and head circumference all falling below the fifth percentile on a growth chart. The extremities were mildly wasted with meconium staining of the skin and nails. The examination of the head revealed normocephaly with normally situated ears. The eyes were closed but pupils were midsized and reactive to light. The palate was intact and intubated with a 3.0-mm endotracheal tube. There was a dramatic rise of the chest wall with ventilator breaths. Breath sounds were equal in all lung fields with inspiratory crackles. The cardiac impulse was easily seen two intercostal spaces below the left nipple.

The child was tachycardiac with an accentuated second sound. No murmurs were appreciated. Weak pulses were present in all extremities with axillary and femoral pulses being equal. The liver was easily palpated 5 cm below the right costal margin, and the spleen not palpable. The kidneys were of normal size. The child had normal female external genitalia, and the urethra was catheterized with a 5-French feeding tube. The ventilatory settings were as follows: F_IO_2 1.0, pressures 34/5 cm H_2O, 60 breaths/min, respiratory time 0.45 seconds; mean airway pressure 16 cm H_2O. Laboratory values revealed arterial blood gases of pH 7.42, Pco_2 30 mm Hg, Po_2 35 mm Hg; a complete blood count revealed a white blood cell count of 6000 (17% bands, 40% segmented, 30% mononuclear, 2% eosinophilic), and platelet count of 149,000. Electrolyte testing demonstrated the following values: sodium 142 mEq/dl, potassium 3.1 mEq/dl, chloride 113 mEq/dl, and serum bicarbonate 19 mEq/dl. Other chemistry values were as follows: glucose 120 mg/dl, blood urea nitrogen 12 mg/dl, creatinine 1.2 mg/dl, serum glutamic oxaloacetic transaminase 34 IU/l, serum glutamic pyruvic transaminase 12 IU/l; and clotting studies showed a prothrombin time 1.2 times that of the control values and a partial thromboplastin time 2 times that of the control values. At the time of admission, the following medications were being administered to the infant: dopamine 10 μg/kg/min, dobutamine 10 μg/kg/min, pavulon 0.20 mg as required with movement, fentanyl 2 μg every 1–2 hours, ampicillin 200 mg every 12 hours, and cefotaxime 100 mg every 12 hours.

MANAGEMENT

Further diagnostic tests were completed soon after arrival in the PICU. These included a chest X-ray showing worsening bilateral patchy infiltrates, an echocardiogram showing a large poorly functioning right ventricle with tricuspid valvular regurgitation, and a right to left shunt at the foramen ovale with no ductal flow or shunting observed and little forward flow into the pulmonary artery. Intracranial ultrasound showed evidence of a grade 1-intraventricular hemorrhage in the right hemisphere with calcification.

After a reasonable trial of continued medical management this infant met our inhouse criteria for ECMO. A decision to offer this therapy was reached and the mother gave consent. The infant was placed on venoarterial ECMO for 5 days after which time ECMO was successfully withdrawn and the infant returned to conventional mechanical ventilation of F_1O_2 of 0.5, peak inspiratory pressures of 18 with a positive end-expiratory pressure of 4 cm H_2O and respiratory rate of 30 breaths/min. She was weaned from conventional mechanical ventilation within 72 hours and discharged from the hospital 10 days later. At that time she was noted to feed slowly and have a slight decrease in tone. A CT scan at the time of discharge was interpreted as normal. When seen in follow-up this infant had grown and developed normally.

DISCUSSION

The primary pathophysiologic problem in the case of this infant was severe hypertension of the pulmonary arterial bed. This hypertension is reversible in most neonatal patients after the first few days of life, but in a case like this, the mortality is quite high with protracted failure of usual maneuvers to bring about resolution. According to chest X-ray evidence, there was also a component of pneumonia most likely to be a chemical one related to the aspiration of meconium.

The first goal of medical therapy is to decrease pulmonary vascular resistance. Hyperoxia, alkalinization (with sodium bicarbonate and/or by hyperventilation), appropriate sedation, decreased handling all may be helpful. A "selective" pulmonary vasodilator would be the most powerful tool but there is not one currently available. An alternative that is receiving much attention is the inhalation of small amounts of nitric oxide gas which can cause pulmonary vasodilatation with no systemic effects. This form of therapy is a number of years from widespread application because of difficulties with safe delivery systems, not to mention the fact that in larger concentrations nitric oxide is a recognized pollutant with known toxic effects.

The second goal of therapy is directed at maintaining adequate oxygen delivery, which includes aggressive support of intravascular volume, hemoglobin, and right and left ventricular function. Avoiding hyperinflation of the lungs may be an important and sometimes unrecognized part of assisting cardiac function, since overinflation further increases pulmonary vascular resistance.

The third goal of therapy—that of minimizing barotrauma—is complicated by the mechanical difficulties caused by the aspirated meconium itself which can cause a chemical pneumonitis and "ball valve" type obstruction of the airways. The most important ventilatory maneuvers are to avoid hyperinflation and ventilator-patient dysynchrony. A new approach has been termed "gentle ventilation." This avoids the use of paralyzation and hyperventilation as the primary mode of alkalinization, arguing that for most patients the aggressive use of mechanical ventilation causes as many problems as it solves. The widespread utility of this approach has yet to be tested in a controlled clinical trial.

The institution of ECMO requires the surgical placement of catheters in an internal jugular vein and usually the accompanying common carotid artery (most often on the right side); most of the time, this means permanent ligation of those vessels. The infant is then systemically heparinized and blood is withdrawn, oxygenated, and returned to the infant with usual flows being 80–100 ml/kg/min, obviously a significant portion of the cardiac output. As long as ECMO is continued the infant is at risk for bleeding, embolus, infection, mechanical failure, and the increased costs of the procedure.

There have been many attempts to assess the success and impact of ECMO as a neonatal therapy. Data from the Extracorporeal Life Support Organization (ELSO) document the successful application of this therapy in more than 70 institutions for thousands of infants, with an overall survival rate of >80% (1). These infants were placed on ECMO when they met institutional criteria that predicted a >80% mortality. The entry criteria used by most institutions have been derived from historical controls. This has generated much controversy, which led to a small prospective randomized trial (2). The trial showed that historical criteria that predicted >85% mortality had a mortality of only 40% in the control (or conventional therapy) group but mortality for the ECMO group was only 3%. Studies done of the financial costs within one institution estimated that because of fewer days in the hospital the actual cost per survivor with ECMO was less than with

conventional therapy once patients reached a level of illness for which ECMO was judged appropriate (3). In terms
of follow-up of ECMO patients, 50–60% appear to function
normally and only a small portion are severely delayed (4).

With the infant we describe, there also was a finding of
particular concern with regard to the use of heparin, that
of a grade 1-intraventricular hemorrhage. The characteri-
zation of that hemorrhage as having calcification suggested it might be older rather than peridelivery, which
reduced the level of concern. At one time ECMO would not
have been offered as a therapy because of the risk that
this hemorrhage might extend with heparinization. With
experience, it has been found that if extremely low doses
of heparin are used most of these infants can be supported
without extension of their bleeding.

Another issue was the HIV-positive serologic status of
the baby's mother. ECMO is a heroic and limited rescue
therapy and there is concern about using it in situations
where the resulting patient outcome is not likely to be ultimately successful. At this time, such concern is dealt with
on a center-to-center basis, but most institutions do not
withhold this heroic therapy because of a positive maternal HIV serology. The risk of transmission from mother to
fetus seems to be about 30% and the outcome for infants
with HIV is changing rapidly. Under these circumstances
the majority of these infants have the capability of doing
relatively well.

COMMENTARY

The excitement of inhaled nitric oxide needs to be tem-
pered by its limited availability, but many prominent peo-
ple in the field believe it may ultimately supplant ECMO
for certain pathologic processes. Until that time, however,
we must find the appropriate population that would most
benefit from this therapy without extraordinary expense
(economically, medically, emotionally, and ethically). For
example, smaller premature neonates do not do well with
ECMO, yet more mature neonates with meconium aspiration syndrome enjoy a great therapeutic success with the
institution of ECMO.

On the horizon are surgical procedures to reconstruct
the carotid artery after decannulation. Low-molecular
weight heparin shows promise in preventing intravascular
clot formation with minimal bleeding complications. Heparin-bonded tubing also promises to reduce the heparin

requirements in these patients, especially for short courses of ECMO.

References

1. Stolar CJH, Snedecor SM, Bartlett RH. Extracorporeal membrane oxygenation and neonatal respiratory failure: experience from the Extracorporeal Life Support Organization. J Pediatr Surg 1990;26: 563–579.
2. O'Rourke PP, Crone RK, Vacanti JP, et al. Extracorporeal membrane oxygenation and conventional medical therapy in neonates with persistent pulmonary hypertension of the newborn: a prospective randomized study. Pediatrics 1989;84:957–963.
3. Pearson GD, Short BL. An economic analysis of extracorporeal membrane oxygenation. J Intensive Care Med 1987;2:116–120.
4. Glass P, Miller M, Short BL. Morbidity for survivors of extracorporeal membrane oxygenation: neurodevelopmental outcome at one year of age. Pediatrics 1989;83:72–78.

Case 21

Satoshi Nakagawa, Hirokazu Sakai, and Katsuyuki Miyasaka
National Children's Hospital
Tokyo, Japan

HISTORY

A 4.6-year-old girl with double-outlet right ventricle, atrial septal defect, ventricular septal defect, and pulmonary stenosis (the so-called criss-cross heart) underwent a modified Fontan procedure. She had had a modified Waterston operation at the age of 5 months. When she was 3.3 years of age, cardiac catheterization was performed in which was revealed a right aortic arch with a longer transverse portion (Fig. 21.1). Subsequently, a modified Fontan operation with fenestrated atrial septum was performed.

After the operation, the child was placed on mechanical ventilation in the ICU. A 5.0-mm inside diameter endotracheal tube was inserted nasally and an appropriate leak around the endotracheal tube was noted. Her cardiovascular status was initially unstable, requiring controlled mechanical ventilation with muscle paralysis for 6 days.

MANAGEMENT

On the 16th postoperative day, when the patient was in the weaning process from the ventilator, her respirator circuit was found to be filled with blood. Sudden circulatory collapse followed marked cyanosis. The central venous pressure did not change, remaining at about 12 mm Hg. The arterial blood gas analysis showed the following: pH 7.16, pO_2 50 mm Hg, pCO_2 74 mm Hg, base excess -2.9,

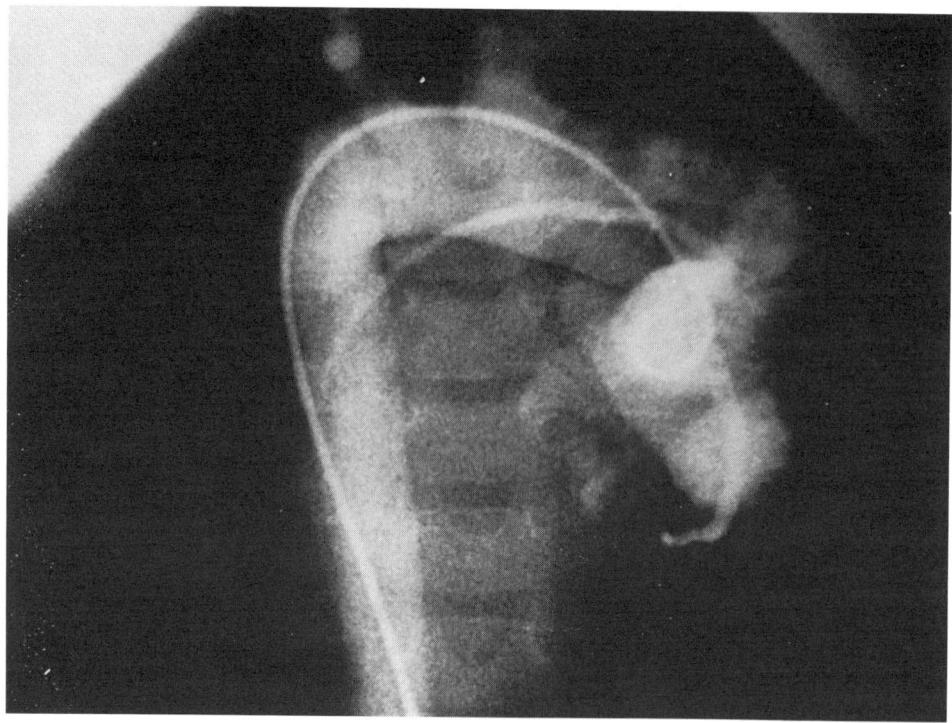

Figure 21.1. Aortography before the modified Fontan operation. Aortic arch is right-sided, and its transverse portion is longer than usual.

SaO$_2$ 56%, and hemoglobin level 7.8 g/dl. The child's chest X-ray is shown in Figure 21.2.

Significant bradycardia was treated with atrioventricular sequential pacing. A blood transfusion was given for the hypotension and anemia. The patient required catecholamine support with dopamine and dobutamine, both at 30 μg/kg/min, to maintain the blood pressure. Peak inspiratory pressure and positive end-expiratory pressure were increased from 25 and 5 cm H$_2$O to 55 and 17 cm H$_2$O, respectively. Fiberoptic bronchoscopy was performed, demonstrating a small-sized granulation at the tracheal lumen just below the tip of the endotracheal tube. Three hours later, a second episode of bleeding occurred suddenly. The bleeding was massive and the patient became hypotensive and hypoxic. Resuscitation was not successful and the child was pronounced dead.

Autopsy findings revealed that there was a fistula between the trachea and transverse aorta. The fistula was located just at the level of the tip of the endotracheal tube. Ulceration of the trachea was also noticed around the fistula (Fig. 21.3).

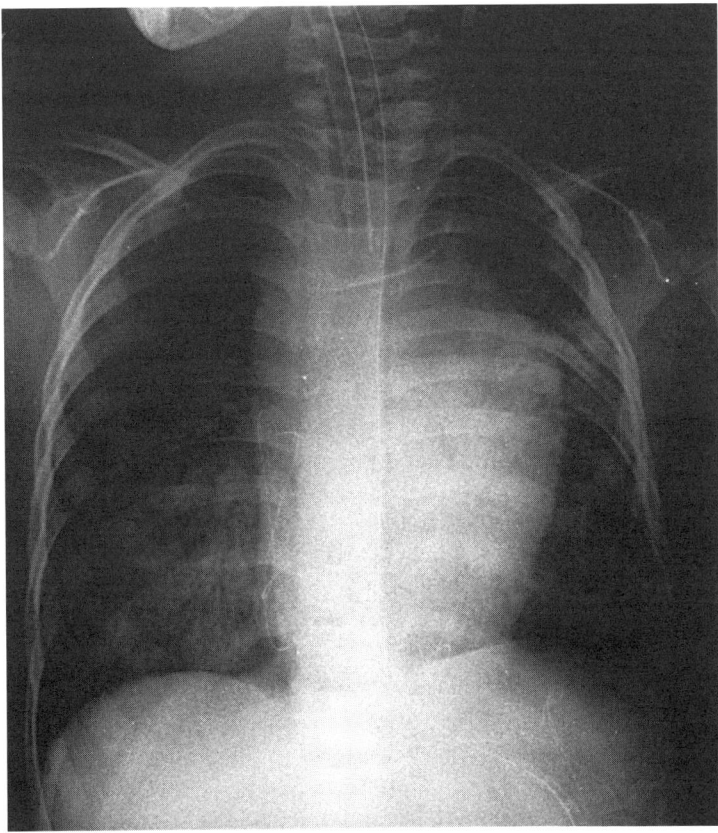

Figure 21.2.   Chest X-ray film soon after the massive airway bleeding.

DISCUSSION

We describe the case of a very rare but fatal complication of endotracheal intubation. There are some descriptions of tracheoinnominate artery fistula as a complication of long-term use of a tracheostomy tube. However, a tracheoaortic fistula has not been reported with the usual use of an endotracheal tube. In our hospital, we employ mechanical ventilation for more than 150 patients a year and have never previously encountered a fatal complication until the case of this child.

Possible reasons this complication occurred are the following: (1) the abnormal shape and size of the aortic arch and (2) tracheitis.

This patient had congenital cyanotic heart disease. The aortic arch was right-sided and the transverse aorta was longer than normal. The tip of the endotracheal tube was located at the level of the transverse aorta.

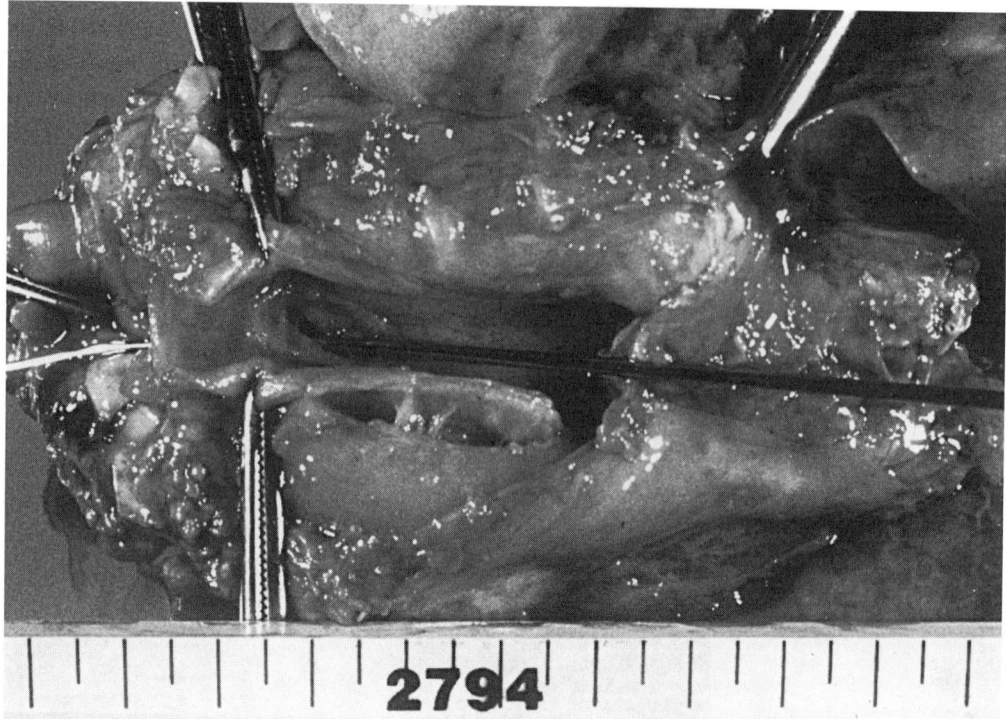

Figure 21.3   Autopsy findings. The fistula is between the trachea and the transverse aorta. A metal probe is passed through the fistula.

This patient was suspected to have had *Pseudomonas* sepsis since the culture of the central venous catheter tip was positive for *P. aeruginosa*. From the evidence of the tracheal ulceration around the fistula, the patient may have had tracheitis.

Fiberoptic bronchoscopy is essential in diagnosing this fatal complication. The reason for failure to detect the bleeding site may be the location of the endotracheal tube—its tip might have covered the fistula. The granulation that was noted with fiberoptic bronchoscopy might be the lower edge of the tracheal ulcer around the fistula.

If we had detected this rare complication at the time of bleeding, the management would have been difficult. The only way for this patient to have survived might have been immediate surgical repair.

In conclusion, whenever bleeding from the airway is noticed with mechanically ventilated patients, we have to consider tracheoaortic fistula as a complication of endotracheal tube management.

COMMENTARY

Fistulas between the airway and great vessels are uncommon but deadly. They usually have a multifactorial etiology, including proximity of the airway and great vessel, prolonged artificial airway placement, and some degree of infection. As a temporizing maneuver prior to surgery, a cuffed endotracheal tube can be placed at the bleeding site and the cuff can be inflated, thus tamponading the bleeding. For bronchial bleeding in older children, a double-lumen endotracheal tube can be used to tamponade the bleeding.

Suggested Reading

1. Cooper JD. Trachea-innominate artery fistula: successful management of 3 consecutive patients. Ann Thorac Surg 1977;24:439–447.

Case 22

Juerg Pfenninger, Mauri Leijala, and Markus Mauderli
University Children's Hospital
Bern, Switzerland

HISTORY

A 6-month-old infant boy was admitted to the PICU of our hospital for management of severe respiratory distress. The infant was the 2070-g product of 34 weeks' gestation. His neonatal period was complicated by respiratory distress, hyperbilirubinemia, and late-onset streptococcal group B sepsis and meningitis. At the age of 1 month, the boy was discharged from the hospital in good health. Because of prematurity, oral iron supplementation had been ordered at that time. The drug was given in the form of coated tablets (Bebe-Tardyferon). Two months prior to admission, the infant aspirated an iron pill into the left mainstem bronchus, which was removed by rigid bronchoscopy. Because of difficulties during extraction, the pill had to be broken and at the end of the procedure a blackish discoloration of the bronchial mucosa was noted. After 3 days, the boy was discharged home again. A chronic cough developed 1 month prior to admission, which was thought to be due to a viral respiratory tract infection. One day prior to admission, an acute deterioration with respiratory distress occurred, and the baby was readmitted to the hospital. Chest radiography showed complete atelectasis of the left lung, and bronchoscopy revealed a blocked left mainstem bronchus.

PHYSICAL EXAMINATION

The child's vital signs were unremarkable, and he was paralyzed (pancuronium) with a nasotracheal tube in

129

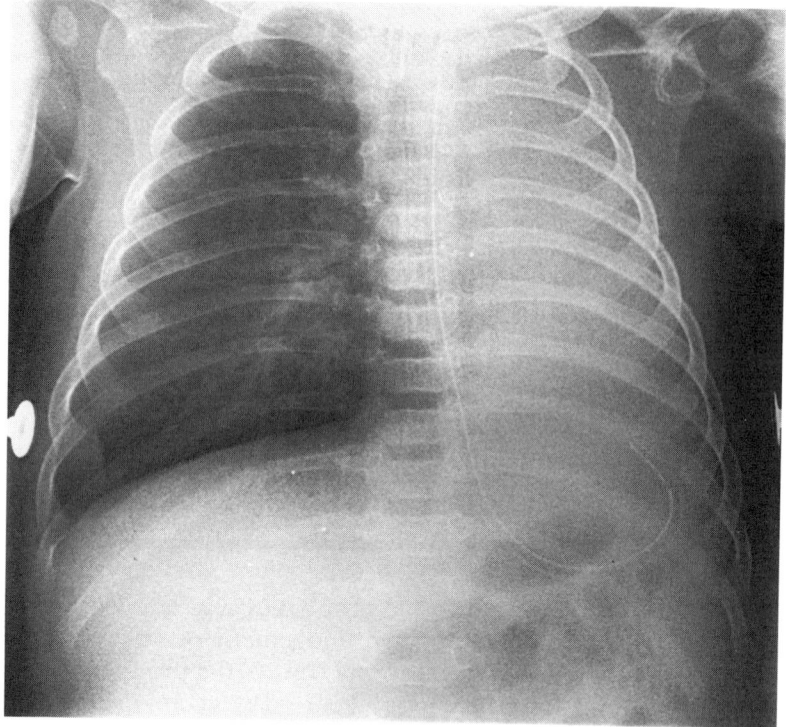

Figure 22.1. Chest radiography at admission, showing complete atelectasis of the left lung.

place and continuous positive pressure ventilation was administered (peak inspiratory pressure [PIP] 26 cm H_2O, positive end-expiratory pressure [PEEP] 5 cm H_2O, respiratory rate 22 breaths/min, and F_IO_2 0.32).

LABORATORY DATA

The infant's $PaCO_2$ was 44 mm Hg; O_2 saturation was 91%. The chest X-ray is shown in Figure 22.1.

MANAGEMENT

Two hours after admission, bronchoscopic examination was repeated. Complete left mainstem bronchus closure by edema and inflammation was confirmed; however, the stenosis could be passed by the optics (2-mm outer diameter) and pus and inflammation were found distally. A coronary artery dilatation catheter (3.5-mm outer diameter during inflation) was introduced into the left mainstem bronchus and repeatedly inflated. This created a lumen of about 3-mm diameter at the end of the procedure. Nasotracheal intubation and continuous positive pressure ventilation were continued postoperatively, but with high PIP (34 cm H_2O) and long inspiratory (TI = 2 seconds) and expiratory times (TE = 4 seconds) and high PEEP (12 cm H_2O), resulting in a $PaCO_2$ of 39 mm Hg and a PaO_2 of 143 mm Hg (F_IO_2 of 38%). Chest radiography shortly after the procedure showed complete resolution of atelectasis of the left lung (Fig. 22.2). In order to allow the infant to maintain coughing, muscle relaxation was discontinued. Steroids (prednisone 3 mg/kg/d for 7 days) and antibiotics (gentamicin/amoxicillin for 3 days) were started.

After this initial successful reopening of the left lung, further management was discussed with several interna-

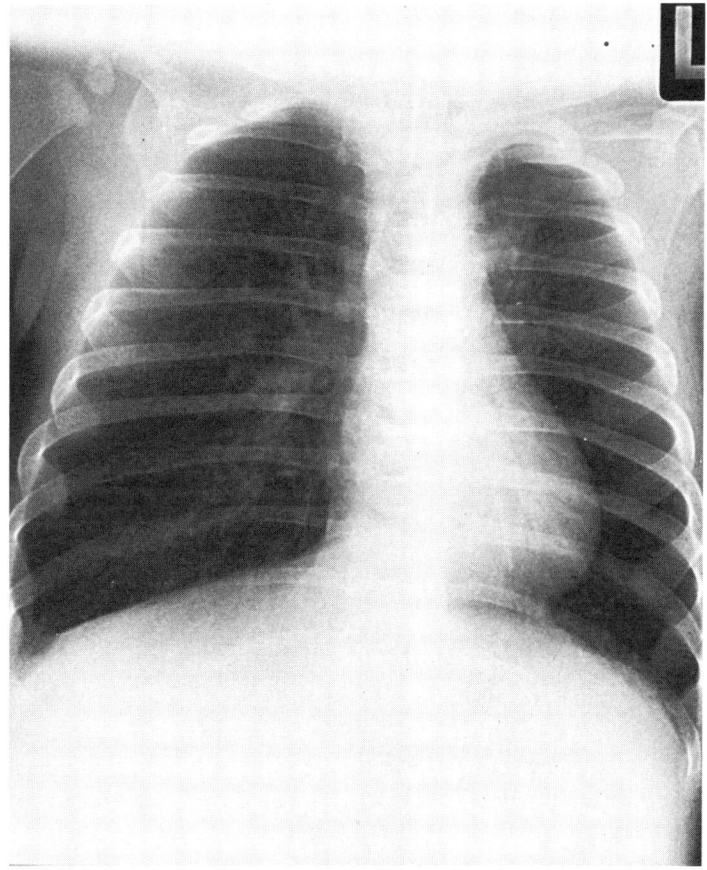

Figure 22.2. Chest radiography after first dilatational treatment and on continuous positive pressure ventilation with deliberately high peak inspiratory pressure, positive end-expiratory pressure, and long inspiratory and expiratory times. The left lung is reexpanded; the right lung shows overexpansion due to high airway pressure.

tional experts. It was decided to continue as long as possible with repeated dilatation and continuous positive pressure ventilation in order to avoid surgery in an acutely inflamed area. Surgery (with resection of the stenotic area or left pneumonectomy) was considered as an eventuality, however. To allow a better surgical judgement of the local changes, bronchography was performed 3 weeks after admission to the hospital (Fig. 22.3).

Dilatational treatment was repeated nine times, either because of recurrent atelectasis or severe air trapping. Figure 22.4 shows the acute effect of dilatation on one of these

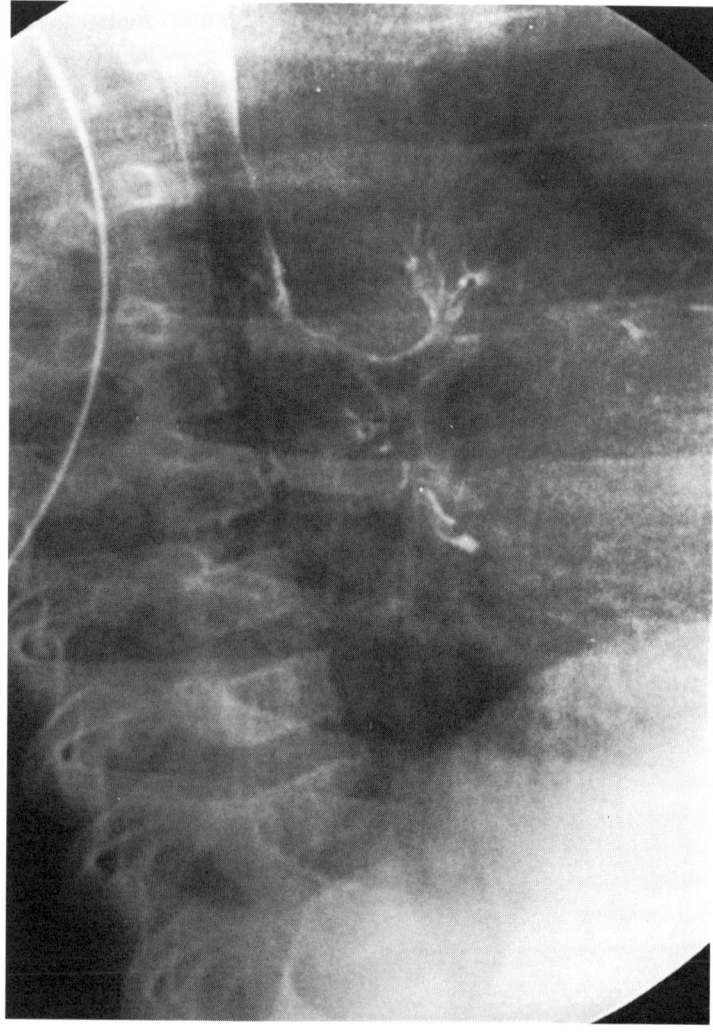

Figure 22.3. Bronchographic examination of the lower segment of the trachea and the left mainstem bronchus. Note the narrow segment that starts near the bifurcation and ends before the separation into the lobar bronchi.

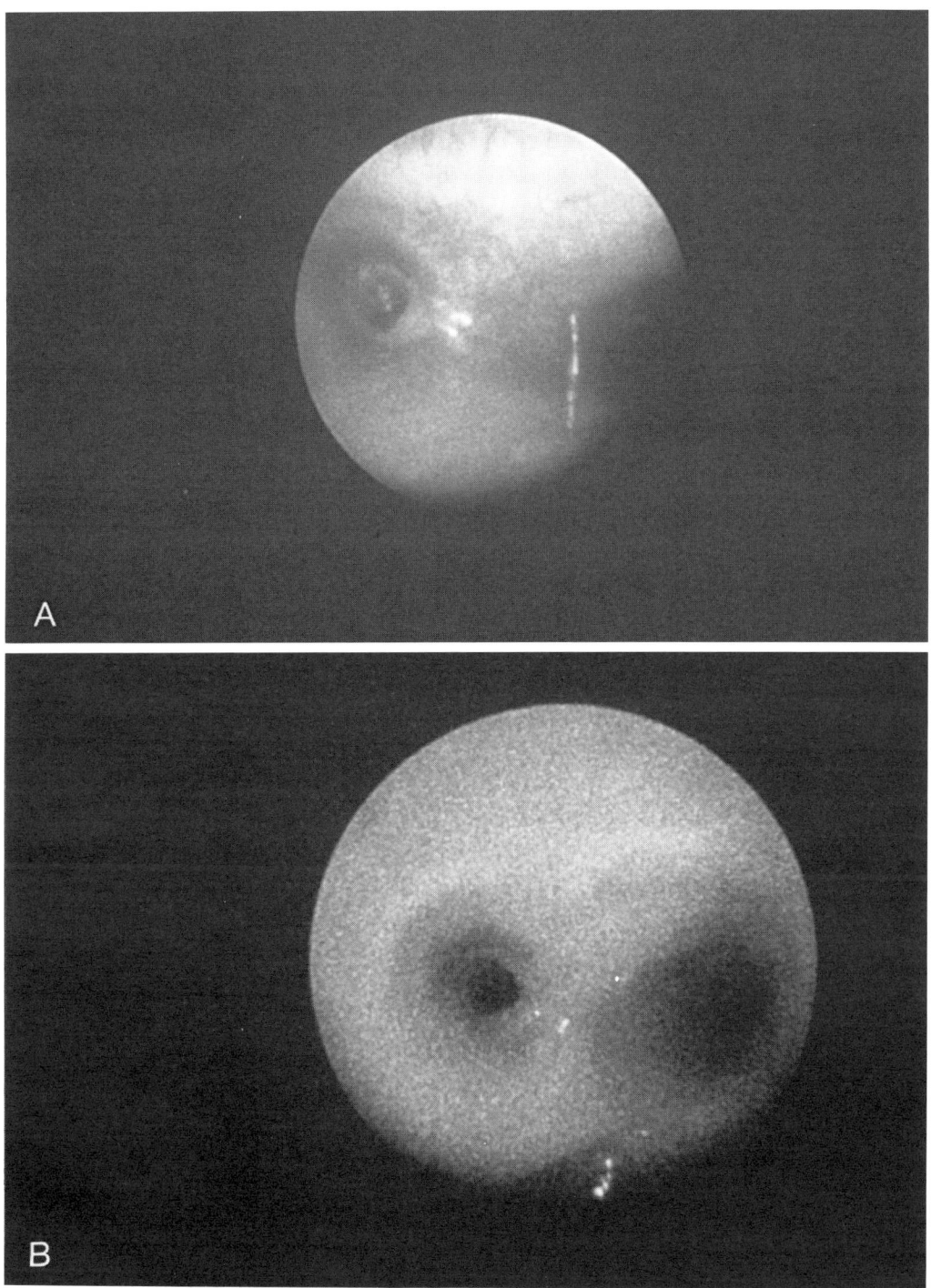

Figure 22.4. Bronchoscopic view of both mainstem bronchi before (*A*) and after (*B*) dilatation of the left mainstem bronchus by means of a Gruentzig coronary artery dilatation catheter.

occasions. (During one of these sessions we also learned the dangers of such a treatment: instead of a Gruentzig coronary artery dilatation catheter, a Fogarty catheter was used. The balloon ruptured during inflation, causing a small tear in the posterior wall of the distal trachea with consequent pneumomediastinum. Fortunately, this complication was not followed by further problems.)

With the evershortening duration of successful dilatations and increasing difficulties in ventilatory management, the decision to perform surgery was made. A left-sided thoracotomy with resection of the stenotic segment and a side-to-end tracheobronchial anastomosis were performed. General anesthesia consisted of ketamine, fentanyl, midazolam, and pancuronium, with selective intubation of the right mainstem bronchus. In order to ventilate the right upper lobe, a side hole was cut into the distal end of the tube. The surgical technique used was an initial cut in the middle of the lesion and further slicing proximally and distally until healthy tissue was met. Figure 22.5 shows the excised slices which, on later microscopic analysis, showed severe inflammatory changes and iron deposits.

Three days postoperatively, paralysis was allowed to

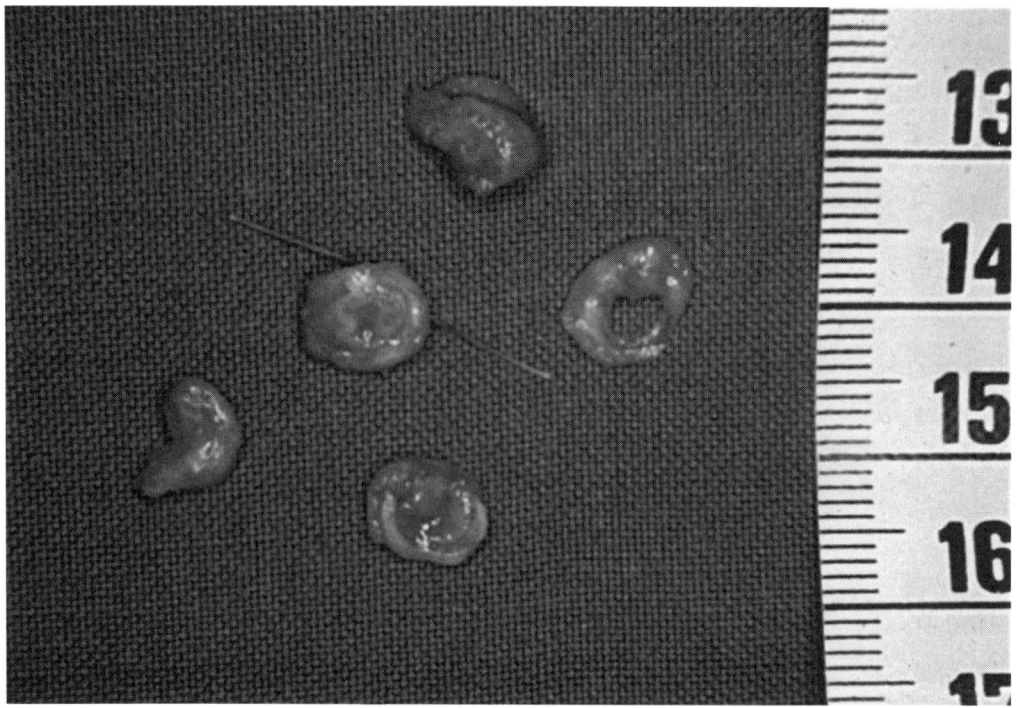

Figure 22.5. Slices of the resected left mainstem bronchus, showing nearly total occlusion.

wear off and the trachea was extubated. Perioperative antibiotic coverage with gentamicin and ticarcillin/clavulanic
acid continued for 5 days. Endoscopic examination 2
weeks postoperatively revealed discrete granulation tissue
on the vocal cords and in the region of the tear in the low
trachea. The area of the anastomosis was perfect and the
left lobar bronchi were free from obstruction. The infant
was discharged from the hospital 14 days postoperatively
in perfect health and with a normal chest radiograph. Further endoscopic examinations 3, 6, and 12 months after
surgery revealed normal results, except for a very short left
mainstem bronchus.

DISCUSSION

This is an instructive case showing the importance of
close cooperation among the various medical and surgical
specialties. For us as intensive care physicians, the greatest challenge was "how to ventilate." The problem was a
respiratory system with two lungs with very different time
constants. The approach chosen was to apply high PIP and
PEEP in order to keep the airways open and to use long
TI and TE. These variables were titrated with chest films
and by means of auscultation of the chest. Although this
approach led to overexpansion of the right lung and also
some cardiovascular compromise, necessitating the use of
diuretics, it probably helped to save the left lung. Other
theoretical possibilities might have been independent
lung ventilation by selective intubation of the left
mainstem bronchus or earlier surgery. Infection control
and nutrition were also significant concerns. Therefore,
we only used high-dose, potent antibiotics for short periods of time in order to avoid selection of multiply resistant bacteria or fungi.

The question of how this aspiration could happen still
remains. Before this case, we were not aware of the fact
that in some parts of our country, as in other European
countries, oral iron therapy was administered in the form
of sweet, coated tablets. In infancy, coordination of swallowing and breathing might not be completely matured
and protective reflexes less efficient than in older age
groups. Oral administration of coated tablets in this age
group is therefore considered unwise. For this reason, we
notified the drug company about this incident, and the
drug was immediately withdrawn from the market. Another preventive step was to present this information to

the Swiss pediatricians during their annual meeting in 1989. We believe that the message has been well accepted.

COMMENTARY

This is a remarkable system: to have a product removed from the market because of an isolated terrible adverse event speaks to a very responsive and responsible pharmaceutical industry as well as fine liaison with the medical community. The approach of education and prevention as described in this case is likely to avert a repetition of this event. Also of interest is the controversial role of iron administration to children in the physiologic nadir of their hematocrit. It may not be necessary to administer iron replacement to the infant. It is enticing to speculate that, once aspirated, the inflammatory response to the iron may in part be a free radical-mediated injury (via Fenton chemistry).

Case 23

Olubunmi A. Okanlami and Nancy Braverman

The Johns Hopkins Hospital
Baltimore, Maryland, USA

HISTORY

A comatose 21-month-old male child of unrelated parents was transferred from the emergency room (ER) of a community hospital to the PICU at Johns Hopkins Hospital. On the morning of admission he had been found in his bed, unresponsive and breathing irregularly. Paramedics noted agonal breathing and he was taken to a nearby ER. It was not clear for how long he had been unconscious and breathing irregularly. The child had a 3-day history of low-grade fever and decreased appetite. He had been active until the evening before we examined him and the only medication administered at home was Tylenol. He had been vomiting and had diarrhea of 1 day's duration about 2 weeks prior to this admission.

Upon arrival at the referring hospital, the child was intubated and artificially ventilated. He developed generalized seizure activity and was found to have profound hypoglycemia (serum glucose 10 mg/dl), which responded to treatment with lorazepam and intravenous dextrose. Blood and urine cultures were obtained and intravenous ceftriaxone was administered prior to interhospital transport.

Past medical history was significant for chicken pox at age 20 months, with no history of acetylsalicylic acid administration, and minor head trauma at age 15 months with no loss of consciousness and a normal cranial CT scan at that time. He had no previous history of seizures.

PHYSICAL EXAMINATION

This well-developed boy was responsive only to painful stimuli and had no spontaneous respiratory effort. He was intubated and artificially ventilated. His vital signs were as follows: temperature 100.3°F, pulse 145 beats/min, blood pressure 109/60 mm Hg, and weight 11.8 kg. The ventilator was set at a rate of 20 breaths/min, tidal volume 150 ml, and F_IO_2 of 0.6.

The boy was normocephalic with no external signs of trauma. The pupils were small and equal but sluggishly responsive to light. No abnormalities of ear, nose, or throat were seen, and the neck was supple. The chest moved symmetrically with ventilation and the lung fields were clear to auscultation. The pulses were palpable in all extremities, peripheral perfusion was adequate by examination, and heart sounds were normal. The abdomen was soft and undistended with no palpable masses or organomegaly and normal bowel sounds. The patient was comatose (Glasgow coma score = 4) with generalized increase in muscle tone and decerebrate posturing in response to noxious stimuli. Corneal and gag reflexes were present.

LABORATORY DATA

Complete blood count results were as follows: white blood cells 13,800/mm^3, hemoglobin 11.9 g/dl, hematocrit 34.7%, and platelet count 567,000/mm^3. Electrolyte count was: sodium 140 mmol/l, potassium 4.7 mmol/l, chloride 111 mmol/l, bicarbonate 20 mmol/l, and ionized calcium 1.13 mmol/l. Magnesium was 1.6 mEq/l and *glucose 10 mg/dl.* Liver function test showed: alanine aminotransferase 178 U/l, aspartate aminotransferase 173 U/l, alkaline phosphatase 150 U/l, ammonia 104 mg/dl, and uric acid 2.3 mg/dl. Bilirubin count and prothrombin time were normal. Arterial blood gas findings were: pH 7.36, PaCO$_2$ 27, PaO$_2$ 439, HCO3 15 on 100% oxygen; pH 7.31, PaCO2 28, PaO$_2$ 329, HCO$_3$ 14 on 60% oxygen. Results of urinalysis revealed a trace of ketones, and the toxicology screen results were negative. Blood and urine cultures were obtained. Chest X-ray confirmed correct position of the endotracheal tube and no infiltrates. CT scan of the boy's head showed diffuse cerebral edema with no shift in the midline structures.

HOSPITAL MANAGEMENT

The clinical impression was that of a comatose child with signs of elevated intracranial pressure (ICP) and evidence of diffuse cerebral edema on CT scan. The possible etiologies included meningitis/encephalitis, Reye's syndrome, toxic encephalopathy, and inborn error of metabolism.

Immediate management was directed toward monitoring and reduction of the elevated ICP and increasing the serum glucose concentration. Mechanical ventilation with hyperventilation was performed, keeping arterial $PaCO_2$ between 25 and 30 mm Hg. ICP was monitored via an intraventricular monitoring device and jugular bulb catheterization was done for trending of jugular bulb oxygen saturation. Continuous arterial blood pressure monitoring was done and vasopressors infused as needed to maintain adequate mean arterial pressures and cerebral perfusion pressures. Intravenous fluids were administered judiciously and diuretics (including mannitol) given as needed to maintain the serum osmolality around 300 mOsm/l. Phenytoin was maintained at therapeutic levels for control of seizure activity. In spite of aggressive therapy, intermittent spikes of ICP as high as 40 mm Hg occurred and continuous pentobarbital infusion was instituted with good response. Broad-spectrum antimicrobial coverage was provided with ceftriaxone, oxacillin, and acyclovir. Blood, urine, and cerebrospinal fluid (CSF) cultures all grew no pathogens.

Urine organic acid analysis, plasma and urine acylcarnitine profiles, and plasma carnitine measurements were done as part of the diagnostic evaluation when the boy was admitted to the PICU. Results were diagnostic of medium-chain acyl-CoA dehydrogenase (MCAD) deficiency. The diagnosis was confirmed by DNA analysis. Definitive therapy with intravenous dextrose (8–10 mg/kg/min) was provided to ensure adequate calories and prevent further lipolysis, and insulin was required to control hyperglycemia. Carnitine, 100 mg/kg/dose, given every 6 hours, was administered via nasogastric tube to enhance the excretion of accumulated acyl-CoA derivatives. Serial measurements of serum electrolytes and liver function studies, electroencephalographic studies, and repeat cranial CT scans were used to monitor the efficacy of therapy and the patient's slow progress. ICP monitoring was discontinued on hospital day 6, and the child was extubated on day 8 and transferred out of the PICU on day 11. During his course in the PICU, he was noted to have developed moderate hepatomegaly and his neurologic examinations (Glasgow coma scale = 10) and electorencephalogram remained abnormal, although his urine organic acid profile and serum transaminases returned to normal levels.

The child remains severely neurologically impaired and is undergoing rehabilitation therapy at the Kennedy Kreiger Center.

DISCUSSION

The findings of hypoglycemia with hypoketosis in a comatose child should make one suspicious of medium-chain acyl-CoA dehydrogenase (MCAD) deficiency, a disorder of fatty acid oxidation. The clinical spectrum of MCAD deficiency includes cases of sudden infant death syndrome, Reye-like illnesses, and asymptomatic individuals (1). However, most children seen with these findings in the 1- to 2-year-old age group have a history of an intercurrent illness leading to decreased oral intake and increasing lethargy. Vomiting and seizures can occur. Patients would previously have appeared healthy, with normal growth and development. It is the occurrence of prolonged fasting that triggers the expression of MCAD deficiency. This may explain why infants, who are frequently fed, are less likely to be seen with MCAD deficiency. Laboratory findings frequently reveal a mild hyperammonemia, moderate elevation of transaminase levels, elevated uric acid level, and a hyperchloremic metabolic acidosis. Blood glucose is often reduced but may be at normal level (2). Further diagnostic evaluation is best understood following a review of the relevant biochemical pathway.

The normal response to fasting includes mobilization of fatty acids from adipose tissue and increased fatty acid oxidation in the liver. Hepatic fatty acid oxidation provides energy for gluconeogenesis and produces ketone bodies as a normal end product. Deficiency of MCAD disrupts fatty acid oxidation, leading to reduced hepatic production of glucose and ketone bodies, and accumulation of toxic intermediates. Fatty acid oxidation occurs in mitochondria of liver and other tissues through a sequence of enzymatic steps (Fig. 23.1). Long-chain fatty acids (mainly C16) enter mitochondria after being esterified to carnitine. They are subsequently converted to acyl-CoA derivatives that then enter the fatty acid oxidation pathway. With each turn of the cycle, the original fatty acyl-CoA becomes two

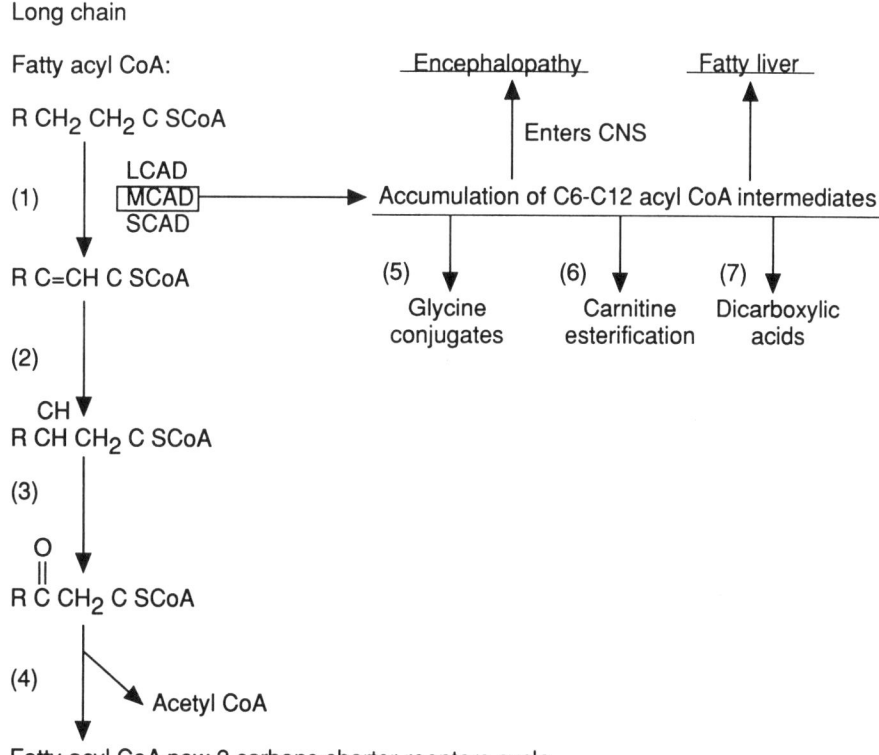

Figure 23.1. Schematic diagram showing mitochondrial fatty acid oxidation (*left side*) and biochemical sequelae of MCAD deficiency (*right side*). Enzymes represented are as follows: (*1*) chain specific acyl-CoA dehydrogenases (*LCAD*, long-chain acyl-CoA dehydrogenase, *MCAD*, medium-chain acyl-CoA dehydrogenase, *SCAD*, short-chain acyl-CoA dehydrogenase); (*2*) enoyl-CoA hydratase; (*3*) 3-hydroxyacyl-CoA dehydrogenase; (*4*) 3-ketoacyl-CoA thiolase; (*5*) mitochondrial glycine N-acylase; (*6*) mitochondrial carnitine acyltransferase; (*7*) microsomal and peroxisomal oxidation pathways.

carbons shorter, acetyl CoA is released, and adenosine triphosphate (ATP) is generated. Ketones are derived by condensation of acetyl-CoA or directly from the last cycle of oxidation. There are three acyl-CoA dehydrogenases, which differ in their chain length specificities. MCAD is most active with C6–C12 carbon chains. Thus, a deficiency of MCAD results in the accumulation of medium-chain fatty acyl-CoAs. These metabolites may be converted to their dicarboxylic and hydroxy acid derivatives via microsomal and peroxisomal pathways, or conjugated to glycine or carnitine in mitochondria. These derivatives are excreted and can be detected in the urine.

When MCAD deficiency is suspected, organic acid analysis of urine by capillary gas chromatography/mass spectrometry should be done early. The characteristic pattern is a medium-chain dicarboxylic aciduria, and the presence of superylglycine, hexanoylglycine, and phenylpropionyl-glycine. The glycine conjugates are more specific for MCAD deficiency (3). Ketones are present in small amounts relative to the degree of dicarboxylic aciduria. The urine organic acid abnormalities are most apparent in samples obtained during the acute phase of illness. Samples obtained after recovery may show no abnormalities. Total plasma carnitine is usually reduced, with an increase in the esterified fraction, representing the acylcarnitine derivatives. Plasma acylcarnitine profiles (using various methodologies) show a predominance of medium-chain carnitine esters with an increased ratio of octanoylcarnitine to acetylcarnitine. This profile is considered diagnostic (4,5) and is abnormal even in asymptomatic individuals. Further confirmation of the diagnosis can be done by enzymatic or molecular studies.

MCAD deficiency is inherited as an autosomal recessive trait. Because affected persons may be asymptomatic, it is important to test all siblings of an affected patient. There is a single point mutation that may account for 90% of alleles (6). Polymerase chain reaction (PCR)-based assays are now available for identification of this point mutation. MCAD deficiency is found predominantly in whites, and most cases reported to date have been from northern Europe and the United States. The true incidence is not yet defined, but investigations support this disorder as being one of the more common inborn errors of metabolism (6). Systemic consequences of MCAD deficiency are not clearly defined. The encephalopathy is thought to be partly due to the toxic effect of octanoate on the CNS. Thus, return to baseline mental status usually lags behind correction of the hypoglycemia. Hepatomegaly occurs secondary to fat accumulation in the liver.

The mainstay of acute therapy is the provision of calories in the form of glucose to prevent further lipolysis. Close attention should be paid to correction of fluid and electrolyte abnormalities. Carnitine is administered orally to enhance the excretion of accumulated acyl-CoA derivatives. When the disorder is recognized and appropriate treatment is instituted early, complete recovery usually occurs and the prognosis is good. Maintenance therapy is dependent on the avoidance of fasting. Carnitine supplementation (50–100 mg/kg/d) and restriction of dietary fat (25% of total calories) are often prescribed but have not been proven to be efficacious. Children with MCAD deficiency require close observation during usual childhood illnesses and may need hospitalization for intravenous fluid and glucose support.

COMMENTARY

As always, early establishment of airway, breathing, and circulation with treatment of hypoglycemia treats much of the acute pathology in this disease. Diagnosing these types of diseases are gratifying because once identified they are often successfully treated.

References

1. Touma EH, Charpentier C. Medium chain acyl-CoA dehydrogenase deficiency. Arch Dis Child 1992;67:142–145.
2. Roe CR, Coates PM. Acyl-CoA dehydrogenase deficiencies. In: Scriver CR, Beaudet AL, Sly WS, Valle D, eds. Metabolic basis of inherited disease. 6th ed. McGraw-Hill 1989:889–914.
3. Duran M, Wadman SK. Chemical diagnosis of inherited defects of fatty acid metabolism and ketogenesis. Enzyme 1987;38:115–123.
4. Millington DS, Terada N, Chase DH, et al. The role of tandem mass spectrometry in the diagnosis of fatty acid oxidation disorders. In: Coates PM, Tanaka K, eds. New developments in fatty acid oxidation disorders. Wiley-Liss 1992:339–354.
5. Schmidt-Sommerfield E, Penn D, Duran N, et al. Detection and quantitation of acylcarnitines in plasma and blood spots from patients with inborn errors of fatty acid oxidation. In: Coates PM, Tanaka K, eds. New developments in fatty acid oxidation disorders. Wiley-Liss 1992:355–362.
6. Matsubara Y, Narisawa K, Tada K. Medium chain acyl-CoA dehydrogenase deficiency: molecular aspects. Eur J Pediatr 1992;151:154–159.

Case 24

Randall C. Wetzel
The Johns Hopkins Hospital
Baltimore, Maryland, USA

HISTORY

A 20-month-old male child was transferred to our hospital from the PICU at another university. The reason for the transfer was to further investigate an underlying metabolic disorder, characterized by documented carnitine deficiency and resembling cytochrome *c* oxidase deficiency. The transfer was arranged by a senior geneticist.

An additional factor in this transfer was that the child had apparent refractory, undiagnosable, life-threatening, gastrointestinal hemorrhage. After numerous episodes and an exhaustive diagnostic work-up, no diagnosis or bleeding site had been found. Over the 2 weeks prior to transfer, there had been seven 100- to 150-ml blood transfusions administered to replace losses from a gastrointestinal bleed. The child had bled again 24 hours prior to transfer and was on a constant Pitressin infusion to prevent further bleeding.

The patient was the product of a full-term, uncomplicated gestation and delivery. He was in the NICU for 7 days with transient tachypnea. During his first year of life he reached normal milestones and had just begun to stand and take his first steps. During this first year he had the usual childhood illnesses, complete immunizations, and normal growth. At 10 months of age, his mother reported that he had generalized, tonic-clonic seizures and episodes of staring, blinking, and repetitive movements. An extensive work-up at that time revealed no abnormalities, with a normal electroencephalogram (EEG) reading for age. He was placed on phenytoin (Dilantin) for his seizures. The mother continued to report seizure activity and his anticonvulsants were increased. Eventually he was receiving phenobarbital, sodium valproate, and phenytoin, with apparent periods of control. At 12 months of age, he was seen with a prolonged seizure. He was noticed to have lost weight and was anemic with a hematocrit of 22%. An extensive work-up revealed biochemical carnitine deficiency and he was given iron and carnitine supplementation. During this hospitalization, he had an early episode of high-spiking fever and apparent sepsis syndrome. Culture results were negative and the fever resolved with antibiotics. He then developed recurrent nasal bleeding, occasional hematemesis, and, by his mother's report, bright red blood in his stools. He continued to lose weight, developed feeding intolerance, and remained anemic. The decision was eventually made to start him on hyperalimentation for which a broviac catheter was placed. He was managed at home with frequent admissions for seizures, fevers, and bleeding.

He had several sepsis-type episodes following the insertion of his central line, and on four separate occasions *Acinetobacter*, *Staphylococcus epidermidis*, *Escherichia coli*, and *Staphylococcus aureus* were cultured from his catheter. Bleeding continued with episodes of bright red blood being found on his bib and in his mouth, and occasional episodes of passage of bright red blood in his diaper. An exhaustive work-up included upper and lower gastrointestinal series, multiple upper and lower endoscopies, recurrent technetium scans, and an angiogram of the mesenteric circulation, all of which were negative. During these months he remained on hyperalimentation, received no nutrition by mouth, had recurrent episodes of febrile illness, and required chronic transfusion. There were reports of his diaper filling up with bright red blood. These episodes were accompanied by alarm from the medical and nursing staff, as well as from the boy's parents. The patient's condition deteriorated, and he became a withdrawn and chronically hospitalized child who failed to continue to develop. Eventually an exploratory laparotomy was done and a small section of bowel resected, which ultimately was histologically normal. At the time that the patient was transferred to our PICU, he had undergone 18 admissions for respiratory problems, diarrhea, vomiting, failure to thrive, seizures, sepsis, recurrent equipment failure when at home, difficulty with parenteral feeding and with medication, and presumptive diagnosis of carnitine deficiency and cytochrome *c* oxidase deficiency and recurrent gastrointestinal bleeding of an unknown etiology.

This child had a sibling who, 5 months prior to this patient's conception, died unexpectedly at 20 months of age at home following a similar history. The sibling's name was the same as this patient's.

PHYSICAL EXAMINATION

On arrival in our PICU, the boy was a pale, lethargic, withdrawn child breathing spontaneously in room air who appeared to be in no apparent acute distress. A broviac catheter was in place, through which he was receiving hyperalimentation. He did not interact with hospital personnel. His heart rate was 110 beats/min, his respiratory rate was 18 breaths/min, his blood pressure was 105/65 mm Hg, and his oxygen saturation was 100%. He was less than the third percentile for both height and weight. His head circumference was in the 50th percentile for age. He appeared warm, well-perfused, and hemodynamically stable with no active bleeding occurring at the time. He was receiving hourly Maalox, cimetidine, valproate, Dilantin, phenobarbital, Valium, and Pitressin. A review of his laboratory studies showed essentially negative results except for normochromic normocytic anemia, with a hematocrit of 22%. No other biochemical abnormalities were detected. The angiograms were reviewed and were normal. An exhaustive review of the medical records from the referring university demonstrated that "no stone had been left unturned in the diagnostic evaluation of this child."

Consultations were obtained from physicians in the following specialties: gastroenterology, pediatric surgery, hematology, and genetic diseases. Preparations were made for an immediate technetium-99 scan in the event of bleeding. The pediatric surgery department was notified and prepared to perform an urgent laparotomy, if necessary, to detect the bleeding site. A radiologist was consulted to provide the best diagnostic tests to identify a bleeding site. Hematologically, no abnormalities were detected and there was no evidence of coagulopathy. The gastroenterology department wanted to wait for an event, as did the pediatric surgery department.

Hyperalimentation was continued, along with the boy's supplements; however, Pitressin, antacids, and all medications except for phenobarbital were discontinued. For 2 days the child remained hemodynamically stable with no evidence of bleeding. Late on the third day after admission, the mother presented the child's bib with bright red blood, and, at the same time, a small (3–5 ml) spot of bright red blood in his diaper. A technetium scan was performed immediately and repeated at 12 hours. Both examinations failed to detect bleeding. Rectal examination revealed soft brown stool without blood. No further episodes of bleeding occurred, and there was no change in the boy's hematocrit. On the following evening this episode and sequence of events was repeated.

At this stage, the consulting services and the PICU staff raised the question of fictitious gastrointestinal bleeding. All medicines were stopped, enteral feeds established, and the child was very cautiously monitored. Over the next 3 days, full enteral feedings were instituted without setback. Hyperalimentation was discontinued. No seizures were observed. The child remained hemodynamically stable. Serial guaiac stools were negative. The child began to thrive, gain weight, and become alert and interactive. Subsequently the child was transferred to a routine nursing unit, where on two further occasions a 3- to 5-ml spot of blood was found in the boy's diaper by his mother. Gastrointestinal lavage and repeated technetium scans were negative. Of note, the bleeding only occurred when the parents were rooming in or with the child. During a medical staff meeting, when the child's further disposition was being discussed, the mother arrived and said she was going to take her child home because we believed that there was nothing wrong with him and the hospital staff members were unable to discover the cause for his multiple problems. The diagnosis of Munchausen's syndrome by proxy had not been mentioned to the family as yet.

Arrangements were made for obtaining a court order and protective custody for the child. The PICU staff has appeared on his behalf in two custody trials. Over the past 2 years, while the child has remained in custody, he has regained all of his milestones and is an active and alert child who is thriving with no medical problems. He is taking no medicine and is for all intents and purposes perfectly healthy.

DISCUSSION

Although Munchausen's syndrome by proxy was considered early in this patient, it was considered necessary to rule out underlying medical conditions. Consulting services and results of laboratory investigations revealed no underlying disease. An exhaustive review of the records was performed. An anticipatory diagnostic posture was maintained to discover, diagnose, and treat any underlying bleeding problem. On meticulous review of the referring hospital's records and by direct question, no one had ever seen this child seize, nor had bleeding occurred in the absence of circumstances where it could have been fictitiously induced by the parents. In the final analysis, it was thought that the mother was removing blood from the broviac catheter and placing it in the child's upper gastrointestinal tract or in his diaper. This resulted in the recurrent fictitious episodes of bleeding and almost certainly in the recurrent episodes of febrile illness and sepsis. Prolonged hospitalization and exhaustive diagnostic work-ups had led to infantilization and withdrawal of the child. Satisfactory improvement in the child with removal from his parents has confirmed the diagnosis. The diagnosis of Munchausen's disease by proxy in this case was made based on the criteria listed in Table 24.1.

In addition to this, the previous death of a sibling, and renaming and replacement of that sibling with the present child were highly suggestive of the diagnosis of Munchausen's disease by proxy.

In retrospect, the diagnosis of this case seems obvious. Nevertheless, a leading university hospital did not consider this diagnosis. Many at our institution doubted it. The family continues to reject it. The courts continue to debate it. In the ICU, diagnosis of Munchausen's syndrome by proxy must be considered in complex patients, but not to the exclusion of exhaustive investigation and detailed, conclusive documentation. This disease represents a seriously deranged parent-child interaction and is fatal in the cases of about 10% of patients. Therefore, great care is necessary to protect the children. In addition to making the diagnosis, the PICU staff has acted several times over the past 2 years to assure this child's safety.

Table 24.1. Criteria for the Diagnosis of Munchausen's Syndrome

1 Persistent and recurrent illness despite therapy that could not be explained
2 History, symptoms, and signs that were at variance with the apparent healthiness of the child
3 Serious problems that caused senior physicians to say "I've never heard of anything like this."
4 Symptomology that was not reported in the parents' absence
5 Prolonged contact with an overattentive parent, who was very concerned with the detailed minutia of the child's therapy and the medical techniques
6 The child's poor tolerance of his various therapies
7 Very rare diagnoses, which had no apparent support (such as carnitine deficiency and cytochrome c oxidase deficiency)
8 Apparent lack of grave parental concern for the child's condition
9 History of seizures (undocumented by medical personnel) and unresponsive to anticonvulsants
10 Unlikely symptoms: e.g., simultaneous, bright red blood from both ends of the gastrointestinal tract

COMMENTARY

As medicine becomes more sophisticated, so do the parents of victims of this disease. Technology-dependent children are particularly vulnerable to this terrible form of abuse. Diagnosis requires an awareness as well as an ability to step back in order to differentiate the forest from the trees.

Suggested Readings

1. Alexander R, Smith W, Stevenson R. Serial Munchausen syndrome by proxy. Pediatrics 1990;86:581–585.
2. Meadow R. Munchausen syndrome by proxy. Arch Dis Child 1982; 57:92–98.
3. Rosenberg DA. Web of deceit: a literature review of Munchausen syndrome by proxy. Child Abuse Negl 1987;11:547–563.
4. Sigal M, Gelkopf M, Meadow RS. Munchausen by proxy syndrome: the triad of abuse, self-abuse, and deception. Compr Psychiatry 1989; 30:527–533.
5. Sullivan CA, Francis GL, Bain MW, Hartz J. Munchausen syndrome by proxy: 1990. A portent for problems? Clin Pediatr 1991;30: 112–116.

Case 25

Elizabeth W. Kelley, Lauren R. Widner, Salvatore R. Goodwin, Alan S. Klein, and Sharon M. Dabrow

Shands Hospital at the University of Florida Gainesville, Florida, USA

HISTORY

A 16-year-old girl was admitted to the PICU for treatment of a theophylline overdose. The patient had a long history with intermittent albuterol inhalers and sustained-release theophylline. After her parents' divorce, she experienced sexual and physical abuse by her stepfather, and made three suicidal gestures between ages 6 and 9 in the form of nontoxic ingestions (bleach, Tylenol, and over-the-counter cold medications). Custody was given to her father and stepmother.

A fight with her boyfriend precipitated a suicide attempt on the day of admission. She ingested 15–300 mg Slobid tablets (69 mg/kg). She vomited twice at home and admitted the attempt, prompting her parents to take her to a local emergency room (ER). Her theophylline level $2\frac{1}{2}$ hours after the ingestion was 52.3 µg/ml. She was described as alert and oriented (Glasgow coma scale = 15) with a heart rate of 120 beats/min. Electrolyte analysis showed: sodium 139 mEq/l, potassium 2.6 mEq/l, chloride 100 mEq/l, HCO_3 17 mEq/l, blood urea nitrogen (BUN) 12 mg/dl, creatinine 1.0 mg/dl, and glucose 169 mg/dl. She received ER treatment with the placement of a peripheral intravenous line and an 18-Fr orogastric evacuation tube

151

through which she received ipecac and two 50-g doses of charcoal, followed soon after by a cathartic (Go-Lytely).

She was then transported to our ER where she was briefly evaluated and begun on a continuous charcoal gastric infusion. En route to radiology, she experienced a grand mal seizure, which was treated by the ER staff with diazepam and phenobarbital.

PHYSICAL EXAMINATION

On arrival to the PICU, she was obtunded and confused, with marked respiratory distress due to partial airway obstruction. She was disoriented to place and time, and her speech was intermittently incoherent. Her memory was vague and inconsistent for the event. Glasgow coma scale was 9. Cranial nerve examination results were normal. Deep tendon reflexes were brisk. Her vital signs were as follows: weight 65 kg, temperature 36.8°C, pulse 154 beats/min, respiration 18 breaths/min, and blood pressure 157/67 mm Hg.

LABORATORY DATA

Arterial blood gas values were as follows: pH 7.29, pCO_2 35, pO_2 133, HCO_3 13.7, BE -6.6, SaO_2 99% on F_IO_2 0.4, lactic acid 13 mmol/l. The liver function test results were within normal limits. Complete blood count showed the following: white blood cells 27,000/mm^3, hemoglobin 11.8 g/dl with a platelet count of 233,000, K^+ 3.7 mEq/l, glucose 267 mg/dl, initial theophylline level in the PICU was 139.3 with a peak level of 159 μg/ml 5 hours after ingestion.

MANAGEMENT

The patient's trachea was intubated on arrival to the PICU for management of partial airway obstruction and severe acidosis. She received 10 mg propranolol intravenously to control her sinus tachycardia, and a continuous charcoal slurry via an orogastric tube. Shortly after arrival, she had another tonic-clonic generalized seizure for which she received midazolam and a loading dose of phenobarbital (20 mg/kg). A radial arterial line and a femoral venous dialysis catheter were placed. The nephrology service was notified and she received continuous charcoal hemoperfusion beginning 4 hours after admission. Heparin infusion

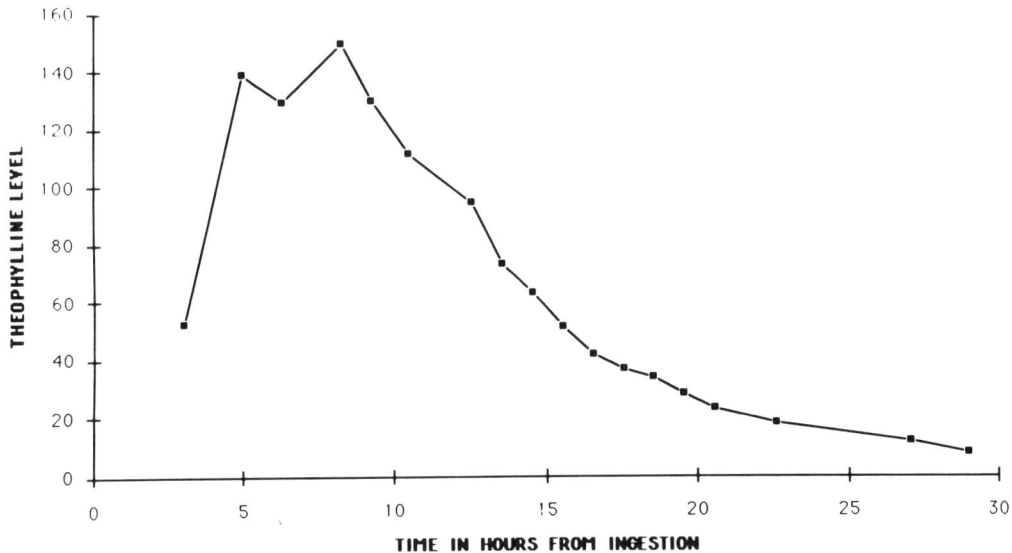

THEOPHYLLINE CLEARANCE BY HEMOPERFUSION

Figure 25.1. Measured theophylline levels from our patient (*y* axis) plotted against the hours postingestion (*x* axis) show the almost linear extraction rate allowed by charcoal hemoperfusion.

was used to maintain bedside activated coagulation times at twice her baseline value. Hemoperfusion continued for approximately 9 hours, with nearly linear reductions in theophylline serum levels (Fig. 25.1). It was discontinued because of hemorrhage from the gastrointestinal (GI) tract, the urinary tract, and the endotracheal tube. Protamine (1 mg/100 U of heparin) was administered to reverse the heparin effect. She continued to have increasing seizure activity despite an adequate phenobarbital level, and received two additional 10-mg/kg loading doses of phenobarbital. Between seizures, her mental status became progressively combative, then obtunded, and it was decided to place her in a pentobarbital coma to control her seizures. She received 5 mg/kg pentobarbital as a loading dose, and was maintained on a continuous infusion of 5 mg/kg/hr, with a level of 46 mg/dl. She was monitored initially for 16 hours with serum drug levels and blood pressure monitoring. An electroencephalogram (EEG) later demonstrated subclinical seizures and daily EEGs were done to document burst suppression and monitor seizure activity. Intermittent seizure activity was documented by EEG for the first 48 hours. After 48 hours, she began exhibiting brainstem dysfunction, with pupils becoming midposition and fixed. She had no response to ice water calorics, abnormal doll's eye examination, absent gag and

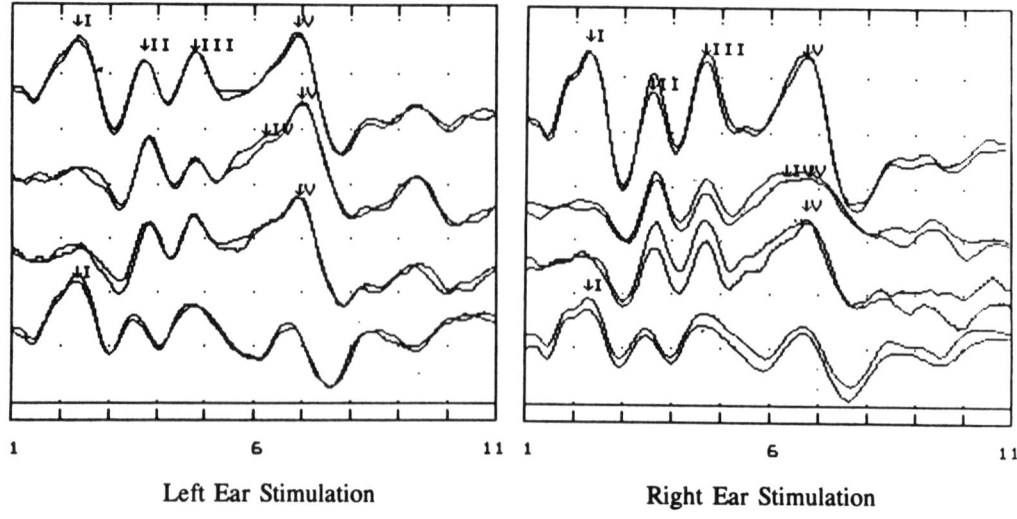

Left Ear Stimulation   Right Ear Stimulation

S.J. 16 Y.O.F Theophylline Overdose
Day 3 of Pentobarb Coma

Figure 25.2.   Left and right ear stimulation: brainstem auditory-evoked potentials obtained on the third day of pentobarbital coma.

corneal reflexes, as well as bizarre EEG findings. She developed diabetes insipidus for which she received desmopressin acetate intranasally. A CT scan demonstrated mild cerebral edema. Results of brainstem auditory and somatosensory-evoked potential tests were essentially normal (Figs. 25.2 and 25.3). On the fifth day of hospitalization, her EEG improved but still demonstrated some residual slowing from medications. She was given additional phenobarbital and pentobarbital was discontinued. She awakened slowly over the next 8 days. While extubation was initially attempted on day 5, she subsequently required reintubation due to the development of *Staphylococcus pneumonia*. She was successfully extubated on hospital day 8.

She began seeing an adolescent psychiatrist 1 day after extubation and was described as confused and hallucinatory, with amnesia for the events surrounding the ingestion. She continued to improve and was transferred out of the PICU on the 14th hospital day.

On hospital day 24, she was transferred to the inpatient psychiatric unit with a diagnosis of severe depression with psychosis and organic amnestic syndrome. She received extensive testing and therapy in the course of a 62-day inpatient stay, and was placed in an appropriate ongoing outpatient program. Cranial CT and magnetic resonance

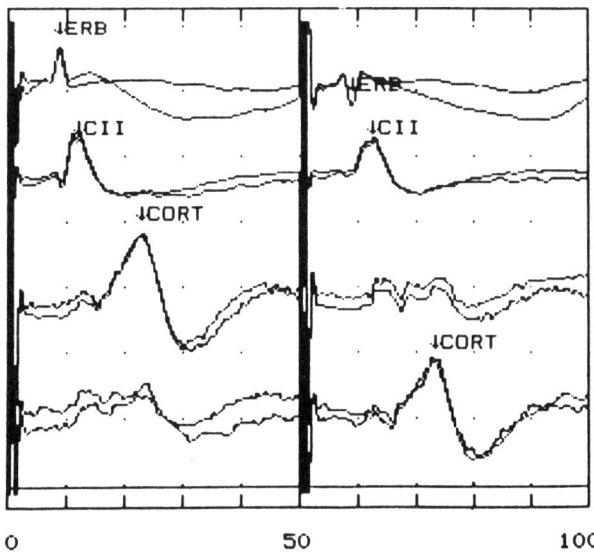

S.J. 16 Y.O.F Theophylline Overdose
Day 3 of Pentobarb Coma

Figure 25.3. Bilateral sequential median nerve somatosensory-evoked potential recordings obtained on the third day of pentobarbital coma.

imaging (MRI) scan results prior to discharge were within normal limits. Follow-up as an outpatient 4 months post-discharge shows her only residual neurologic deficit to be memory loss and poor attention.

DISCUSSION

Theophylline is a commonly used medication with an extremely low therapeutic index (1–4). Accidental or deliberate overdose may lead to life-threatening consequences. Although mild to moderate overdose ingestions are relatively straightforward in their treatment, severe ingestions require aggressive, multidisciplinary interventions to improve the chance for a good outcome. This case demonstrates the more serious neurologic sequelae of one such severe ingestion, and permits discussion of the toxicity of theophylline (1,2,4–6). We discuss charcoal hemoperfusion for removal of the drug (7–11), pentobarbital coma for treatment of status epilepticus (2,8,12), and the recently described multimodality evoked potentials to predict neurologic outcome in comatose children (13,14).

Theophylline is clinically useful in asthma, pulmonary

edema, and as a respiratory stimulant. Dilatation of the bronchial smooth muscle is its primary action in asthma treatment. When used for the treatment of pulmonary edema, it exerts a positive inotrope and positive chronotrope effect through catecholamine release with improved cardiac output. It is also a peripheral vasodilator. It has direct stimulatory effect on the vasomotor center with resultant increased rate and depth of breathing. Theophylline is believed to be helpful in weaning because it decreases fatigue by increasing diaphragmatic strength. Its use for apnea treatment is considered to be as a central respiratory stimulant.

Central Nervous System Toxicity

At levels >20 µg/ml, respiratory alkalosis may occur as a result of tachypnea from stimulation of the respiratory center (1). Central nervous system stimulation leads to nausea, emesis, wakefulness, headaches, agitation, psychosis, irritability, seizures, and coma. The mechanism of seizures is unknown, but postulations include cerebral hypoperfusion due to hypotension, and cerebral vasoconstriction, often causing a refractory state of ischemia (1). Benzodiazepines as single agents are the most effective in these often refractory seizures. Phenytoin is ineffective as a single agent (1). Often multiple anticonvulsants are needed, and, as in our patient, at times neuromuscular paralysis and pentobarbital coma may be needed. In patients chronically taking theophylline, seizures may be seen at theophylline levels as low as 25 µg/ml, but are more often associated with levels exceeding 40 µg/ml. Seizures are occasionally, but not uniformly, preceded by mild symptoms of tachycardia, poor oral intake, and irritability (1). Seizures are usually easily treated when levels are less than 40 µg/ml, but may be refractory at higher levels.

In acute overdoses, as with our patient, seizures are seen at levels of 80–100 µg/ml, are often refractory to multiple drug regimens, and are reportedly associated with a 50% mortality (12). The onset of the syndrome of severe status epilepticus is reportedly the most important determinant of serious sequelae because of associated hypoventilation, hyperthermia, cardiovascular stress, and metabolic derangements (i.e., acid-base, electrolyte, and glucose abnormalities). Failure to terminate status epilepticus may result in acute and fatal cerebral edema.

Pentobarbital, a short-acting barbiturate, has a rapid onset of action in the emergent treatment of seizures and may be given as a constant infusion. If the seizure cannot be eliminated by benzodiazepines and bolus infusions of long-acting barbiturates (i.e., phenobarbital), titrating pentobarbital while monitoring for burst suppression on EEG can rapidly suppress the seizure's focus, and terminate the status episode.

Gastrointestinal Toxicity

Nausea and emesis are partially due to local effects on the gastrointestinal mucosa, but may also be due to central effects. One may also see cramps with diarrhea, increased gastric acid secretion, ileus, and even necrotizing enterocolitis in infants (1,2).

Cardiac Toxicity

Increased production of catecholamines with their decreased uptake in the brain leads to tachycardia, decreased cardiac output, peripheral vasodilatation, and hypotension, with resultant myocardial ischemia and lactic acidosis. Lactic acidosis is partially due to stimulation of the gluconeogenesis and glycogenolysis from increased catecholamines (15). Both lactic acidosis and arrhythmias are seen as an end result of these changes in increased catecholamine levels. The hypotension is fairly refractory to volume and pressors (1,2,6,16). Arrhythmias are mainly sinus tachycardia followed by supraventricular, premature ventricular contractions, with ventricular tachycardia and fibrillation being uncommon. Arrhythmias are seen more commonly in patients who take theophylline chronically and have concurrent respiratory failure while receiving an intravenous bolus of theophylline (2). In acute overdoses, one may not see minor symptoms prior to the onset of seizures or arrhythmias. Cardiorespiratory collapse is seen at levels over 80 μg/ml in acute overdoses (2). Rhabdomyolysis may be seen as a result of seizures or hypokalemia (4).

Toxic symptoms occur 75% of the time in patients with theophylline levels >20 μg/ml. Of those with a level >15 μg/ml, 30% have toxic symptoms. Toxicity varies with the type of preparation (2). There is prolonged toxicity with the sustained release preparations as they peak in 1–24 hours with a mean of 11 hours and a duration of 12–24 hours. Short-acting preparations peak at 2 hours and have a duration of 7 hours. The volume of distribution is constant at 0.45 ml/kg, but the elimination rate and half-life vary by age, disease state, individual, and environmental factors (2,3,5).

Acute versus Chronic Toxicity

There are major differences in theophylline toxicity in acute versus chronic overdose (1,2,17). A chronic overdose usually results from accidental excessive dosing over time. Arrhythmias occur mainly in those with preexisting heart disease (5). Toxicity in older patients is more often chronic and deaths may occur at levels of 30–46 mg/l (2). Acute overdoses are usually suicide attempts or large one-time accidental ingestions. They often have symptoms of hyperthermia, leukocytosis, metabolic acidosis, hypokalemia, hyperglycemia, hypocalcemia, hypophosphatasemia, and hypomagnesemia (1,2,17). Patients with acute overdoses are usually younger, and deaths occur at levels of 138–228 μg/ml (2). Acute overdoses are associated with higher peak theophylline levels, higher mortality, and younger age (4). Patients with life-threatening arrhythmias, status epilepticus, and hepatic dysfunction are considered to be at high risk for death (1). The mortality rate for theophylline overdose has been reported as 10%. During 1987, 15 cases of fatal theophylline toxicity were reported. Theophylline toxicity was the condition most treated with charcoal hemoperfusion in 1986 (4).

Treatment is supportive, and decontamination in the form of lavage is initiated. Activated charcoal in dosages of 0.5–1 g/kg followed by a cathartic every 2–4 hours is given to prevent absorption and decrease the half-life by increasing theophylline excretion (1,2,7). Symptomatic electrolyte imbalances are corrected with particular emphasis on correction of the metabolic acidosis with sodium bicarbonate. β Blockers such as propranolol and esmolol have been used to treat the dysrythmias ((1,2,6,16). The hypotension in theophylline overdose is felt to be attributable to stimulation of the β_2 receptor, with resultant peripheral vasodilatation and decreased diastolic filling due to tachycardia from β_1 stimulation. Propranolol and esmolol were speculated to work by increasing peripheral vascular resistance and by decreasing the tachycardia (16). In the cases of those acute patients in whom a poor outcome is expected, one may choose to use charcoal hemoperfusion, as we did. Peritoneal or hemodialysis, and multiple oral doses of activated charcoal may also be used (7,9). This method of treatment consists of a loading dose of 2 g/kg of activated charcoal followed by 1 g/kg every 2–6 hours with a cathartic. The method was also called gastrointestinal dialysis by Lev in his reports. The half-life of theophylline decreases by 39–46% because of increased clearance resulting from adsorption of the theophylline to the charcoal (2,18).

Charcoal hemoperfusion has been used for rapid removal of theophylline in both acute and chronic overdoses since 1978 (11). Criteria have been advocated to identify patients who might benefit from this technique, namely those with:

1. Serum theophylline levels >60 μg/ml or >40 μg/ml if associated with renal, hepatic, or congestive heart failure;
2. Serum theophylline levels >50 μg/ml and intolerance of oral activated charcoal, or if older than 60 years of age with hepatic disease or congestive heart failure;
3. Serum theophylline levels >40 μg/ml if younger than 6 months of age, older than 60 years of age, or >60 μg/ml if between 6 months and 60 years of age (19).

The recommendation in acute overdoses has been levels >80–100 μg/ml, and in cases where life-threatening symptoms of seizures, intractable arrhythmias, hypotension, or progressive deterioration occur despite adequate supportive care (4,6,7).

In a review by Paloucek and Rodvold of 26 patients treated with charcoal hemoperfusion, 5 patients treated prior to severe toxicity recovered, and in 15 patients in whom treatment was initiated after the onset of severe symptoms, 10 quickly improved and 3 died of renal failure or anoxic brain injury. In all patients, heart rate decreased, hypotension improved, seizures stopped, and neurologic grading scales improved in most of the treated patients (6).

Side effects of the hemoperfusion are rarely clinically significant, but include thrombocytopenia lasting 24–72 hours, hypocalcemia, hypotension, coagulopathy, chills, hyperpyrexia, anemia, and leukopenia (6,19). Earlier problems of charcoal embolization were solved by coating or embedding the charcoal onto a column (19). Clotting problems have been treated with heparinization (7,10). The use of prostacyclin may reduce the thrombocytopenia (7). Hemolysis may occur because of the mechanics of hemoperfusion (19).

Reported duration of hemoperfusion has been from 90 minutes to 5 hours (6). Our patient received 9 hours, and termination was due to a coagulopathy manifested by elevated activated coagulation times and clinical bleeding (11). Efficacy depends on the extraction ratio (er), which is determined by the formula: er = (arterial theophylline level-venous theophylline level)/arterial theophylline level. The published er range for hemoperfusion is $0.082 - 1$ (6). The cartridges needed to be changed every 2 hours to counter the decrease in extraction rate due to cartridge saturation. The mean baseline theophylline half-life was 21 hours, mean half-life during hemoperfusion was 1.5–2 hours, and mean half-life was 10.3 hours after hemoperfusion stopped. Symptomatic rebound is rarely problematic. Our patient had decreased her level from 159 to 33.8 µg/ml at the end of her 9-hour hemoperfusion run.

Sessler concluded that he and his team could predict which of the acute cases would benefit from charcoal perfusion using certain predictive criteria for need (4). This was not true for chronic overdoses. The use of an invasive procedure that is costly, has serious side effects, and at times requires hospital transfer made the authors reluctant to recommend its use for cases of chronic overdose unless life-threatening symptoms were present.

Evoked Potentials

It is very difficult to predict outcome in children who are comatose from any cause. While diazepam and then pentobarbital coma seemed to control our patient's seizures, as evidenced by the lack of tonic-clonic activity, she remained comatose and EEGs documented continued spiking waves or subclinical status epilepticus activity. Because of the high mortality associated with theophylline-induced seizures (12), the refractory nature of her seizures, and her diabetes insipidus, we were pessimistic regarding her outcome. However, her brainstem auditory-evoked potentials and somatosensory-evoked potentials were normal (Fig. 25.2). We have found this technology to be exceedingly helpful as an adjunct to clinical, radiologic, and laboratory information in predicting outcome.

COMMENTARY

In this report, the pharmacology and pathophysiology of theophylline overdose are reviewed. Charcoal hemoperfusion is not used as frequently in the United States as in Europe. The European experience with this therapy for a wide variety of conditions is encouraging. Scattered reports as well as case series are documenting the predictive value of SSEPS in a variety of pathologies.

References

1. Albert S. Aminophylline toxicity. Pediatr Clin North Am 1987;34: 61–73.
2. Ehlers S. Theophylline. In: Haddad, LM, Winchester JF, ed., Clinical management of poisoning and drug overdose. 2nd ed. Philadelphia: WB Saunders, 1990:1407–1418.
3. Eshleman SS, Leslie S. Massive theophylline overdoses with atypical metabolic abnormalities. Clin Chem 1990;36(2):398–399.
4. Sessler C. Theophylline toxicity: clinical features in 116 consecutive cases. Am J Med 1990;88:567–576.
5. Emerman C, Devlin C, Connors A. Risk of toxicity in patients with elevated theophylline levels. Ann Emerg Med 1990;6:643–648.
6. Paloucek F, Rodvold K. Evaluation of theophylline overdoses and toxicities. Ann Emerg Med 1988;17(2):135–142.
7. Katona B, Siegel E, Cluxton RJ. The new black magic: activated charcoal and new therapeutic uses. J Emerg Med 1987;5:9–18.
8. Sahney S, Abarzua J, Sessums L. Hemoperfusion in theophylline neurotoxicity. Pediatrics 1983;71(4):615–619.
9. Shannon M, Amitai Y, Lovejoy F. Multiple dose activated charcoal for theophylline poisonings in young infants. Pediatrics 1987;80(3): 368–370.
10. Stegmayr B. On-line hemodialysis and hemoperfusion in a girl intoxicated by theophylline. Acta Med Scand 1988;223:567–577.
11. Woo O, et al. Benefit of hemoperfusion in acute theophylline intoxication. Clin Toxicol 1984;22(5):411–424.
12. Zwillich C, et al. Theophylline-induced seizures in adults. Ann Intern Med 1985;82(6):784–787.
13. Goodwin SR, Friedman WA, Bellefleur M. Is it time to use evoked potentials to predict outcome in comatose children and adults? Crit Care Med 1991;19:518–524.
14. Goodwin SR, Toney KA, Mahla ME. Sensory evoked potentials accurately predict recovery from prolonged coma caused by strangulation. Crit Care Med 1993; in press.
15. Leventhal L, et al. Lactic acidosis in theophylline overdose. Am J Emerg Med 1989;7(4):417–418.
16. Seneff M, et al. Acute theophylline toxicity and the use of esmolol to reverse cardiovascular instability. Ann Emerg Med 1990;19(6): 671–673.
17. Shannon M, Frederick L. Hypokalemia after theophylline intoxication: the effects of acute vs. chronic poisoning. Arch Intern Med 1989;149:2725–2729.
18. Berlinger W, et al. Enhancement of theophylline clearance by oral activated charcoal. Clin Pharmacol Ther 1983;3:351–354.
19. Gallagher EJ, Howland M, Greenblatt H. Hemolysis following treatment of theophylline overdose with coated charcoal hemoperfusion. J Emerg Med 1987;5:19–22.

Case 26

Edward E. Conway, Jr., H. Michael Ushay, and Anthony L. Palomba

Children's Medical Center at Montefiore
Bronx, New York, USA

HISTORY

A 14-year-old boy with congenital hydrocephalus was seen at our hospital with diplopia and increasing ataxia. Hydrocephalus was first diagnosed at age 2 years and was attributed to "a forceps delivery and birth trauma." The patient had been in school until approximately 2 years prior to this admission, at which time he slowly began to develop diplopia, unsteady gait, and left-sided weakness. The patient was admitted for a ventriculoperitoneal shunt.

PHYSICAL EXAMINATION

The patient was a well-appearing boy with a heart rate of 82 beats/min, blood pressure of 112/62 mm Hg, respiratory rate of 16 breaths/min, and a temperature of 37°C. Physically, he had horizontal nystagmus, left sixth nerve palsy, and no papilledema. His chest was clear to auscultation with no rales, rhonchi, or wheezes. Results of cardiac examination revealed a 2/6 systolic ejection murmur heard best along the left upper sternal border. There was no organomegaly and the patient was a Tanner 5 male. Neurologically, in addition to the eye findings, he had a slight decrease in motor strength (4/5) in the left upper and lower extremities. The deep tendon reflexes were normal throughout and the plantar response was down—going bilaterally. The patient had an ataxic gait, and he had diffi-culty in repeating the finger-to-nose task.

LABORATORY DATA

The patient's admitting serum chemistry values, liver profile, coagulation study results, and hematologic evalua-tion were all normal. The admitting chest radiograph did not reveal any abnormalities and the electrocardiogram (ECG) demonstrated a normal sinus rhythm. An echocar-diogram was performed to evaluate the murmur and did not reveal any structural or functional heart disease. A CT scan of the head was significant for moderate bilateral dilatation of the lateral ventricles and a dilatated third ventricle as well. There was both cerebral and cerebellar atrophy.

MANAGEMENT

The patient had a ventriculoperitoneal shunt placed via a right occipital approach. He was extubated in the operat-ing suite and was transferred from the recovery area to the pediatric ward. He complained of a diffuse, nonradiating headache for which he was given acetaminophen. On the morning following surgery, the patient was lethargic and an emergent cranial CT scan was arranged. The patient was electively intubated and hyperventilated. The CT scan demonstrated a moderate to large right-sided epidural he-matoma with a slight midline shift. A craniotomy was per-formed and the epidural hematoma was removed. Repeat hematologic and coagulation profile results were normal. The patient was transferred to the PICU. On postoperative day 1, the patient was weaned to a T-piece; arterial blood gas (ABG) values drawn while he breathed F_IO_2 .40 re-vealed pH 7.37, $PaCO_2$ 35 torr (4.6 kPa), and a PaO_2 of 180 torr (23.9 kPa). The patient's trachea was extubated without event. Approximately 6 hours later, he developed an acute, severe episode of respiratory distress with an oxygen desaturation of 85% detected by pulse oximetry while he was breathing F_IO_2 1.0 and his trachea was emer-gently intubated. The patient had been lying in a midline position with his head elevated to 30°. A large volume of pink frothy tracheal secretions were suctioned from the endotracheal (ET) tube. Physical examination revealed a decrease in breath sounds and rales noted only on the left

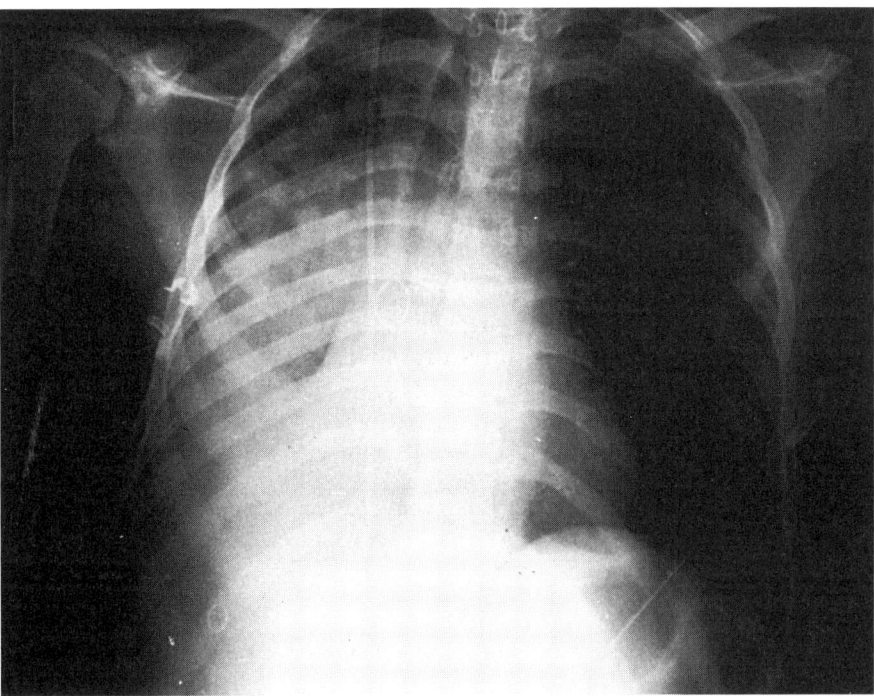

Figure 26.1. Chest radiograph obtained on postoperative day 1 demonstrating a diffuse left-sided alveolar infiltrate.

side. A chest radiograph (Fig. 26.1) was obtained and demonstrated a diffuse alveolar infiltrate localized only in the left chest. The clinical picture and radiograph were consistent with pulmonary edema. Therefore, the patient was placed on a mechanical ventilator (Servo 900C) with a tidal volume of 600 ml, intermittent mandatory ventilation (IMV) 18, positive end-expiratory pressure (PEEP) of 6 torr, and he received a dose of furosemide to which he quickly responded. The patient was started on clindamycin and cefuroxime to protect against the possibility of aspiration, although no acute episode was documented. The patient was again extubated on postoperative day 6, and a normal chest radiograph was obtained (Fig. 26.2). Approximately 4 hours following extubation, the patient developed post-extubation stridor, which initially responded to racemic epinephrine and intravenous dexamethasone.

However, 3 hours later the boy's distress grew worse. ABG values demonstrated pH 7.51, $PaCO_2$ 33 torr (4.4 kPa), and PaO_2 51 torr (6.8 kPa) while the boy was breathing F_IO_2 .80, and his trachea was again reintubated. Physical examination revealed rales and decreased breath sounds on the right. A chest radiograph was obtained (Fig.

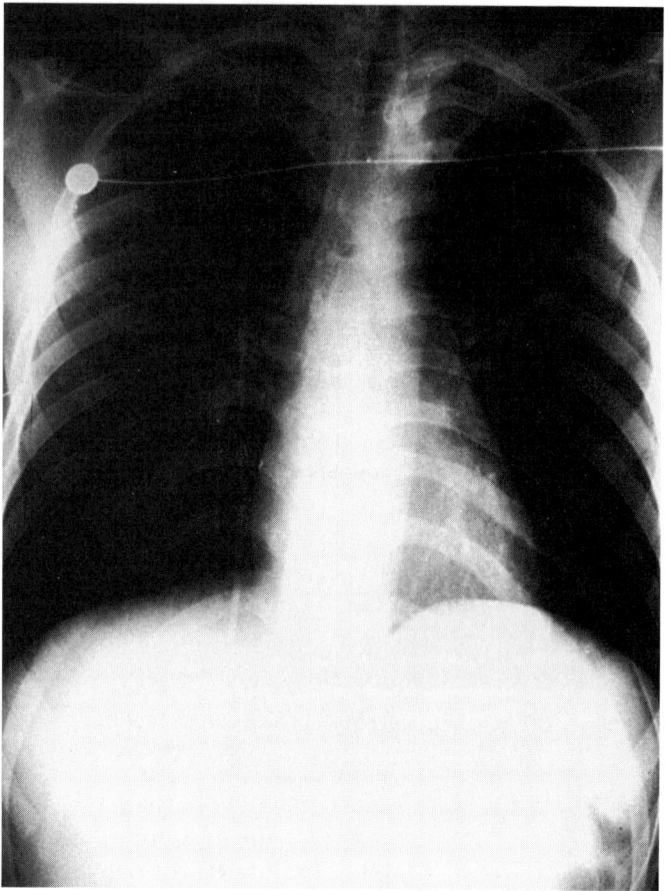

Figure 26.2.   Chest radiograph obtained on postoperative day 6 demonstrating clear lung fields bilaterally. The ventriculoperitoneal shunt tubing can be seen on the right.

26.3), which showed a diffuse alveolar infiltrate localized only to the right chest. Copious amounts of pink frothy material were obtained from the ET tube and the patient again responded to furosemide, mechanical ventilation, and PEEP.

On postoperative day 12, the patient underwent a flexible fiberoptic bronchoscopy through which was noted a small amount of granulation tissue in the supraglottic area. The subglottic area and major bronchi were normal in appearance, however, and the patient was extubated. He appeared to be doing well until postoperative day 15 when he developed a third episode of respiratory distress attributed to probable upper airway obstruction which required reintubation. A chest radiograph at this time was normal. On postoperative day 24, two large supraglottic

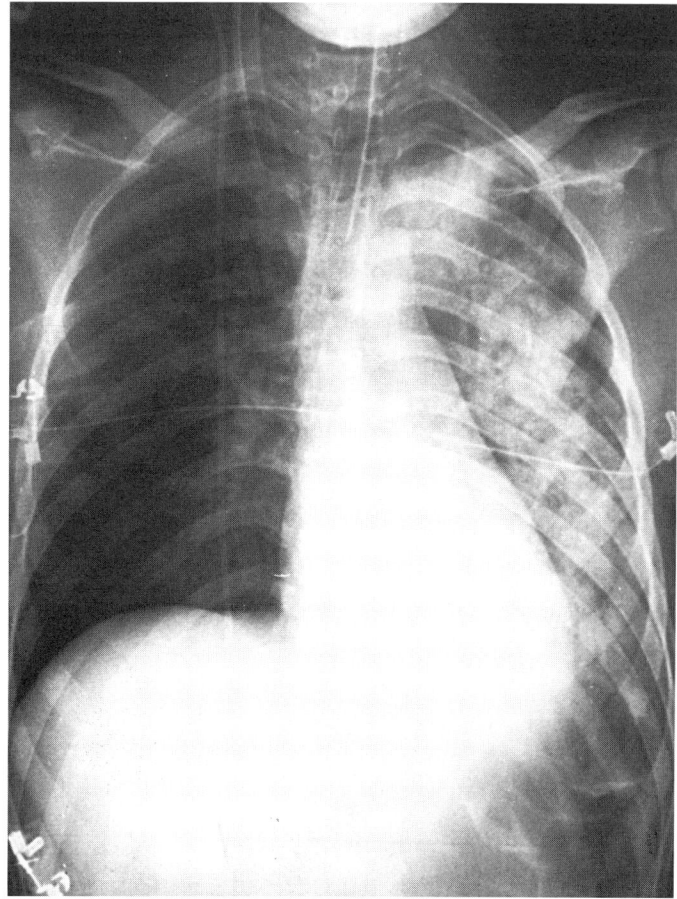

Figure 26.3. Chest radiograph obtained on postoperative day 6 demonstrating a diffuse right-sided alveolar infiltrate.

granulomas were removed and a tracheostomy was performed. The patient was easily weaned from the ventilator and his trachea was eventually decannulated. His neurologic status and strength improved, and he was able to return to his native country.

DISCUSSION

Acute pulmonary edema has many possible etiologies. These may include cardiogenic pulmonary edema of ischemic or valvular origin, pulmonary embolism, laryngeal obstruction, bronchial aspiration, naloxone use, acute respiratory distress syndrome, and postcardiopulmonary bypass (1). Acute postobstructive pulmonary edema usually appears bilaterally and has been associated with laryngospasm, epiglottis, croup, laryngotracheobronchitis, foreign body aspiration, tumor, upper airway trauma, strangulation, Ludwig's angina, angioedema, adenoidal or tonsillar hypertrophy, obstructive sleep apnea, and nasopharyngeal masses. The pathophysiology of the obstructive pulmonary edema involves the generation of a markedly negative intrapleural pressure initiated by a forceful inspiratory effort against an obstructed extrathoracic airway (Muller maneuver). This allows the exudation of fluid across the capillary and alveolar membranes. Acidosis, hypoxic vasoconstriction, increased sympathetic outflow, and tissue hypoxia may also play a contributory role in the pathogenesis of the edema.

Unilateral pulmonary edema is a very uncommon entity. Most cases of unilateral pulmonary edema occur following the reexpansion of a pneumothorax. Acute unilateral pulmonary edema is also referred to as reexpansion pulmonary edema. The etiology of reexpansion pulmonary edema is unclear but is usually related to the (1) chronicity of collapse (usually >48–72 hours), (2) the amount of air or fluid (i.e., usually >2 l) evacuated, and (3) the rapidity of reexpansion of the affected lung (2). The most accepted theory of its pathophysiology is that there is an increase in the permeability of the alveolar capillary membrane. This may be due to mechanical deformation of endothelial pores allowing fluid and protein flux into the interstitium, tissue hypoxia, decreased pulmonary blood flow, and decreased alveolar ventilation leading to possible reperfusion injury with toxic oxygen radicals and possible alterations in surfactant activity. Reexpansion pulmonary edema is usually rapid in onset; however, it may be seen as late as 24 hours following the inciting event.

Unilateral pulmonary edema has also been shown to occur in the setting of systemic to pulmonary artery shunts, unilateral veno-occlusive disease, prolonged lateral decubitus position, pulmonary contusion, congenital absence or hypoplasia of a pulmonary artery, Sawyer-James syndrome, pulmonary thromboembolism, localized emphysema, lobectomy, pleural disease, and following a Pott's procedure (3). Recent reports have included unilateral pulmonary edema occurring with epileptic seizures, neurogenic pulmonary edema following head trauma, acute subglottic edema, and following an atrial septal defect repair where the patch occluded the right pulmonary veins leading to rapid increase in the hydrostatic pressure of the right lung.

The case we describe is unusual in that the unilateral pulmonary edema alternated and the patient did not appear to have any of the previously described clinical associations. Unilateral pulmonary edema should be suspected in any patient who has any of the predisposing conditions listed above in whom there is sudden onset of dyspnea, tachypnea, hypoxemia, hypercapnia, and pink-frothy secretions are produced. This clinical deterioration usually occurs rapidly, but may be delayed by as much as 24 hours. Prompt recognition is essential because unilateral pulmonary edema is reversible with timely and aggressive support. That support should include endotracheal intubation, mechanical ventilation, and the use of positive end-expiratory pressure.

COMMENTARY

Unilateral pulmonary edema appears to be more common in children as compared with adults. This phenomenon is not well documented in the literature, however. The first consideration is always directed at straightforward mechanical explanations as in surgical repairs of the pulmonary veins obstructing venous return, and broken ventriculoperitoneal shunt catheters draining fluid into a hemithorax. The relationship between upper airway obstruction and pulmonary edema is a multifactorial one. The negative intrathoracic pressure demands that the left ventricle produce enough work (i.e., pressure) to drive the blood into the descending aorta (which is approximately at atmospheric pressure). From the perspective of the left ventricle, this necessary change in driving pressure is no different from a huge rise in afterload by an increase in systemic blood pressure. This increased work explains in part the paradox of pulsus paradoxus: during a Muller maneuver the heart sounds like it is working harder (it is), yet the blood pressure falls. This increased work can cause left ventricular failure and consequent pulmonary edema. This does not completely explain the fascinating observation of alternating unilateral pulmonary edema. With a heightened awareness of this pathology, it is hoped that the physiology will be elucidated.

References

1. Schiff GA, Simpson JI. Unilateral pulmonary edema after atrial septal defect repair. Anesthesiology 1991;74:785–786.
2. Timby J, Reed C, Zeilender S, Glauser FL. Mechanical causes of pulmonary edema. Chest 1990;98:973–979.
3. Calenoff L, Kruglik G, Woodruff A. Unilateral pulmonary edema. Radiology 1978;12:19–24.

Case 27

Waldemar Storm
Children's Hospital
Madison, Wisconsin, USA

HISTORY

On a farm in central Wisconsin, a previously healthy 3-year-old boy was found lying unconscious in a barn stall with a cow and calf, apparently having been kicked or butted by the larger animal. He was taken to the emergency room of the local hospital.

PHYSICAL EXAMINATION

The patient had spontaneous respirations. There was increased extensor tone. He was responsive to noxious stimuli, but was highly variable, alternating between periods of agitation and periods of flaccidity with apnea. Initial Glasgow coma score was approximately 6. There were large subgaleal hematomas of the right parietal and left temporal scalp, and blood draining from the left ear. There were abrasions of the forehead and left side of the face. The pupils were equal and reactive to light, but eye movements were disconjugate. No significant extracranial injuries were found. The neck was stabilized in a cervical collar. Intravenous mannitol 1 g/kg was given. The child was orally intubated and flown by helicopter to University of Wisconsin Children's Hospital. Vital signs during transport included heart rate 150 beats/min, blood pressure 125/59 mm Hg, respiratory rate 30 breaths/min (with Ambu bag), and temperature 37°C.

LABORATORY DATA

Laboratory data at the time of admission were as follows: sodium 134 mEq/l, potassium 3.4 mEq/l, chloride

104 mEq/l, total CO_2 16 mEq/l, blood urea nitrogen (BUN) 16 mg/dl, creatinine 0.4 mg/dl, glucose 308 mg/dl, amylase 74 U/l, hemoglobin 12.3 g/dl, white blood count $26.4 \times 10^3/\mu l$, prothrombin time 13.7 seconds, and partial thromboplastin time 23.2 seconds. Urinalysis indicated specific gravity of 1.010, pH of 5.0, and was negative for blood. Cervical, thoracic, and lumbar spine radiographs and abdominal and pelvic CT scans showed no abnormalities. A cranial CT scan obtained when the boy arrived at the hospital showed a large right parieto-occipital skull fracture and diastasis of the lambdoid suture, and subarachnoid blood surrounding the brainstem and filling the superior cerebellar cistern (Fig. 27.1). Parenchymal hemorrhage involved the left brachium pontis (Fig. 27.2). The ventricles appeared normal.

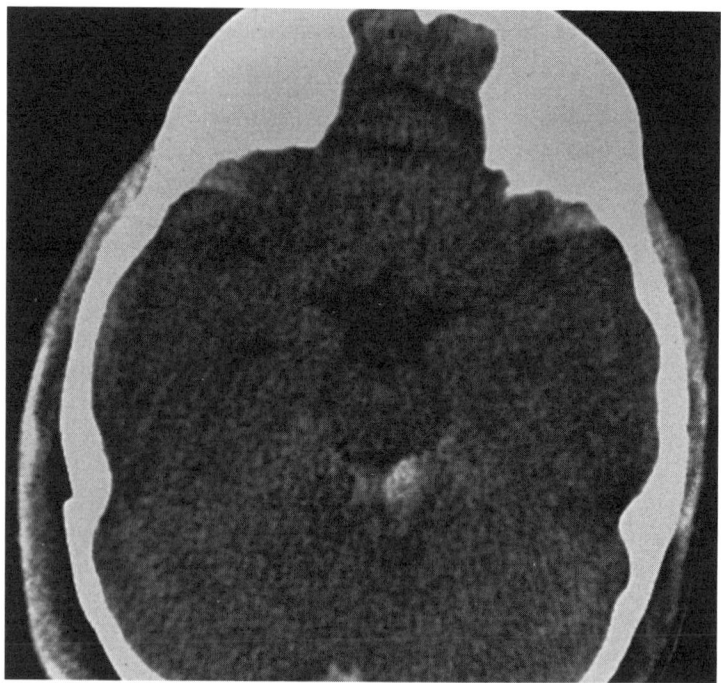

Figure 27.1. Hemorrhage fills the subarachnoid space around the brainstem and the superior cerebellar cistern. Note parietal skull fracture.

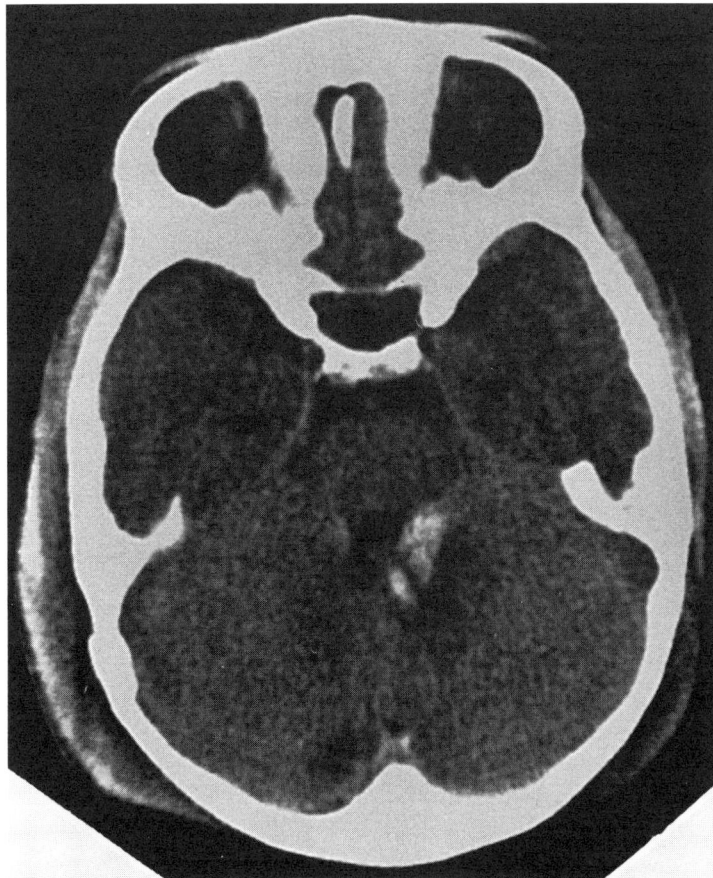

Figure 27.2. Hemorrhage has involved the left cerebellar parenchyma. Low density changes have developed in the cerebellar hemispheres.

MANAGEMENT

The child was admitted to the PICU. An epidural pressure monitor was placed and the patient received hyperventilation to a $PaCO_2$ of 25–28 mm Hg. Initial intracranial pressure ranged between 6 and 10 mm Hg. The pressure gradually increased to a maximum of 40 mm Hg on the fourth hospital day, necessitating intermittent osmotic therapy. Lorazepam was given for sedation. Serial CT scans demonstrated evolving changes of cerebral edema, large bilateral cerebellar contusions, and intraventricular hemorrhage. A cerebrospinal fluid (CSF) leak from the left ear gradually resolved by 1 week after injury.

Fluids were initially restricted to approximately two-thirds of maintenance requirements. There was early sus-picion of syndrome of inappropriate antidiuretic hormone secretion (SIADH) when sodium decreased to 129 mEq/l by the third day, with simultaneous serum osmolarity of 269 mOsm/l, and urine osmolarity 677 mOsm/l. This rap-idly resolved with additional fluid restriction. Enteral tube feedings were begun on the fourth hospital day and were quickly advanced, with added Lipomul (cottonseed oil) and Propac (1). A fever of 38.5°C developed on the fifth hospital day. *Escherichia coli* was cultured from the urine, and the patient was started on trimethoprin/sulfamethoxazole via nasogastric tube. No antibiotics had been used prior to this infection.

One week after injury, the intracranial pressure re-mained in the 20 mm Hg range without osmotic agent intervention. Moderate sedation with morphine was con-

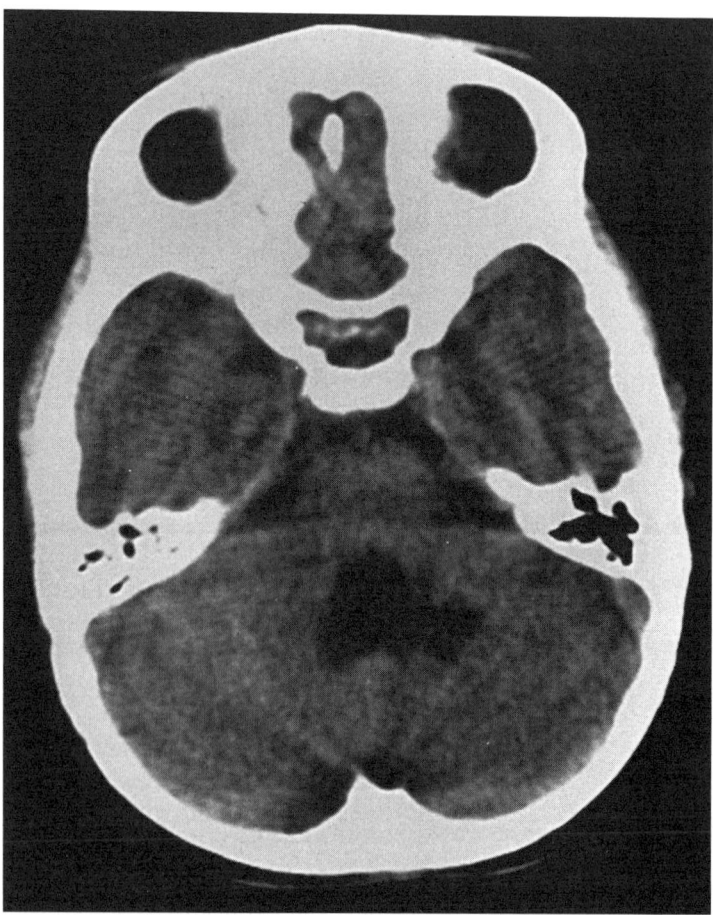

Figure 27.3. After 6 weeks, changes of encephalomalacia are present in the cerebellum.

tinued. At this time the patient demonstrated spontaneous movement of all extremities (with weakness of the left upper and lower extremities), localized stimuli, and showed some purposeful movement. The pupils were equal in size and light response. Corneal reflexes demonstrated a partial deficit of the left eye. Cough and gag reflexes were present. Facial grimacing demonstrated complete left facial paralysis. The Glasgow coma score had gradually improved to a level of 9 (eyes = 3, verbal = 1, motor = 5). The boy continued to show gradual improvement. He was weaned slowly from the ventilator and was extubated on the 11th hospital day. The intracranial pressure monitor was also discontinued. Physical, occupational, and speech therapy were initiated shortly thereafter. The child became gradually more responsive and active, and was transferred to the rehabilitation service 1 month after admission. Results of a swallow study were normal. Oral food intake was advanced rapidly. The left facial paralysis gradually improved. Left upper and left lower extremity weakness and impaired coordination were present but also improving. By 6 weeks postinjury, the patient was walking with assistance. Receptive and expressive language tested within normal limits. Behavioral problems of impulsivity and distractibility were noted. A follow-up CT scan at that time showed areas of encephalomalacia in the cerebellum and left brachium pontis (Fig. 27.3). The patient was discharged to continued outpatient speech and rehabilitation therapy.

DISCUSSION

Trauma is the leading cause of death and injury in children older than 1 year of age (2,3). Farm-related injuries are a significant problem in agricultural areas (4). In Wisconsin, the mean annual farm-related injury death rate for children ages 0–9 years is 3.2 per 100,000 rural children (5,6). Nearly 300 children and adolescents die each year from farm injuries and 23,500 sustain nonfatal trauma (7). More than half of the children who die never reach a physician, and about 20% die en route to a hospital. Only 7.4% of the children who ultimately die live long enough to receive inpatient care (7). The most common cause of these injuries is farm machinery (4,6). Less commonly, injuries are caused by farm animals (8).

Subarachnoid hemorrhage is common in pediatric head trauma (9). It rarely requires surgical intervention but may produce obstructive or communicating hydrocephalus. Intraparenchymal hemorrhages are often small and usually do not require surgical treatment, but larger intraparenchymal hematomas may cause a mass effect and require evacuation. Contusional hemorrhages are usually associated with some degree of parenchymal damage. Basilar skull fractures are commonly associated with CSF otorrhea and rhinorrhea, cranial nerve palsies (as in this patient), hearing loss, and vascular lesions (10).

Primary brain injury as a result of the direct traumatic insult is generally not treatable (11). Treatment for head trauma is directed at prevention of secondary brain injury (3,11). Hyperemia, cerebral edema, intracranial hypertension, decreased cerebral blood flow, decreased systemic blood pressure, hypoxia, and hypercarbia may all contribute to secondary ischemic injury. Children may be predisposed to early hyperemic brain swelling (3). The dynamic processes involved are complex and have been extensively investigated (9,12–14). The traditional mainstay of treatment consists of airway control and hyperventilation to decrease cerebral blood volume in response to decreased $PaCO_2$. Head elevation, sedation, intracranial pressure monitoring, use of osmotic agents, control of seizures and fever (which increase cerebral oxygen requirements), and surgical intervention for evacuation of mass lesions are also helpful (11). Recent investigations have raised new questions about the usefulness of prophylactic hyperventilation, which could possibly promote ischemia (12,15). Clearly, further investigation in this area is needed. The goal of therapy is to permit sufficient cerebral blood flow to deliver oxygen and glucose to the brain, while minimizing the deleterious effects of elevated intracranial pressure. Future therapies may include biochemical methods to suppress the local inflammatory process-mediated cytotoxic and vasogenic edema (16).

Numerous systemic changes may occur in response to brain injury. Some of these such as immediate systemic hypertension, neurogenic pulmonary edema, and hyperglycemia are probably secondary to catecholamine release (17). Vagally mediated mechanisms may lead to hypotension. Hypothalamic and pituitary dysfunction may occur, resulting in diabetes insipidus or SIADH. Traumatic release of brain thromboplastin into the circulation may result in disseminated intravascular coagulation. Related to the increased catecholamine levels, as well as elevated serum cortisol levels following severe head injury, the metabolic rate may be dramatically increased, resulting in a profoundly catabolic state with markedly increased caloric and nutritional requirements (18–23). Failure to supply sufficient nitrogen and calories may result in immunoincompetence and systemic organ failure (24). Nutritional support for the acutely head-injured patient has traditionally been delayed until return of gastrointestinal function and then provided by the enteral route (25). Frequently, no nutritional support is provided for as long as a week after the injury, despite the widespread recognition of potential nutritional deficiency. Increased survival of head-injured patients has been demonstrated with early administration of total parenteral nutrition, apparently as a result of decreased susceptibility to sepsis (25).

The Glasgow coma scale is helpful in estimating prognosis (26). Children with an initial Glasgow coma scale τ8 generally do well and make a complete recovery, while those with a Glasgow coma score of 3–5 have a high incidence of death and severe neurologic sequelae (9). Those with a score of 6–8 often do well with aggressive treatment, although deterioration and poor outcome may occur; the main determinant in these patients may be related to the amount of primary diffuse impact injury to the white matter (9). The presence of a lucid interval predicts a more favorable prognosis than immediate, sustained unconsciousness following head injury.

Head injuries are the most common cause of late sequelae and persistent disability in pediatric trauma victims. Some degree of disability persisting at 6 months has been reported in >50% of children hospitalized with severe head injuries (27), emphasizing the need for rehabilitation services after the initial recovery period. Although some residual disability is probable, the patient we describe demonstrated remarkable recovery at the time of discharge.

COMMENTARY

Head trauma is a common cause for admission to the PICU everywhere in the world. What differs is the mechanism by which the trauma occurs. In the Midwestern United States, it is often due to farm machinery and animals. We are on the verge of a new era when effective treatment of brain-injured patients will be possible after the insult has occurred. The biochemical manipulations to intervene in late secondary injury will be moved forward by the great amount of basic science research in this area. As always, prevention of injuries is the most important way to approach the problems of trauma.

References

1. Twyman D, Young AB, Ott L, et al. High protein enteral feedings: a means of achieving positive nitrogen balance in head-injured patients. JPEN 1985;9:679.
2. Haller JA, Jr. Pediatric trauma, the number one killer in children. JAMA 1983;249:47–53.
3. Kissoon N, Dreyer J, Walia M. Pediatric trauma: differences in pathophysiology, injury patterns and treatment compared with adult trauma. Can Med Assoc J 1990;142:27.
4. Swanson JA, Sachs MI, Dahlgren KA, Tingvely SJ. Accidental farm injuries in children. Am J Dis Child 1987;141:1276.
5. U.S. Bureau of the Census. 1980 census of population, Vol 1: Characteristics of the population, ch B: General population characteristics. Pt 51: Wisconsin. US Department of Commerce, Government Printing Office, 1982:317–322.
6. Salmi RL, Weiss HB, Peterson PL, et al. Fatal farm injuries among young children. Pediatrics 1989;83:267.
7. Rivara FP. Fatal and nonfatal farm injuries to children and adolescents in the United States. Pediatrics 1985;76:567.
8. Cogbill TH, Busch HM, Stiers GR. Farm accidents in children. Pediatrics 1985;76:562.
9. Bruce DA, Alavi A, Bilaniuk L, et al. Diffuse cerebral swelling following head injuries in children: the syndrome of "malignant brain edema." J Neurosurg 1981;54:170.
10. Thomas LM. Skull fractures. In: Wilkins RH, Rengacharey SS, eds. Neurosurgery. New York: McGraw-Hill, 1985:1623–1626.
11. Jaffe D, Wesson D. Emergency management of blunt trauma in children. New Engl J Med 1991;324:1477.
12. Bouma GJ, Muizelaar JP. Cerebral blood flow, cerebral blood volume, and cerebrovascular reactivity after severe head injury. J Neurotrauma 1992;9:S333.
13. Fishman RA. Brain edema. New Engl J Med 1975;293:706.
14. Prough DS, Rogers AT. Physiology and pharmacology of cerebral blood flow and metabolism. Neurol Crit Care 1989;5:713.
15. Muizelaar JP, Marmarou A, Ward JD, et al. Adverse effects of prolonged hyperventilation in patients with severe head injury: a randomized clinical trial. J Neurosurg 1991;75:731.
16. Chan PH, Longar S, Fishman TA. Protective effects of liposome-entrapped, superoxide dismutase on posttraumatic brain edema. Ann Neurol 1987;21:540.
17. Rosner MJ, Newsome HH, Becker DP. Mechanical brain injury: the sympathoadrenal response. J Neurosurg 1984;61:76.
18. Andrassy RJ, Dubois T. Modified injury severity scale and concurrent steroid therapy: independent correlates of negative nitrogen balance in pediatric patients. J Pediatr Surg 1985;20:799.
19. Clifton GL, Robertson CS, Grossman RG, et al. The metabolic response to severe head injury. J Neurosurg 1984;60:687.
20. Drew JH, Koop CE, Grigger RP. A nutritional study of neurosurgical patients with special reference to nitrogen balance and convalescence in the postoperative period. J Neurosurg 1947;4:7.
21. Kolpek JH, Oh LG, Record KE, et al. Comparison of urinary urea nitrogen excretion and measured energy expenditure in spinal cord injury and nonsteroid-treated severe head trauma patients. JPEN 1989;13:277.
22. Phillips R, Ott L, Young B, Walsh J. Nutritional support and mea-

sured energy expenditure of the child and adolescent with head injury. J Neurosurg 1987;67:846.

23. Schiller WR, Long CL, Blakemore WS. Creatinine and nitrogen excretion in seriously ill and injured patients. Surg Gynecol Obstet 149: 561, 1979.

24. Touho H, Karasawa J, Shishido H, et al. Hypermetabolism in the acute stage of hemorrhagic cerebrovascular disease. J Neurosurg 1990;72:710.

25. Rapp RP, Young B, Twyman D, et al. The favorable effect of early parenteral feeding on survival in head-injured patients. J Neurosurg 1983;58:906.

26. Jennett B, Bond M. Assessment of outcome after severe brain damage: a practical scale. Lancet 1975;1:480.

27. Wesson DE, Williams JI, Spence LJ, et al. Functional outcome in pediatric trauma. J Trauma 1989;29:589.

Case 28

Brian R. Krafte-Jacobs, Ann Marie LeVine, and James D. Wilkinson
Children's National Medical Center Washington, DC, USA

HISTORY

A 10-week-old infant girl was in good health until 4 days prior to admission at which time she had an episode of crying associated with a distended abdomen. The episode resolved and she remained asymptomatic until 1 day prior to admission when, 2 hours after a diphtheria-pertussis-tetanus (DPT) immunization, she became tachypneic and cried inconsolably. A visit to an emergency room (ER) resulted in the diagnosis of "DPT reaction" and she was discharged home. The symptoms continued, however, and the baby was brought to the ER at Children's Hospital.

Her birth history was notable for an episode of tachypnea at 24 hours of age associated with hypoglycemia that resolved with a regimen of glucose and intravenous fluids. Results of a sepsis work-up at the time were negative.

The family history was notable for multiple cases of sudden infant death syndrome on the maternal side.

PHYSICAL EXAMINATION

At the time of admission, the infant was noted to be in respiratory distress with tachypnea, grunting, and flaring. Her vital signs were as follows: temperature 38.6°C, pulse rate 186 beats/min, respiration 64 breaths/min, and blood pressure 112/58 mm Hg.

The baby was pale, her lips were dry, and her anterior fontanel was flat. There were no exanthems, and capillary refill was 2 seconds, with the liver appreciated 11 cm below the right costal margin. There were no additional physical abnormalities.

LABORATORY DATA

Results of laboratory tests were as follows: arterial blood gas on room air pH 6.99, pCO_2 12.8 mm Hg, pO_2 104 mm Hg, base deficit -27.5; carboxy hemoglobin 2.6 mm Hg; sodium 143 mEq/l, potassium 3.3 mEq/l, chloride 109 mEq/l, bicarbonate 7 mEq/l; anion gap 27 mEq/l, blood urea nitrogen (BUN) 16 mg/dl, glucose 96 g/dl, calcium 9.2 mg/dl, ammonia 182 μg/dl, bilirubin 1.2/0.4 mg/dl, lactate 6.9 mmol/l, serum glutamic oxaloacetic transaminase 1065 U/l, serum glutamic pyruvic transaminase 323 U/l, lactic dehydrogenase 2761 U/l, alkaline phosphatase 175 U/l, triglyceride 688 mg/dl, white blood count: 13,200/mm^3 with 48% polymorphs, 11% bands, 36% lymphocytes, hemoglobin 9.2 g/dl, hematocrit 26.8%, platelets 582,000/mm^3, prothrombin time 12.7 seconds, partial thromboplastin time 78.1 seconds, UA specific gravity 1.024, pH 5, 3+ protein, and 3+ ketones. A urine toxicology screen was negative.

MANAGEMENT

The patient was intubated and required assisted mechanical ventilation. A sepsis work-up was performed, and the patient was treated with antibiotics. Despite administration of 40 ml/kg of intravenous fluid and 2 mEq/kg of bicarbonate, repeat arterial blood gas values still reflected a severe metabolic acidosis (pH 6.79, pCO_2 26 mm Hg, pO_2 190 mm Hg, and base deficit -32). Upon arrival at the PICU, the infant was mottled, with cool extremities, had tachycardia to 195 beats/min, and was hypotensive with systolic pressures of 30–40 mm Hg. Arterial and central venous lines were placed. Additional fluid boluses and a dopamine infusion titrated from 10–25 μg/kg/min failed to improve the baby's blood pressure, and an epinephrine infusion was titrated to 1 μg/kg/min, resulting in improved blood pressure and perfusion. During the first day of admission, the patient continued to have cardiovascular instability, as well as persistent severe metabolic acidosis with abnormally high lactate levels despite giving the infant multiple bicarbonate boluses and a continuous bicarbonate infusion. The patient developed hypernatremia secondary to the bicarbonate and was changed to a tromethamine infusion for continuing treatment of the metabolic acidosis. The initial hyperammonemia resolved spontaneously, and the coagulopathy was corrected with fresh frozen plasma. Approximately 24 hours after the infant was admitted, the metabolic acidosis had resolved and the tromethamine infusion was discontinued. The patient's cardiovascular status stabilized and the inotropic support was discontinued as well. The patient was subsequently extubated and did not require supplementary oxygen therapy.

On the third hospital day the infant was inadvertently fed a milk-based formula and several hours later developed tachypnea, grunting, and a metabolic acidosis with elevated lactate levels, which was treated with tromethamine. The acidosis and respiratory distress resolved promptly and the patient was changed to a nonprotein formula because of presumptive diagnosis of a urea cycle abnormality. Cultures from the time of admission remained negative. Liver function abnormalities returned to normal. Serum and urine organic acid and urine metabolic screens were negative. The patient remained free of acidosis.

A glucagon challenge test was performed that resulted in a lactic acidosis. This result was strongly suggestive of a glycogen storage disease. Liver and muscle biopsies were performed that were consistent with the diagnosis of glycogen storage disease type 1A (von Gierke's disease). The patient was discharged home and continues to do well on continuous nasogastric feedings of a milk-based formula along with supplemental oral feedings. She has had no recurrent episodes of acidosis or respiratory distress.

DISCUSSION

This 10-week-old infant girl was first seen with respiratory distress, severe metabolic acidosis with an elevated anion gap, hepatomegaly with evidence of hepatocellular dysfunction, and hypertriglyceridemia. Elevated anion gap acidoses generally fall into one of four categories: ingestions, renal failure, ketoacidosis, and lactic acidosis. The lactate levels in this patient placed the diagnosis in the latter category. Lactic acidoses has been further divided into two categories: type A, or conditions associated with impaired cellular oxygen delivery (i.e., shock), and type B, or disorders not associated with impaired tissue oxygen delivery (i.e., liver disease, diabetes mellitus, hypoglycemia, and inborn errors of carbohydrate metabolism) (1).

In type A lactic acidosis, cellular hypoxia favors conversion of pyruvate to lactate as normal pyruvate metabolism via the tricarboxylic acid cycle is suppressed in the absence of oxygen (Fig. 28.1). When oxygen delivery is restored at the cellular level, this process is allowed to reverse, and lactate is no longer produced. In von Gierke's disease, a type B lactic acidosis, the conversion of glucose-6-phosphate to glucose is impaired because the enzyme glucose-6-phosphatase is deficient. Lactic acid produced by red cells and muscle cannot be converted to glucose by the liver. In addition, glycogen and other molecules customarily degraded to glucose in the liver are instead converted to lactate. As a result of the above processes, serum lactate levels reach up to ten times normal in von Gierke's disease, particularly during the fasting state in which there is no exogenous glucose to prevent glycogenolysis (2).

The typical age of presentation in von Gierke's disease and other glycogen storage diseases is between 1 month and 1 year. Most of these patients will be seen with hepatomegaly, lactic acidosis, hypoglycemia, hypertriglyceride-

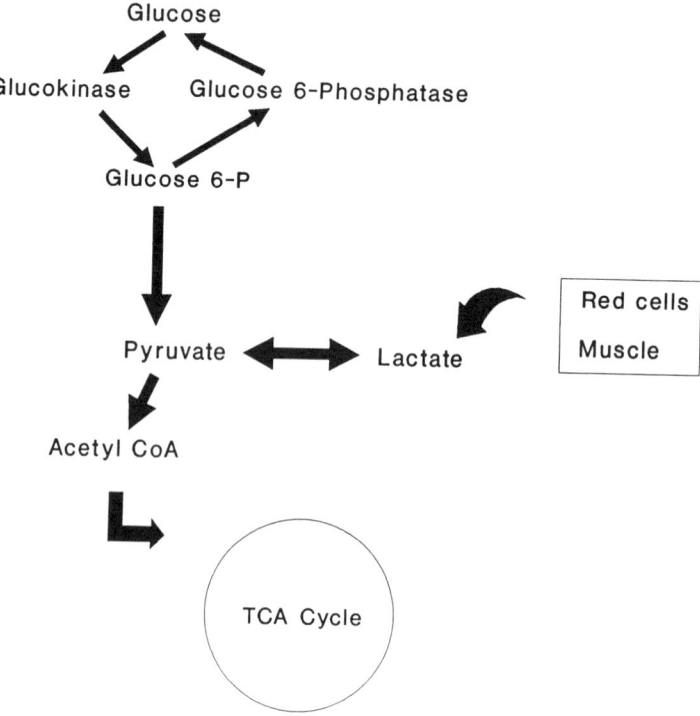

Figure 28.1. Pathways in glucose and lactate metabolism.

mia, and abnormal liver function tests. Prognosis has improved with the use of frequent daytime meals, eating of starch, and nighttime infusions of glucose-containing formulas.

Treatment of lactic acidosis involves correction of the base deficit with sodium bicarbonate, tromethamine, dichloroacetate, or equimolar mixture of sodium carbonate and sodium bicarbonate (Carbicarb). Studies in animals with lactic acidosis indicate that sodium bicarbonate decreases cardiac output and may adversely affect survival (3). Sodium bicarbonate has also been shown to increase lactate production in some cases (4). There is divergence of opinion concerning the most optimal base to use. In addition to treating the base deficit, patients with von Gierke's disease require a constant source of glucose parenterally until the acidosis is corrected. Feedings are then advanced enterally as tolerated.

COMMENTARY

Patients with metabolic derangements come to the PICU frequently. Often they are seen with multisystem involvement. We are often faced with focusing in on the "triggering event" that precipitated the first decompensation. Whether that event was an infection or, as in the case of the patient we describe, an immunization leading to sufficient irritability to decrease food intake, we frequently find it difficult to tease out the derangement to come upon the correct diagnosis.

References

1. Kreisberg RA. Lactic acidosis: an update. J Intensive Care Med 1987; 2:76–84.
2. Scriver CR, Beaudet AL, Sly WS, Valle D, eds. The metabolic basis of inherited disease. New York: McGraw-Hill, 1989:425–448.
3. Park R, Arieff AI, Leach W, Lazarowitz V. Treatment of lactic acidosis with dichloroacetate in dogs. J Clin Invest 1982;70:853–862.
4. Fraley DS, Adler S, Bruns FJ, Zett B. Stimulation of lactate production by administration of bicarbonate in a patient with a solid neoplasm and lactic acidosis. N Engl J Med 1980;303:1100–1102.

Case 29

Herwig P. Stopfkuchen
Universitaetskinderklinik
Mainz, Germany

HISTORY

A 1900-g newborn girl was admitted to the PICU because of complications of prematurity. The child was born at 33 weeks by cesarean section because of premature rupture of fetal membranes to a 39-year-old gravida 1 woman. The mother had immigrated from the Philippines 3 years prior to the pregnancy and the father was a native of Germany. Their first child was 2 years of age and was in good health. During the first 2 weeks of life, the infant developed hyperbilirubinemia, failure to suck, and failure to thrive. On day 9, a chest radiograph obtained because of a systolic murmur was interpreted as normal (Fig. 29.1). On the 27th day of life, a chest radiograph was again ordered because the baby had episodes of bradycardia/tachycardia, apnea, and cyanosis. This radiograph (Fig. 29.2) with bilateral patchy infiltrates was diagnosed as being consistent with pneumonia. Because cultures were not helpful at this time, ampicillin, penicillin, and gentamicin were initiated intravenously. No clinical response resulted from this regimen; therefore erythromycin was added as treatment for possible chlamydial pneumonia. The child continued to deteriorate during the next 2–3 weeks.

LABORATORY DATA

Cranial ultrasound revealed a normal brain and normal ventricles. A CT scan of the head confirmed the results of the ultrasound. Results of an electroencephalogram (EEG) were normal for age. Lumbar puncture was performed; the cerebrospinal fluid (CSF) examinations showed no cells

187

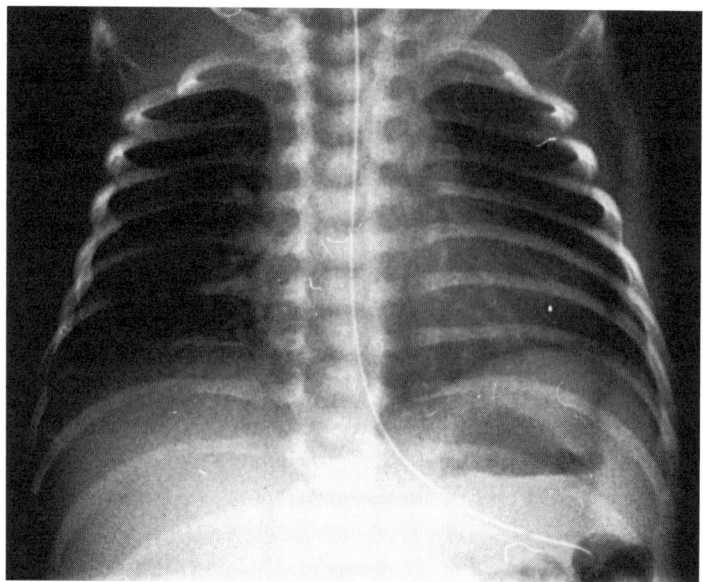

Figure 29.1.   Radiograph of the chest showing normally inflated lungs. The cardiac silhouette is normal (day 9).

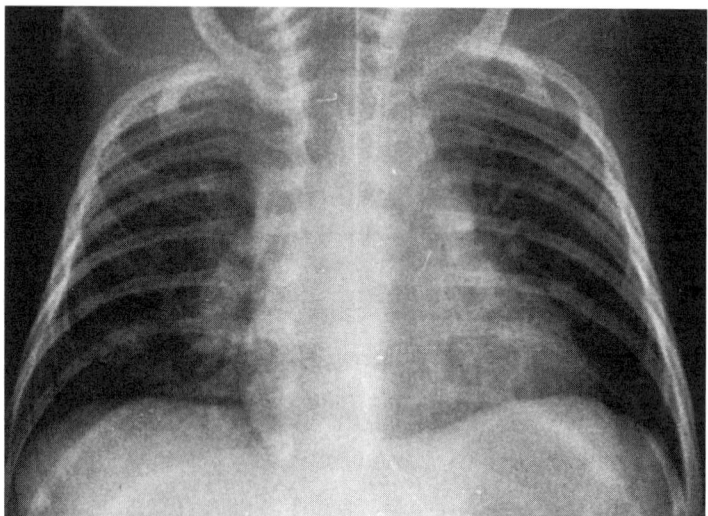

Figure 29.2.   Radiograph of the chest revealing bilateral patchy pulmonary infiltrates (day 28).

and normal glucose and protein concentrations. An ECG revealed normal rhythm and normal configuration. A cardiac catheterization revealed a mild left to right shunt at the atrial level and normal pulmonary artery pressures. Anomalous pulmonary venous return was not observed. Cultures of blood, CSF, and tracheal secretions were negauve for common pathogens. Results of serologic tests for *Candida* and for *Aspergillus* antigen showed were negative. Results of tests evaluating cell-mediated immunity were also normal.

MANAGEMENT

On the 44th day of life, the infant's respiratory distress worsened, with the development of respiratory acidosis, and the infant was admitted to the PICU. Endotracheal intubation and mechanical ventilation were initiated, and a chest X-ray was obtained (Fig. 29.3). Tracheal aspirate from endotracheal suctioning was sent to the laboratory for mycobacteria and fungi. Antibiotic therapy was changed to moxalactam, gentamicin, ketoconazole, and doxycycline. On the 64th day of life, a closed lung biopsy was performed. The culture of lung biopsy material revealed the presence of *Mycoplasma homines*. The child's condition continued to deteriorate and another chest X-ray was obtained (Fig. 29.4). On the 77th day of life, the cultures from the gastric aspirate revealed *Mycobacterium tuberculosis*. In addition, by means of the Ziehl-Neelsen technique, we found acid-fast bacilli in the endotracheal aspirate. Using dosages thought to be appropriate for neo-

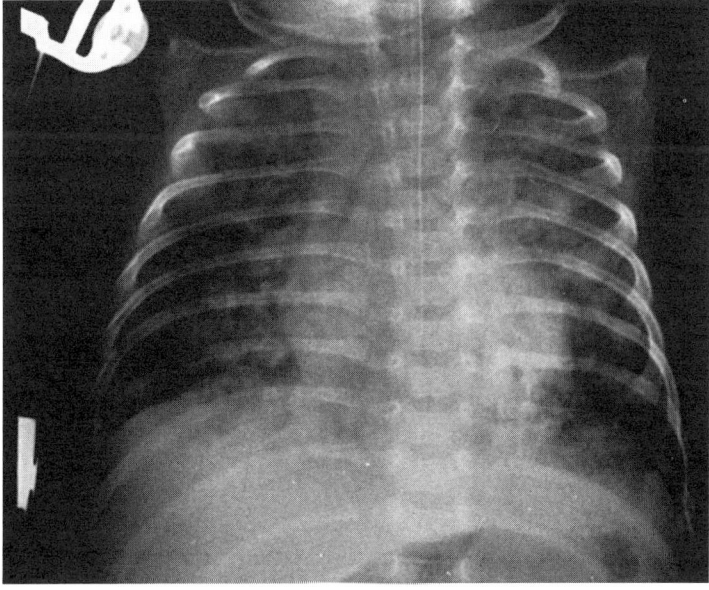

Figure 29.3. Radiograph of the chest showing irregularly distributed bilateral patchy pulmonary infiltrates (day 44).

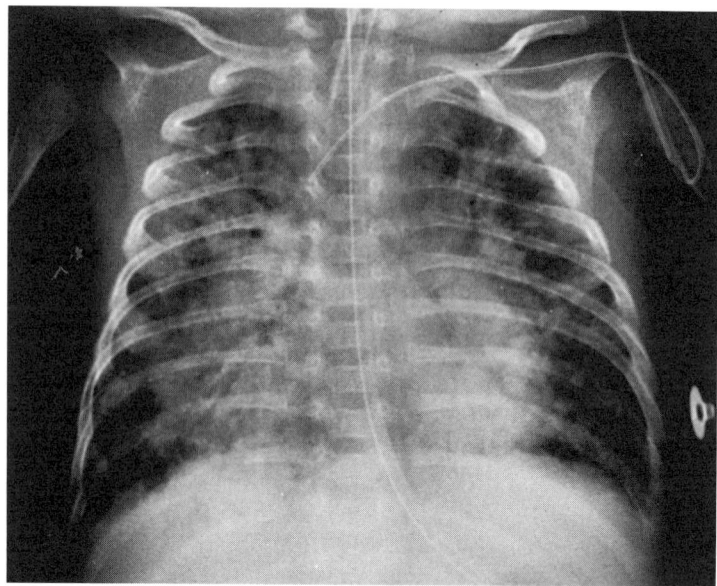

Figure 29.4. Radiograph of the chest revealing irregularly distributed extensive bilateral pulmonary infiltrates. The right cardiac edge is obscured. Endotracheal tube, central venous catheter, and nasogastric tube are in place (day 64).

nates, we began to administer isoniazid, rifampin, and streptomycin. At this time, we discovered that the mother had developed miliary tuberculosis. Over the next weeks, the respiratory status of the infant improved. On the 134th day of life the child was successfully extubated. On the 210th day of life, the infant was discharged with mild respiratory distress. A chest X-ray at that time demonstrated some improvement (Fig. 29.5).

DISCUSSION

Tuberculosis in a neonate could either be congenital, that is, acquired in utero by inhalation or ingestion of infected amniotic fluid, or neonatal, that is, acquired at birth. Tuberculosis acquired in utero from an infected placenta seemed to be unlikely in this case since the histologic examination of the placenta after birth did not show signs of amnionitis. Because tuberculosis in the newborn is an extremely rare event in Germany today, performance of the specific diagnostic procedures was delayed. This case of this infant emphasizes that, at least in neonates of women from areas of the world where tuberculosis is highly preva-

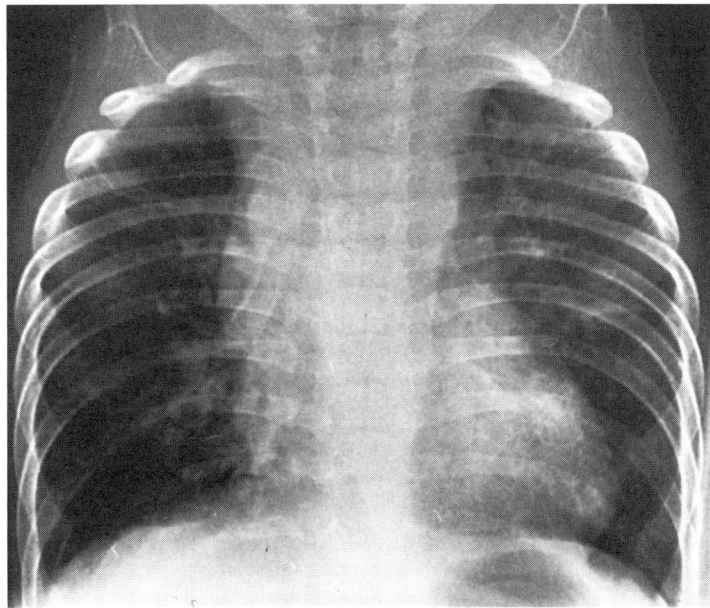

Figure 29.5. Radiograph of the chest showing bilateral hilar and peritracheal adenopathy. The patchy pulmonary infiltrates have disappeared. There are strands of increased density between the hilar nodes and the lung periphery, and there is peripheral hyperaeration of both lungs (day 210).

lent, one has to be alert for this disease even though mothers are thought to be well at the time of delivery.

COMMENTARY

Tuberculosis has become an increasingly prevalent disease once again. Unfortunately, it is not restricted to third world countries; rather it is becoming more common in inner cities in the United States. We therefore have raised our sensitivity to this disease and we are expecting more admissions to the PICU for pulmonary tuberculosis. In addition to that, the incidence of tuberculosis in patients with acquired immunodeficiency syndrome (AIDS) has increased. Our colleagues who are treating the adult population see it with increasing frequency, and it is quite likely that we will see more and more cases of tuberculosis in children with AIDS. Of even greater public health concern is the tuberculosis that is emerging as resistant to our customary medications. If that form reaches epidemic proportions, there could be a more severe health crisis. Therefore we must all consider the diagnosis of tuberculosis and anticipate aggressive diagnosis and treatment for our patients.

Suggested Readings

1. Hageman JO, Shulman ST, Schreiber MI, Luck SU, Yogev RA. Congenital tuberculosis: critical reappraisal of clinical findings and diagnostic procedures. Pediatrics 1990;66:980–984.
2. Myers JO, Perlstein PA, Light IR, Towbin RI, Dincsoy HO, Dincosoy ME. Tuberculosis in pregnancy with fatal congenital infection. Pediatrics 1981;67:89–94.
3. Remington JA, Klein JE. Infectious diseases of the fetus and newborn infant. Philadelphia: WB Saunders, 1990.

Case 30

Jana A. Stockwell, Frank H. Kern, Jon N. Meliones, Scott R. Schulman, and William J. Greeley

Duke Univerity Medical Center
Durham, North Carolina, USA

HISTORY

A previously healthy 9-year-old boy developed cough and upper respiratory tract symptoms. He was diagnosed with bronchitis and sinusitis and treated with trimethoprim-sulfamethoxazole (TMP-SMX). One week later he developed fever, facial erythema, and diffuse rash. TMP-SMX was discontinued and amoxicillin begun. The rash progressed and 2 days later measles was diagnosed. By the 12th day of treatment, he had blisters on his lips, face, chest, and extremities. He was admitted to the emergency department for further evaluation and treatment.

PHYSICAL EXAMINATION

When the boy was first examined, his vital signs were as follows: heart rate 96 beats/min, respiratory rate 14/min, and blood pressure 105/55 mm Hg. His temperature was 38.5°C, orally, his weight was 30 kg, and his body surface area was 1.1 m².

The child was alert and cooperative, but experiencing pain with any movement. He was diffusely erythematous with large bullae and denuded areas on his face, neck, chest, and upper extremities, totaling about 80% of his body surface area. His lips and buccal mucosa were denuded. Target lesions were observed on his trunk. Bilateral conjunctivitis without corneal involvement was noted. His lungs were clear with equal breath sounds, and respirations were unlabored. Cardiac rhythm was normal with no murmurs. Capillary refill was <2 seconds and pulses were normal distally. Bowel sounds were present and the abdomen was soft and nontender.

LABORATORY DATA

With arterial saturation on room air of 96% by pulse oximetry, the following values were obtained: sodium 123 mmol/l, potassium 6.1 mmol/l, bicarbonate 25 mmol/l, chloride 94 mmol/l, glucose 119 mg/dl, and ionized calcium 1.06 mmol/l, blood urea nitrogen (BUN) 15 mg%, and creatinine 0.9 mg%. Hemoglobin was 13.2 g/dl with a hematocrit of 38%. White blood count was 7,500 cells/mm^3 (51% segments, 9% bands, 26% lymphocytes). Total protein was 4.9 g/dl, and albumin was 2.4 g/dl. Chest radiograph revealed no air space disease.

MANAGEMENT

The patient was placed on sterile sheets over an air-fluidized mattress with warmth provided as needed by a radiant heater. Fluid resuscitation was initiated based on one-half the Parkland burn formula (4 ml/% burn/kg) estimating 75–80% affected body surface area. Intravenous fluids consisted of Ringer's lactate with 12.5 g albumin/l at 10 ml/kg/hr for 8 hours, then decreased to 5 ml/kg/hr, and concurrent crystalloid replacement with 5% dextrose plus ¼ normal saline plus 20 mEq KCl/l at 800/ml/m^2/d. Fluids were titrated to keep urine output >2.0 ml/kg/hr. Wounds were cleansed with saline soaks, and topical antibiotic lubricating ointments were applied. Reverse isolation was begun. A nasogastric tube was placed for the purpose of bolus enteral feeds. Pain was managed using morphine via a patient-controlled anesthesia delivery system. No antibiotics or steroids were administered. A skin punch biopsy was obtained.

On the second hospital day, the patient developed fever, respiratory distress, an oxygen requirement, bilateral lung crackles, and intermittent desaturation by pulse oximetry. A chest radiograph showed alveolar opacities and interstitial edema. The patient was sedated and intubated, and mechanical ventilation was initiated using synchronized volume-limited ventilation with the following parameters:

F_IO_2 0.35, tidal volume = 16 ml/kg, respiratory rate 12 breaths/min, peak end-expiratory pressure (PEEP) 5 cm H_2O, P_{aw} 10 cm H_2O, and I:E = 1:2 yielding a peak inspiratory pressure (PIP) of approximately 39 cm H_2O. Urine output remained >2 ml/kg/hr despite massive fluid losses from the skin wounds. Skin biopsy revealed marked necrosis of the basal and upper layers of the epidermis and follicular epithelium with sparse superficial perivascular lymphocytic infiltrate, confirming the suspected diagnosis of toxic epidermal necrolysis (TEN).

The patient was taken to the operating room on the third hospital day for removal of bullae and debridement of his neck, back, upper chest, arms, buttocks, and upper legs. A synthetic biologic membrane was applied to the affected areas to decrease fluid and heat losses. The chest radiograph showed increasing perihilar opacification suggestive of early adult respiratory distress syndrome (ARDS). Because of an increasing alveolar-arterial (A-a) gradient and decreasing dynamic lung compliance, the patient was paralyzed. The mode of ventilation was changed to pressure control with the following settings: F_IO_2 = 0.35, PIP = 35 cm H_2O, PEEP = 8 cm H_2O, I:E = 1:3, and respiratory rate = 12 breaths/min. After a period of cardiovascular instability and decreased urine output suggestive of sepsis, nafcillin and ceftazidime were begun.

The patient's lung compliance decreased further and the chest radiograph showed increased opacification. A pulmonary artery thermodilution catheter revealed initial values as follows: systemic vascular resistance index = 1100 dyne/sec/cm^5/m^2, pulmonary vascular resistance index = 290 dyne/sec/cm^5/m^2, cardiac index (CI) = 6.6 l/min/m^2, and pulmonary artery occlusion pressure = 18 mm Hg. A continuous infusion of low-dose dopamine and furosemide 2 mg/kg/d was begun. The patient developed ileus. Therefore, enteral feedings were discontinued and parenteral nutrition initiated to provide approximately twice his estimated basal energy expenditure. Over the next several days, the patient developed multiple pneumothoraces. Mean airway pressure increased significantly, to 41 cm H_2O, with a dynamic compliance of 20.4 ml/cm H_2O (0.68 ml/cm H_2O/kg). Extracorporeal membrane oxygenation was considered but not implemented because of a lack of adequate cannulation sites as a result of the epidermal necrosis.

On the 11th day, the patient was febrile to 38.9°C, hyperdynamic (CI = 7.9 l/min/m^2), and had a white blood cell count of 26,000 cells/mm^3 with a left shift. Nafcillin was discontinued and vancomycin and gentamicin were added to the ceftazidime regimen. A chest radiograph revealed recurrent bilateral pneumothoraces and progression of the bilateral opacities. Tracheal specimens showed heavy polymorphonuclear cell infiltrates but no bacterial growth. Amphotericin B was begun empirically, and soon thereafter two previous wound cultures (obtained on days 8 and 10) grew *Candida parapsilosis*. Dynamic pulmonary compliance was greatly diminished by this point, 6.6 ml/cm H_2O or 0.22 ml/cm H_2O/kg on F_1O_2 0.80, PEEP = 14 cm H_2O, PIP = 60 cm H_2O, and I:E = 1:1. Attempts to improve pulmonary function using inverse ratio ventilation, higher or lower PEEP, and altered inspiratory time did not result in improvement. A brief trial of isoproterenol only increased the ventilation/perfusion mismatch. Vancomycin and ceftazidime were stopped and imipenem begun.

Despite the impressive improvement in his skin, his lung disease and presumed sepsis proved overwhelming. After discussion with his parents, no further resuscitative measures were attempted and he died on the 20th hospital day. Permission for postmortem examination was not granted.

DISCUSSION

Toxic epidermal necrolysis (TEN) is a severe exfoliative disease of the skin and mucous membranes requiring comprehensive intensive, but largely supportive, care. It is a rare idiopathic or dose-independent drug-induced disease with a mortality rate of 20–70% (1,2). Most deaths occur as the result of secondary infection. TEN can occur at any age. Many drugs have been associated with TEN (3), but most frequently implicated are phenytoin, phenobarbital, carbamazepine, sulfonamides, and nonsteroidal anti-inflammatory agents. Pathogenic mechanisms are unclear and possibilities include delayed hypersensitivity reactions (4), circulating toxic drug metabolites (5), genetic predisposition (6), virus- or drug-mediated cytotoxic antibodies (7).

Drug-related cases become symptomatic within 3 weeks of drug ingestion and with drug re-exposure symptoms may become evident within hours (8). A prodrome consists of fever, malaise, and pharyngitis. The acute phase is heralded by the sudden development of an erythematous morbilliform or confluent rash with tenderness (similar to sunburn pain), typically first noted on the face and limbs. Target lesions may be seen. The acute phase is followed rapidly by widespread blistering and formation of fragile bullae, positive Nikolsky's sign, and extensive necrosis of the epidermis with sloughing of sheets of skin. Mucous membranes (oral, conjunctival, bronchial, tracheal, esophageal, and urethral) are frequently involved, and stricture formation may occur with healing. Systemic toxicity also may be observed. The recovery phase is marked by re-epithelialization from epidermal elements within the hair follicles in 10–28 days.

Diagnosis of TEN is based on clinical appearance, with the differential diagnosis of exfoliative skin disorders typically including staphylococcal scalded-skin syndrome and Stevens-Johnson syndrome (see Table 30.1). Skin biopsy is diagnostic, demonstrating full-thickness epidermal necrosis, subepidermal blistering, and basement membrane vacuolization. Staphylococcal scalded-skin syndrome is particularly seen in young children. It is caused by a staphylococcal exotoxin that is specific for the subgranular layer keratinocytes. Because of this high epidermal splitting, patients tend to heal without scarring. Mucous membranes are rarely involved. Stevens-Johnson syndrome can affect any age. That syndrome also has mucous membrane involvement and bullae formation, but the skin biopsy shows a lymphocytic infiltrate around dermal blood vessels.

Bullae and loose and necrotic skin should be removed and protection from drying and bacterial colonization provided with homografts, porcine xenografts, or synthetic biologic dressings (9,10). Fluid losses through the de-

Table 30.1. Differential Diagnosis of Toxic Epidermal Necrolysis

	Toxic Epidermal Necrolysis (TEN)	Staphylococcal Scalded Skin Syndrome (SSSS)	Stevens-Johnson Syndrome (SJS)
Age	All	<5 years old	All
Mortality	25–70%	<30%	<10%
Rash	Painful diffuse erythema of face and limbs, progressing to coalescing bullae	Tender macular erythema, prominent around mouth and nose, progressing to bullae	Erythema progressing to localized bullae
Skin biopsy	Epidermal necrosis, subepidermal blistering, basement membrane vacuolization	Intraepidermal splitting	Lymphocytic infiltrate around blood vessels in upper dermis
Mucous membranes	Involved	Rare involvement	Involved (prominent)
Target lesions	±	−	+
Etiology	?	*Staphylococcus* exotoxin	?

nuded areas are massive, though reported to be less than that observed in burns affecting equal body surface area (2,11). Fluid management requires close observation of intravascular volume status, urine output, and perfusion. Fluid losses are typically difficult to accurately assess because of the widespread distribution of the lesions. Placement of the patient on an air-fluidized mattress in order to decrease skin trauma has been reported to result in hypothermia from increased evaporation (12,13). Attention must be paid to maintaining a neutral thermal environment through humidification of warm gases and use of radiant heat.

Antibiotic therapy should be withheld until an infectious focus or strong clinical suspicion of infection is present. Sepsis develops in 40% of TEN patients; early infection is typically with *Staphylococcus aureus* and later with *Pseudomonas aeruginosa*, *Klebsiella pneumoniae*, or *Escherichia coli*. More than 50% of deaths result from sepsis (14). Use of corticosteroids is limited to the early acute stage before extensive bullae have formed. Steroids may increase the risk of sepsis and mortality in these patients and therefore their use is not recommended (2). Topical treatment of denuded areas with antibiotic and/or hydrating agents may be helpful. Sulfa-containing topical agents such as Silvadene (silver sulfadiazine) and Sulfamylon (mafenide) should be avoided. Reverse isolation is required until the skin re-epithelializes.

Pneumonia and pneumonitis occur in 30% of patients (15). Mucus retention and sloughing of tracheobronchial mucosa not only provide a nidus for infection, but also result in focal areas of atelectasis, leading to increased pulmonary insufficiency. Development of ARDS, as in this patient, significantly increases the risk of mortality.

Ophthalmologic evaluation should be obtained early in the disease process. Conjunctivitis and photophobia are seen in the acute phase with possible formation of pseudomembrane, symblepharon, or vascularization of the cornea (16). Topical ocular antibiotics and lubricants are instilled multiple times per day. Of the survivors, 5–9% have chronic visual changes (11).

Oral and/or esophageal mucosal lesions, present in 90% of TEN patients, and parotitis may prevent oral feeding, necessitating an oro- or nasogastric tube. Ileus may preclude enteral feedings. Approximation of caloric needs with a pediatric burn formula overestimates the caloric needs in children affected with TEN (17). Use of indirect calorimetric measurements is the most accurate way to evaluate the nutritional needs of the patient. Hypoalbuminemia is the result of massive seepage of protein-containing fluid from the denuded body surfaces.

Hematologic manifestations include leukopenia, neutropenia, and bandemia. Neutropenia occurs 2–5 days after appearance of the rash. Persistence of neutropenia is a poor prognostic sign. Normochromic, normocytic anemia may be seen. Elevated d-dimers can be present in the absence of a coagulopathy, although disseminated intravascular coagulation is not rare.

Patients with TEN experience moderate to intense pain of the affected areas. In the alert and cooperative patient, patient-controlled anesthesia often provides adequate relief. Patients with extensive lesions may be unable to physically manipulate the control device, however, and parenteral analgesia be required. Protection of the denuded areas with grafts or synthetic biologic membranes often results in significant pain relief.

The use of plasmapheresis to remove circulating toxins or antibody complexes has been evaluated. In two uncontrolled studies of five patients each, rapid clinical improvement occurred in nine of the ten patients (18,19). In another study, five patients with TEN were treated with cyclophosphamide, an inhibitor of cell-mediated cytotoxicity, and demonstrated rapid recovery (4). The response to these therapies is supportive of a circulatory cytotoxic factor as the cause of TEN. Further investigation into these treatment modalities is necessary.

In summary, TEN is a severe exfoliative disease that has a high mortality rate as a result of secondary multisystem impairment. Care of patients with TEN requires a multidisciplinary assessment and comprehensive treatment plan.

COMMENTARY

The case of this boy presents many issues to the intensivist. The multidisciplinary approach to TEN requires coordinated efforts by the departments of surgery, nutrition, and intensive care. This case also illustrates the painful dilemma of "when to stop." With theoretically limitless possible avenues of therapy, admitting that more aggressive therapy would be futile is one of the most difficult decisions pediatric intensivists and parents have to make.

Another interesting aspect of this case was the diagnosis of measles. As failure in immunization programs and vaccines has become obvious, the prevalence of this disease has increased, reaching epidemic proportion in some areas of the country. This epidemic demands that we reacquaint ourselves with the diagnosis of the disease and familiarize ourselves with the potential role of vitamin A in measles.

References

1. Adzick N, Kim S, Bondo C, et al. Management of toxic epidermal necrolysis in a pediatric burn center. Am J Dis Child 1985;139: 499–502.
2. Revuz J, Roujeau J-C, Guillaume J-C, Penso D, Touraine R. Treatment of toxic epidermal necrolysis: Creteil's experience. Arch Dermatol 1987;123:1156–1158.
3. Avakian R, Flowers F, Araujo O, Ramos-Caro F. Toxic epidermal necrolysis: a review. J Am Acad Dermatol 1991;25:69–79.
4. Heng M, Allen S. Efficacy of cyclophosphamide in toxic epidermal necrolysis. J Am Acad Dermatol 1991;25:778–786.
5. Hensen E, Claas F, Veermer B. Drug-dependent binding of circulating antibodies in drug-induced toxic epidermal necrolysis. Lancet 1982;2:151–152.
6. Roujeau J-C, Huynh T, Bracq C, et al. Genetic susceptibility to toxic epidermal necrolysis. Arch Dermatol 1987;123:1171–1173.
7. Halebian P, Madden M, Finkelstein J, et al. Improved burn center survival of patients with toxic epidermal necrolysis managed without corticosteroids. Ann Surg 1986;204:503–512.
8. Chan H-L, Stern R, Arndt K, et al. The incidence of erythema multiforme, Stevens-Johnson syndrome, and toxic epidermal necrolysis. Arch Dermatol 1990;126:43–47.
9. Sowder L. Biobrane wound dressing used in the treatment of toxic epidermal necrolysis: A case report. J Burn Care Rehabil 1990;11: 237–239.
10. Ward D, Krzeminska E, Tanner N. Treatment of toxic epidermal necrolysis and a review of six cases. Burns 1990;16:97–104.
11. Heimbach D, Engrav L, Marvin J, et al. Toxic epidermal necrolysis: a step forward in treatment. JAMA 1987;257:2171–2175.
12. Chosidow O, Delcher J-C, Chaumette M-T, et al. Intestinal involvement in drug-induced toxic epidermal necrolysis. Lancet 1991;337: 928.
13. Timsit J, Mion G, LeGulluche Y, Corsin H. Hypothermia and air-fluidized beds during toxic epidermal necrolysis management. Intensive Care Med 1991;17:506–509.
14. Revuz J, Penso D, Roujeau J-C, et al. Toxic epidermal necrolysis: clinical findings and prognosis factors in 87 patients. Arch Dermatol 1987;123:1160–1165.
15. Pruitt B. Burn treatment for the unburned. JAMA 1987;257:2207.
16. Leahey A, Wulc A, Day D, Uberti-Benz M, Katowitz J. Canalicular obliteration from toxic epidermal necrolysis. Am J Ophthamol 1991; 112:469–470.
17. Hildreth M. Caloric needs of pediatric patients with toxic epidermal necrolysis. J Am Diet Assoc 19906l.9.
18. Kamanabroo D, Schmitz-Landgraf W, Czarnetzki B. Plasmapheresis in severe drug-induced toxic epidermal necrolysis. Arch Dermatol 1985;121:1548–1549.
19. Sakellariou G, Koukoudis P, Karpouzas J, et al. Plasma exchange (PE) treatment in drug-induced toxic epidermal necrolysis (TEN). Int J Artif Organs 1991;14:634–638.

Case 31

Robert Henning
Royal Children's Hospital
Melbourne, Victoria, Australia

HISTORY

A 24-month-old child was admitted to the ICU of the Royal Children's Hospital, Melbourne, from a suburban general hospital with a provisional diagnosis of meningococcal septic shock. She had been previously well, but at approximately 3 p.m. on the day of admission she had become febrile and vomited. Over the next 3 hours her skin became cool, she developed rigors, and her conscious state deteriorated. At about 7 p.m., a rash developed on her, and at 8 p.m., the drowsy child was admitted to the suburban general hospital with cool mottled skin, a rash typical of early meningococcemia, and moderately severe metabolic acidosis. Blood was taken for culture and biochemical and hematologic tests. Penicillin and ceftriaxone were given intravenously, and resuscitation commenced with colloid solution, sodium bicarbonate, and dobutamine infusion.

The Pediatric Emergency Transport team arrived at the referring hospital at 9 p.m. (time = 0 in Fig. 33.1). At this point, the patient was receiving oxygen by mask and dobutamine 10 µg/kg/min. Her condition remained stable during transfer by road to the Royal Children's Hospital.

PHYSICAL EXAMINATION

On arrival at Royal Children's Hospital, the child was again noted to be drowsy and pale with mottled skin and cool limbs. Her blood pressure was 98/45 torr, her heart rate was 198 beats/min, and her rectal temperature was 38.9°C. She had a few hemorrhagic spots on the skin of

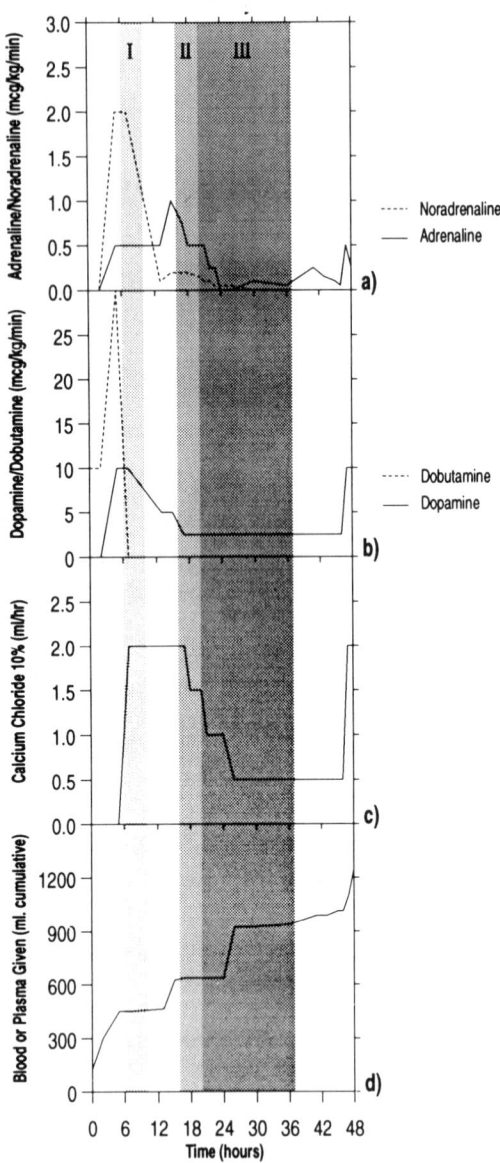

Figure 31.1. Requirements for inotropic drugs (*A*, *B*), calcium chloride (*C*) and plasma expansion (*D*) during the 48 hours after first contact with the Royal Children's Hospital ICU. Periods I and II represent 1200-ml plasma exchanges. During period III, plasmafiltration continued at 8 ml/kg/hr.

her back, chest, and inner thigh. She was hypotonic with symmetrically brisk reflexes, flexor plantar responses, and normal fundi.

MANAGEMENT

Shortly after arrival, the child had a grand mal seizure lasting 10 minutes that stopped after intravenous administration of clonazepam 0.4 mg. She was given an intravenous loading dose of phenytoin 10 mg/kg and 150 ml of 5% albumin in saline over a 1-hour period.

One hour later (time = 3.5 hours in Fig. 31.1), her rash became more marked, her skin perfusion deteriorated, and her pulse decreased. At this point, her trachea was intubated and she was mechanically ventilated with a rate of 20 breaths/min, peak inspiratory pressure of 24 cm H_2O, and a positive end-expiratory pressure (PEEP) of 2 cm H_2O in 70% oxygen. This gave a pH of 7.28, $PaCO_2$ of 37 torr, PaO_2 of 68 torr, and base excess of -8. She was sedated with midazolam 4 µg/kg/min and paralyzed with pancuronium.

At 2 a.m. (time = 5 hours in Fig. 31.1), her blood pressure decreased to <35 torr despite administration of dobutamine 30 µg/kg/min and plasma expansion. Infusions of noradrenaline, adrenaline, dopamine, and calcium chloride were commenced (Fig. 31.1). Despite these measures and boluses of adrenaline and noradrenaline, it was difficult to keep her mean arterial pressure (MAP) >35 torr. A decision was therefore made to commence plasmafiltration. An 11.5-French double-lumen Mahurkar catheter (Quinton, Seattle) was inserted percutaneously into a femoral vein. Venovenous pump-assisted plasmafiltration was started at 3.30 a.m. (Fig. 31.1, period I). Blood flow through the filter was 25 ml/min, with a filtrate (and replacement) flow of 400 ml/hr. A two-plasma volume exchange (1200 ml) was performed over a 3-hour period. The first 900-ml filtrate was replaced with Stabilized Plasma Protein Solution (SPPS, Commonwealth Serum Laboratories, Parkville, Victoria, Australia) and the last 300 ml with fresh-frozen plasma. Heparin was infused pre- and postfiltration to keep the activated clotting time at 150–160 seconds. Acid citrate dextrose solution was infused prefiltration at 5 ml/hr.

Hydrocortisone 10 mg/6 hr intravenously was started at 3 a.m. The doses of inotropic drugs and $CaCl_2$ were adjusted to maintain an MAP of 45–60 torr and a urine output >0.5 ml/kg/hr. As Figure 31.1 shows, during the first plasma exchange, the infusion rates of dopamine, dobutamine, and noradrenaline could be reduced. Four hours after completion of the plasma exchange (time = 13 hours), the patient's blood pressure fell to 39 torr, necessitating a bolus of intravenous adrenaline and an increase in the infusion rates of adrenaline and noradrenaline. At this time, the urine output decreased to <0.5 ml/kg/hr despite administration of a large dose of furosemide, and the serum potassium level increased to 7.5 mmol/l, necessitating injection of 50% dextrose (1 ml/kg) and 1 U insulin.

A second two-volume plasma exchange was performed over a period of 4 hours (Fig. 31.1, period II), following which plasmafiltration was continued at 100 ml/hr (8 ml/kg/hr) (Fig. 31.1, period III) for the next 18 hours. During this period, the child remained stable with an MAP between 45 and 60 torr, a heart rate of 160–190 beats/min, and right atrial pressure of 16–18 torr.

At 39 hours, a pleural effusion and tense ascites were drained, resulting in a short period of hemodynamic instability. Plasmafiltration had been discontinued at 37 hours. The urine output remained poor despite adequate blood pressure and plasma volume repletion, and large doses of furosemide (7 mg/kg over 24 hours). Continuous venovenous pump-assisted hemofiltration was therefore commenced at 47 hours to achieve fluid and electrolyte homeostasis and was continued for 8 days. Hemodynamic stability improved gradually during this period, and the serum creatinine level remained in the range of 0.07–0.19 mmol/l. The patient remained in oliguric acute renal failure until day 14 and polyuric renal failure until day 18, when her serum creatinine level returned to normal over a 6-day period.

Adrenaline infusion was ceased on day 4. Dopamine infusion was continued at 2.5 μg/kg/min until day 11. In order to minimize the area of tissue loss from small vessel occlusion, infusion of sodium nitroprusside was commenced on day 2 when a stable adequate blood pressure had been secured, and was changed on day 3 to prostacyclin 5 ng/kg/min for 5 days.

She was discharged from the PICU on day 17. At the time of hospital discharge on day 47, she was starting to walk, was normotensive, and had recently had a skin graft to an area of skin loss on the left forearm. At follow-up examination 10 weeks after her admission, she was neurologically normal and appeared to have made a full recovery.

DISCUSSION

This child had a hemodynamic deterioration that was uncontrolled by plasma expansion and very high doses of inotropic and vasoconstrictor drugs, but responded on two occasions to plasmafiltration. Plasmafiltration may be beneficial in septic shock by removing some substances that interfere with myocardial function, vascular tone, or catecholamine effectiveness.

The use of plasmapheresis to assist in the control of septic shock was suggested in the 1970s (1). Reports of its successful use in small groups of adults with septic shock have appeared since then (2), although no controlled trials of its use have been described (3,4). Plasmafilters have a sieving coefficient of 1.0 for molecules up to 3,000,000 daltons, and hemofilters have a sieving coefficient of 1.0 for molecules up to 10,000 daltons. Thus, it is likely that whole lipopolysaccharide (molecular weight 100,000 daltons) may be removed by plasmafiltration but not by hemofiltration. Two small inconclusive trials in experimental animals with endotoxemia showed a trend toward improved survival, higher blood pressure, and cardiac output and improved myocardial performance in those animals that were plasmafiltered or hemofiltered compared with control animals. Lipid A reproduces in experimental animals many of the pathologic effects of endotoxin and has a molecular weight of 2,000–5,000 daltons. It is filterable by small-pore hemodialysis membranes (5) and presumably also by hemofilter and plasmafilter membranes. It is known that tumor necrosis factor (molecular weight 17,000 daltons) and interleukin-1 (molecular weight 35,000 daltons) are bound to plasma proteins and therefore may be cleared by plasmafiltration but not by hemofiltration. Several other mediators thought to play a part in the pathogenesis of septic shock such as myocardial depressant factor (molecular weight 4–10,000 daltons), platelet-activating factor (molecular weight approximately 550 daltons), and leukotrienes (molecular weight 500 daltons) may be removed by hemofiltration or plasmafiltration.

COMMENTARY

As we increase our understanding of Gram-negative infections, rational therapeutic interventions will increase in number and effectiveness. With cases such as that of this child, utilizing plasmapheresis along with an immunologic approach to the patient with specific monoclonal antibodies, we hope that astounding clinical successes such as this will become commonplace.

References

1. Scharfman WB, Tillotson JR, Taft EG, Wright E. Plasmapheresis for meningococcaemia with disseminated intravascular coagulation. New Engl J Med 1979;300;1277.
2. Barzilay E, Kessler D, Berlot G, Gullo A, Geber D, Ben Zeer I. Use of extracorporeal supportive techniques as additional treatment for septic-induced multiple organ failure patients. Crit Care Med 1989; 17:634–637.
3. Stein B, Pfenninger E, Grunert A, Schmitz JE, Hudde M. Influence of continuous hemofiltration on hemodynamics and central blood volume in experimental endotoxic shock. Intensive Care Med 1990;16: 494–499.
4. Muraji T, Okamoto E, Hoque S, Toyosaka A. Plasma exchange therapy for endotoxin shock in puppies. J Pediatr Surg 1986;21:1092–1095.
5. Passavanti G, Buongiorno E, De Fino G, Fumarola D, Coratelli P. The permeability of dialytic membranes to endotoxins: clinical and experimental findings. Int J Artif Organs 1989;12:505–508.

Case 32

W. Casey Lenox, Jr.
The Johns Hopkins Hospital
Baltimore, Maryland, USA

HISTORY

A nearly 8-year-old boy was transferred to our hospital from a local community hospital for work-up and treatment of evolving left hemiparesis.

Because the patient was adopted, there was no known family history. The patient was 5 weeks premature, but whether he was mechanically ventilated or dependent on oxygen for any period of time was unknown. The boy had developed a "scarlatina-form" rash on three occasions in the past that seemed to be most prominent on the knees and elbows. The rash was associated with a strep throat infection at one point. When the rash first appeared, an arrhythmia was noted. This was evaluated by a Johns Hopkins Hospital cardiologist and was reportedly benign with no follow-up required. The boy was not receiving any medications or allergic to any known medications at the time of hospital admission.

The family had been vacationing 3 days prior to the boy's admission, and the patient appeared to be entirely normal during that time. Two days prior to admission, the patient enjoyed a vigorous roller coaster ride, and thereafter complained of right neck pain and right scalp pain. He appeared otherwise normal and active. One day prior to admission, he began complaining of right-sided headaches and right-sided and posterior neck pain that seemed to be more severe than on the previous day. He vomited one time and continued to complain of increasing neck pain.

On the morning of his hospital admission, the boy was noted to be lethargic and had a left upper extremity weakness that began to worsen. His symptoms evolved over the next several hours to include left lower extremity weakness, and he was brought to a community hospital emergency room (ER). He was unable to walk at that time because of a staggering gait and was carried into the ER. He was afebrile. Immediately after arrival at the outside ER, he vomited once and was noted to be increasingly lethargic. Laboratory values obtained there were as follows: sodium 138 mEq/l, potassium 4.1 mEq/l, chloride 109 mEq/l, total CO_2 20 mEq/l, blood urea nitrogen (BUN) 9 mg/dl, creatinine 0.4 mg/dl, and glucose 119 mg/dl, aspartate transaminase 35 U/l, alanine transaminase 16 U/l, uric acid 3.7 mg/dl, alkaline phosphatase 202 U/l, calcium 9.9 mg/dl, phosphorous 5.4 mg/dl, protein 7.1 g/dl, and albumin 4.7 g/dl. A complete blood count showed a hemoglobin of 13.3 g/dl, hematocrit of 37.4%, white blood cell count of 8900 with two bands, 86 polymorphs, 11 lymphocytes, and 1 monocyte. Ammonia was 42 μg/dl. A noncontrast CT scan was interpreted as normal, as was an ECG. A lumbar puncture was performed following the CT scan that showed two red cells, no white cells, protein level of 27 g/dl, and glucose level of 69 mg/dl. Cultures were obtained. The patient was transported uneventfully by ambulance to the Johns Hopkins Hospital PICU.

PHYSICAL EXAMINATION

At the time of admission, vital signs were as follows: blood pressure 168/92 mm Hg, pulse 70 beats/min, and respiratory rate 20 breaths/min. The patient was afebrile. In general, he was a lethargic, cooperative young boy who opened his eyes in response to the sound of a voice. Head examination revealed a patient preferring his neck turned to the right side, with pupils equal and reactive bilaterally and extraocular movements intact. His left fundus was benign with a sharp disc and no vascular abnormalities, but the right was not visualized well. He complained of neck pain on the right side and an increased amount of pain with flexion of his neck. There were no Kernig or Brudzinski signs. The lungs were clear to auscultation. The skin revealed a café au lait spot on the right thigh 5 × 6 cm, a ½ × ½-cm café au lait spot on the back, and one on the chest. There was no axillary freckling. A cardiac examination revealed a regular heart rate and rhythm with a 2/6 systolic ejection murmur at the left upper sternal border without radiation. The boy's hands and feet were warm and pulses were 2+ in all extremities. The abdomen was nondistended with positive bowel sounds and no hepatosplenomegaly or masses.

Neurologically, the child had a depressed gag and cough reflex. Corneal examination revealed a decreased ipsilateral and consensual corneal reflex on the left with normal examination results on the right. Extraocular movements were intact. There was decreased shoulder shrug on the left. The patient would not turn his chin to his left shoulder, and he was unable to cooperate with finger-to-nose testing. Motor examination results showed his strength to be 2 out of 5 in all groups in the left upper extremity and 2 out of 5 in the left lower extremity in all groups with a triple reflex to pain. The strength of the right lower extremity was 4 out of 5 in all groups and the right upper extremity was 3 out of 5. Deep tendon reflexes were symmetric with upgoing toes bilaterally. Patellar reflex was 1 +, ankles 2 +, and biceps 2 + and symmetric.

Following admission, the patient had a 12-lead ECG that was normal and a normal echocardiogram. Laboratory tests, including a complete blood count, coagulation profile, electrolytes, and liver function tests were repeated and revealed no abnormalities. A CT scan with and without contrast was repeated and initially read as normal. In retrospect, however, there was a small hyperdense area in the area of the posterior left upper medulla. The remainder of the CT scan appeared normal. There were no signs of increased intracranial pressure or any shifts noted.

The patient's gag and cough weakened in the early hours after admission. He was then electively intubated and in spite of low ventilator rates, hyperventilated himself to a pCO_2 of 30 mm Hg. His symptoms rapidly progressed into a dense left hemiparesis and then to a quadriparesis in the 12 hours following admission. Results of magnetic resonance imaging the next morning showed an intraparenchymal posterior medullary hematoma of approximately $1/2 \times 2$ cm. An angiogram revealed no abnormalities. The patient was taken to the operating room where a C1 laminectomy and evacuation of an intraparenchymal clot were performed. The intraoperative findings were that of an organized intraparenchymal clot at the cervical medullary junction with no evidence of an arteriovenous malformation or cavernous angioma. The pathologic specimen showed only hematoma.

The patient received 24 hours of a solumedrol infusion following a bolus in the operating room. During the first 2 postoperative weeks, he slowly regained function of his right lower extremity, then his right upper and left lower extremities, with bulbar function returning to the point where he could be extubated. At nearly 4 weeks postoperatively, the boy's voice was hoarse, but he remains extubated and has residual left upper extremity weakness.

DISCUSSION

Intraparenchymal brainstem hemorrhage in children is a rare occurrence (1,2). Of the 29 reported cases, arteriovenous malformation (AVM) was determined to be responsible in 23 of the 26 cases in which radiologic or pathologic confirmation was possible. The other 3 patients had hemorrhage of uncertain etiology. Hemorrhage into a small AVM or even a small tumor may destroy all evidence of the origin by the time tissue is examined (3).

One quarter of childhood intracranial AVMs are located in the posterior fossa, with half of those found in the brainstem (2). This may contribute to the high mortality rate of pediatric intracranial AVMs, 25% overall but 57% for malformations in the posterior fossa. Most authors agree that immediate surgical management is indicated if hemorrhage has occurred and the patient is showing signs of progressive neurologic deficit or brainstem compression. The risk of recurrent hemorrhage has been reported as 22% in patients managed conservatively or in those in whom only partial resection was possible at first operation (2). The risk for bleeding of an unruptured AVM is inversely correlated with its size and is as great as 52% over 5 years when the AVM is less than 3 cm (4). The overall risk is 2–3% per year (5).

Typically, in childhood, AVMs present acutely, with the signs and symptoms of stroke, following hemorrhage into the mass. Brainstem AVMs are therefore seen with signs of pyramidal tract dysfunction, bulbar palsies, ataxia, disturbances in respiratory and cardiac rhythm, and depressed consciousness. These patients are at great risk of secondary injury and even death because of inadequate airway and ventilatory control. Often deterioration occurs very rapidly over hours or even minutes and will be missed if the clinician attributes the problems to the more slowly growing posterior fossa tumor, which may be the more frequent reason for these symptoms in this age group. Any suspicion of posterior fossa or brainstem involvement necessitates immediate neurosurgical consultation and admission to a PICU.

Strokes, including those of the hemorrhagic variety, may be seen at an early age as a manifestation of congenital disease (5,3,6). These may include anomalies such as an aneurysm or AVM, cyanotic congenital heart disease, renal anomalies, metabolic disease such as homocysteinuria, ornithine transcarbamylase deficiency and meth-

Table 32.1. Causes of Pediatric Stroke

Vascular
  Arteriovenous malformation
  Congenital aneurysm
  Fibromuscular hyperplasia
  Migraine
  Venous thrombosis
    Polycythemia
    Dehydration
    Leukemia
Vasculitis
  Kawasaki's disease
  Systemic lupus erythematosus
  Polyarteritis nodosa
  Takayashu's arteritis
  Giant call arteritis
  Wegener's granulomatosis
Cardiac
  Cyanotic congenital heart disease
  Dysrhythmias
  Cardiopulmonary bypass and ECMO
Coagulopathies
  Congenital
    Protein C deficiency
    Protein S deficiency
    Antithrombin III deficiency
    Hemophilia
    von Willibrand's disease
    Other clotting factor deficiencies
  Acquired
    Idiopathic thrombocytopenic purpura
    Disseminated intravascular coagulopathy
    Iatrogenic
    Hemolytic uremic syndrome
Blood dyscrasias
  Sickle cell disease
Metabolic
  Ornithine transcarbamylase enzymatic defects
  Methylmalonic aciduria
  Homocysteinuria
Infectious
  Pyogenic meningitis
  Encephalitis
  Extensions of head and neck infections
    Tonsillitis
    Mastoiditis
    Sinusitis
    Periorbital cellulitis
    Otitis media
  Subacute bacterial endocarditis
Trauma
  Penetrating oral trauma
  Extremes of cervical motion
  Closed head injury
  Child abuse
  Fat embolism

(continued)

Table 32.1. (*Continued*)

Renal
Congenital anomalies resulting in hypertension
Nephrotic syndrome
Other
Head and neck neoplasms
Syringomyelia/hematomyelia
Familial hyperlipidemia
Neurofibromatosis
Hypertension
Cocaine

ylmalonic aciduria, congenital coagulopathies and blood dyscrasias such as sickle cell disease, protein C and protein S deficiency, and antithrombin III deficiency (6–8) (Table 32.1). Acquired processes sometimes resulting in stroke in pediatric patients include infections of the head and neck (9), oral trauma (10), subacute bacterial endocarditis, and multiple vasculitides (11). An unusual cause of stroke but one that has potential for increasing in frequency is traumatic aneurysm caused by head-banging practices of teenage heavy metal rock enthusiasts (12). Although the patient described above had no radiologic evidence of aneurysm at the time of catheterization, his vigorous roller coaster ride may have resulted in neck injury.

COMMENTARY

Strokes in childhood may be more common than was once thought. Some of the etiologies have changed as the times change (e.g., heavy metal rockers [12]), but most have been around for a long time. We have now become quite sophisticated in diagnosing the cause of strokes. As our colleagues with an adult clientele (who have greater experience with strokes) make use of the basic science research in this area, we will benefit from the inevitable therapeutic advancements in this field. Combined surgical and medical therapy will no doubt help patients with certain types of stroke. The focus upon poststroke morbidity will surely aid in the rehabilitation and recovery of these patients.

References

1. Texier P, Diebler C, Bruguier A, Ponsot G. Hematoma of the brainstem in childhood. Neuroradiology 1984; 26:499–502.
2. Kondziolka D, Humphreys R, Hoffman H, Hendrick E, Drake J. Arte-

riovenous malformations of the brain in children: a forty year experience. Can J Neurol Sci 1992;19:40–45.

3. Humphreys RP. Complications of hemorrhagic stroke in children. Pediatr Neurosurg 1991–1992;17:163–168.

4. Graf C, Perret G, Torner J. Bleeding from cerebral arterio-venous malformations as part of their natural history. J Neurosurg 1983; 58:331–337.

5. Golden GS. Stroke syndromes in childhood. Neurol Clin 1985;3(1): 59–75.

6. Lanska M, Lanska D, Horwitz S, Aram D. Presentation, clinical course, and outcome of childhood stroke. Pediatr Neurol 1991;7: 333–341.

7. Vomberg P, Breederveld C, Fleury P, Arts W. Cerebral thromboembolism due to antithrombin III deficiency in two

8. Israels S, Seshia S. Childhood stroke associated with protein C or S deficiency. J Pediatr 1987;111(4):562–564.

9. Tagawa T, Mimaki T, Yabuuchi H, Iwata Y, Makino A. Bilateral occlusions in the cervical portion of the internal carotid arteries in a child. Stroke 1985;16(5):896–898.

10. Martin N, Warren G. Thrombosis of the internal carotid artery due to intra-oral trauma. South Med J 1969;62:103–107.

11. Moore P, Cupps T. Neurological complications of vasculitis. Ann Neurol 1983;14(2):155–167.

12. Egnor M, Page L, David C. Vertebral artery aneurysm—a unique hazard of head banging by heavy metal rockers. Pediatr Neurosurg 1991–1992;17:135–138.

Case 33

Aaron L. Zuckerberg
The Johns Hopkins Hospital
Baltimore, Maryland, USA

HISTORY

A 2½-year-old girl with no preexisting diseases was playing in the family station wagon while her parents were making final preparations for a trip. Three to four minutes after leaving the child unattended, the family returned to the car and found the child trapped by the neck in the electric car window, which must have been accidentally activated by the child. Following her extrication from the window, the child was apneic, cyanotic, and limp. A pulse was present and mouth-to-mouth resuscitation resulted in the resumption of spontaneous breathing 30–45 seconds later. Air transport to the pediatric trauma center was accomplished with the patient's neck immobilized and the stretcher positioned in a 30° head-up tilt. On arrival at the heliport, the patient was crying robustly.

PHYSICAL EXAMINATION

When we examined her, her vital signs were as follows: weight 15 kg (90th percentile for age), temperature 37.2°C, pulse 145 beats/min, blood pressure 130/palpable mm Hg, respiratory rate 25 breaths/min, and arterial oxygen saturation beginning at 98% and falling to 75% on room air. At the initial examination, the child had a plethora of facial petechiae and a long bright red mark across her laryngeal prominence. There was no evidence of hemoptysis, subcutaneous emphysema, stridor, dysphonia, or alteration of the contour of the anterior neck. She was transported to the emergency department where she became unresponsive to commands or painful stimuli and began extensor

215

posturing. Rapidly, her tongue and perioral tissues became increasingly edematous; air exchange was diminishing with a fall in arterial oxygen saturation increased by pulse oximetry. Despite administration of 100% oxygen by non-rebreathing mask, the pulse oximeter documented a precipitous fall in oxygen saturation.

MANAGEMENT

Following confirmation of intravenous access and the application of slight cricoid pressure, atropine (0.2 mg), lidocaine (15 mg), thiopental (80 mg), and succinylcholine (30 mg) were administered in rapid sequence, while a tracheostomy tray was made available. Direct laryngoscopy during the maintenance of inline cervical traction revealed normal glottic anatomy with an unobscured view of the proximal trachea. A 3.5-mm inside diameter, 28-cm long endotracheal tube (NCC Division, Malinckrodt, Argyle, N.Y.) was gently place through the cords and into the proximal trachea. This endotracheal tube is designed to be longer than the normal 3.5-mm endotracheal tube. The child's chest rose with positive pressure ventilation, bilateral breath sounds were auscultated, and the endotracheal tube was secured. Cricoid pressure was released. The oxygen saturations rapidly increased to 100%.

Cervical spine films confirmed the absence of subcutaneous emphysema. There were no fractures or dislocations of the cervical vertebrae. A chest X-ray demonstrated appropriate endotracheal tube placement. A cranial CT scan appeared normal. Esophagoscopy and bronchoscopy in the operating room demonstrated no disruption of the esophagus, larynx, or trachea.

Neurologically, the girl returned to normal postoperatively. Dexamethasone (7.5 mg every 6 hours) was administered, and she remained sedated, intubated, and fluid restricted for 36 hours. She was then successfully extubated. There was no evidence of dysphonia, dysphagia, or neurologic sequelae. She was discharged from the hospital on the third day.

DISCUSSION

Laryngotracheal trauma is an uncommon injury seen in 1–2% of trauma patients. Blunt anterior neck injury may result in laryngotracheal disruption, which is potentially life threatening. Children may sustain such an injury in falls against bicycle handlebars, horse riding accidents, as unrestrained passengers in vehicular collisions, and in "clothesline" injuries during the use of recreational vehicles (1,2). The initial presentation may be subtle and is often overlooked during the management of other serious injuries that are common in these deceleration accidents.

In blunt neck trauma, the esophagolaryngotracheal complex is violently compressed against the cervical spine. The extent of injuries following this trauma to the anterior neck is dependent on the degree and direction of the force applied and the position of the cervical spine. Extension of the neck fixes the anterior structures, limiting their mobility at the time of impact. Another important determinant is the degree of calcification of the laryngotracheal cartilages. Calcification of these elements begins after the age of 18 (3), and in an experimental model of blunt injury, the severity of fractures corresponded to the extent of calcification, increasing with age. However, severe laryngeal fractures also occurred with an increased incidence in young patients as well (4). The small size, fine structure of the pediatric larynx, and the relative paucity of intervening soft tissues are possible explanations for this finding.

Laryngotracheal disruption is heralded by dyspnea, dysphagia, dysphonia, subcutaneous emphysema, and stridor. Hemoptysis is indicative of an intralaryngeal laceration, which would only occur in this type of injury if the patient had suffered a fractured larynx. Surprisingly, these patients can maintain an airway despite complete airway disruption. A patient who suffered a complete laryngotracheal transection following a motorcycle accident involving a low-hanging cable was "able to get up and walk half a mile to a service station to get assistance" (5).

Establishment and maintenance of a secure airway is of paramount importance. Paralysis and endotracheal intubation may complete a tracheal disruption, induce total airway obstruction, or create a false passage (6,7). The net result would be loss of a previously severely compromised airway. A cricothyroidotomy would be of little utility in these patients. Under the appropriate circumstances, intubation of a distally transected trachea retracted into the mediastinum over a fiberoptic bronchoscope may be beneficial (8). Most authors strongly advocate tracheostomy (2,5,7), emphasizing the low risks in securing the airway. Others point out that orotracheal intubation with a smaller than normal endotracheal tube following direct visualization by the most experienced individual available minimizes the risk of additional damage (9,10).

Simultaneous with activities dedicated to establishment of an airway, efforts must be made to immobilize the cervical spine until a complete evaluation for evidence of ligamentous as well as vertebral injury has been performed. Esophageal disruption and bilateral recurrent laryngeal nerve transection need to be concerns as well.

The little girl in this case suffered a crush injury to the anterior neck. Though the mechanism of injury was not one of high-speed deceleration, the force applied to this young fragile larynx was unestimable, and thus serious consideration was given to the possibility of a laryngotracheal disruption. She had no symptoms that would be suggestive of a laryngotracheal disruption. All illustrative cases in the literature have had at least two symptoms referable to the cervical aerodigestive complex. If the circumstances would have allowed, the ideal management of this patient would have included direct laryngoscopy in the operating room using an anesthetic that allows for spontaneous ventilation.

The rapid decompensation of the airway in this patient was very likely due to development of a tremendous amount of edema, despite appropriate positioning. This serves to emphasize the importance of positioning in this injury (11). Had a head-up position not been maintained during transport, one could only assume that catastrophic airway compromise would have occurred during transport. The neurologic symptoms of unresponsiveness and posturing during this decompensation only served to complicate the situation further. Considerations at that time included hypoxia-induced seizure activity, cervical spine injury, and cerebral edema from venous outflow obstruction.

The decision to proceed with a rapid-sequence intubation was based on the lack of heralding symptoms of airway disruption, the urgency of the decompensation, and concerns about intracranial hypertension and the detrimental effects of laryngoscopy, hypoxia, and hypercarbia in this patient. Preparations for emergent tracheostomy were being made in the event that intubation was impossible.

COMMENTARY

As intensive care deliverers, our prime objective is to maintain airway, breathing, and circulation. Laryngotracheal trauma is a particularly frustrating pathology because routine management of the airway can result in worsening of airway obstruction. A careful tracheostomy with the patient spontaneously breathing may be the most conservative approach, although still fraught with difficulty.

If endotracheal intubation is attempted, long (so-called "epiglottitis") endotracheal tubes are helpful. If normal tubes are used when a smaller outside diameter is necessary in the face of narrowing and swelling of the airway, then the connector ends up inside the patient's mouth. This problem is avoided with longer tubes.

Of more importance is the issue of prevention. Automatic car window closers have no safety mechanism to stop or reverse the window closure when something (or somebody) gets caught in the window. There are standards for automatic garage door closers that reverse or stop if the door closes on something. As pediatricians, we should advocate similar safety standards for automatic car window closers.

References

1. Alonso WA, Pratt LL, Zollinger WK. Complications of laryngotracheal disruption. Laryngoscope 1974;276–1290.
2. Sofferman RA. Management of laryngotracheal trauma. Am J Surg 1981;141:412–417.
3. Yerman HM, Werkhaven J, Schild JA. Evaluation of laryngeal calcium deposition: a new methodology. Ann Otol Rhinol Laryngol 1988;97:516–520.
4. Lee SY. Experimental blunt injury to the larynx. Ann Otol Rhinol Laryngol 1992;101:270–273.
5. Snow JB. Diagnosis and therapy for acute laryngeal and tracheal trauma. Otolaryngol Clin North Am 1984;17:101–106.
6. Schaefer SD, Close LG. Acute management of laryngeal trauma. Ann Otol Rhinol Laryngol 1989;98:98–104.
7. Minard G. Laryngotracheal transection. J Tenn Med Assoc 1990;83:402–403.
8. Grover FL, Ellestad C, Arom VK, et al. Diagnosis and management of major tracheobronchial injuries. Ann Thorac Surg 1979;28:384–391.
9. Gussack GS, Jurkovich GJ. Treatment dilemmas in laryngo-tracheal trauma. J Trauma 1988;28:1439–1444.
10. Casiano RR, Goodwin, WJ. Restoring function to the injured larynx. Otolaryngol Clin North Am 1991;24: 1215–1226.
11. Shumrick KA, Shumrick DA. Laryngeal and tracheal foreign bodies and blunt trauma. In: Callaham ML, ed. Current therapy in emergency medicine. Toronto: BC Decker, 1987:235–238.

Case 34

William R. Hayden
Rush Medical College-
Cook County Hospital
Chicago, Illinois, USA

HISTORY

A 3-month-old infant boy was admitted to the PICU at Johns Hopkins Hospital with respiratory failure and ventricular bigeminy. He was delivered at 37 weeks' gestation weighing 3.06 kg. His mother was a gestational diabetic, and some fetal decelerations were noted in the final stages of labor. A low blood sugar level early in life was treated with feeding and resolved. Shortly after birth, the infant's parents noted occasional episodes of nonprojectile vomiting. Several formula changes were attempted in the first 2 months of life without success, and the infant was lost to follow-up for a month prior to his admission.

On the night of admission he appeared in the emergency room of another hospital. He was weak, emaciated, dehydrated, and barely breathing. His serum potassium was 3.0 mEq/l and an ECG strip revealed many premature ventricular contractions. The child was intubated, given 1 mg/kg lidocaine intravenously, and transferred by helicopter to the Johns Hopkins PICU.

PHYSICAL EXAMINATION

Physical examination revealed an intubated child being mechanically ventilated. Vital signs included a blood pressure of 110/58 mm Hg, pulse rate of 94 beats/min, respiratory rate of 6 breaths/min, temperature of 36.5°C, and an oxygen saturation of 100% in an $F_IO_2 = 1.0$. The baby's head circumference was 38.5 cm (<5%), his weight was 3.7 kg (<5%), and his length was 58.5 cm (<5%). Pertinent

221

physical findings included a depressed fontanel, sunken eyes, poor skin turgor, and easily palpable pulses. The abdomen was scaphoid, and an olive-sized mass was palpated in the right upper quadrant. There appeared to be no other physical abnormalities.

During the physical examination, the ECG monitor demonstrated a sudden conversion from normal sinus rhythm to ventricular bigeminy. A 1 mg/kg-dose of lidocaine was administered intravenously and the rhythm converted to sinus.

LABORATORY DATA

Laboratory values were as follows: hemoglobin 9.2 g/dl, glucose 79 mg/dl, sodium 128 mEq/l, potassium 2.2 mEq/l, bicarbonate 42 mEq/l, blood urea nitrogen 42 mg/dl. The urine pH was 7.0. An assay of arterial blood gas values revealed a pH of 7.9, pCO_2 of 22 torr, base excess of +24 mEq/l.

HOSPITAL MANAGEMENT

The treatment plan included rehydration and correction of the metabolic abnormalities using 5% dextrose in normal saline with 80 mEq/l of potassium chloride. Six hours after admission, arterial blood gas values revealed a pH of 7.70, pCO_2 of 30 torr, and base excess of +11 mEq/l. At 8 hours postadmission, the endotracheal tube became dislodged. Because he appeared to be breathing adequately, the infant was not reintubated and 30 minutes later blood gas values were as follows: pH 7.45 and pCO_2 58 torr. By 12 hours postadmission, he was spontaneously breathing, his weight had increased to 4.1 kg, his serum sodium level was 140 mEq/l, potassium level was 4.3 mEq/l, chloride level was 91 mEq/l, bicarbonate level was 32 mEq/l, pH was 7.51, pCO_2 was 48 torr, and the ventricular dysrhythmia had not recurred. He underwent a successful pyloromyotomy on the third day after admission and was discharged 5 days postadmission in good condition.

DISCUSSION

Pyloric stenosis is a common disorder seen in pediatrics and is usually associated with mild or moderate dehydration. Hypokalemic, hypochloremic metabolic alkalosis of variable severity is also commonly seen. Rehydration with added sodium, potassium, and chloride is effective in reversing the metabolic abnormalities and stabilizing the child for surgery.

Goldring et al. (1) induced chronic metabolic alkalosis in human volunteers with bicarbonate, Tromethamine, or diuretic administration and studied the effects over a period of 6 to 11 days. Progressive hypoventilation characterized by increasing pCO_2, falling minute volume, and depressed ventilatory response to 5% CO_2 inhalation was noted and found to be inversely related to the severity of the metabolic alkalosis. Arterial blood pO_2 fell an average of 17 torr and the pCO_2 rose to levels between 50 and 55 torr in three patients whose alkalosis was induced by ethacrynic acid. The 20% decrease in minute volume was entirely attributable to the reduction of resting tidal volume, which in turn was significantly related to the serum bicarbonate concentration. This study was confirmed by Javaheri et al. (2) in 1982.

Irsigler et al. (3) confirmed a reduced ventilatory response to hypercapnia and hypoxia in a similar group of patients. They also studied changes in cerebrospinal fluid (CSF) chemistry during the alkalosis. Because there were no significant changes in the CSF values for pH, pCO_2, or bicarbonate, they concluded that the changes were most likely mediated by the peripheral rather than the medullary chemoreceptors.

The second important effect of alkalosis on the ventilatory apparatus concerns that of the accompanying hypokalemia on the respiratory musculature. Glaser and Stark (4) studied young rabbits given a potassium-deficient diet for 20–60 days and observed progressive wasting and weakness. Electrophysiologic studies on the paravertebral muscles revealed an increased muscle refractory period time constant in the hypokalemic, alkalotic animals. Pathologic examination revealed segmental degeneration of muscle fibers with loss of striations and invasion by macrophages. The lesions were spotty and associated with apparently normal and regenerating muscle fibers, the latter with numerous proliferating nuclei.

The electrolyte disturbance can be identified as the factor influencing the ventilatory disturbance in this child.

There is controversy about whether underlying pathology of the heart is a prerequisite for ventricular dysrhythmias induced by hypokalemia. Weller et al. (5) studied the effects of acute removal of potassium by dialysis in dogs with normal hearts. They showed consistent changes in the ECG progressing from an increase in the height and width of the P wave, to a prolongation of the atrioventricular conduction time, a widened QRS complex and, finally, a shift in the QRS axis. However, no ventricular dysrhythmias developed at any time in any of their animals in spite of the massive potassium depletion. In contrast, the study by Nordrehaug et al. (6) of patients with myocardial infarcts demonstrated that the incidence of ventricular ectopic beats was inversely related to the serum potassium level at the time of admission.

Follis et al. (7), among others, however, has provided evidence that the hearts of chronically, potassium-deficient animals are not normal. In 1942, his group at Johns Hopkins demonstrated that the hearts of rats fed a diet deficient in potassium developed characteristic pathologic changes. They noted a loss of striations of the individual muscle fibers, nuclear degeneration, and inflammatory cell infiltrate as early as 8 days after the experiment was begun. Between the 8th and 15th days, the lesions increased in size and number and were found in atrial as well as ventricular tissue. Follis and colleagues noted the similarity in appearance of these lesions to myocarditis; some areas even suggested the cardiac involvement of diphtheria. McAllen (8) described similar lesions in two patients who died of diseases associated with severe potassium deficiency, confirming in human counterparts the study by Follis and associates.

Thus, the wasted, weak infant we describe in our report with hypokalemic, metabolic alkalosis may have had poor control of ventilation, weak muscles, and reversible myocardial damage. The conditions were right for the respiratory failure and the ventricular bigeminy that he exhibited. Ventilation, gradual replacement of the fluid and electrolyte deficits, and the timely use of lidocaine in case of a life-threatening ventricular dysrhythmia can result in a successful outcome.

COMMENTARY

The finding in the infant we describe—severe electrolyte disturbances due to vomiting from pyloric stenosis—is an unusual cause for admission to the PICU. This referral is a credit to our general pediatric colleagues in the community in the identification and treatment of this relatively common disease. In the United States, these referrals are almost always to surgeons, whereas in other countries, some of these cases are medically managed. As the etiology of pylorospasm is better elucidated, pharmacologic medical management becomes a more realistic possibility. Recent evidence suggests that nitric oxide synthase dysfunction may cause this problem (9).

Some of the sad irony of what we do as intensivists is correcting problems that are a result of the limitations of primary care. As is true in so many of these cases in pediatrics, an ounce of prevention is worth a pound of cure. When the pediatric intensivist is presented with these challenging multisystem physiologic disturbances, it is gratifying to know that the pound of cure often results in such a success.

References

1. Goldring R, Cannon P, Heinemann H. Respiratory compensation to chronic metabolic alkalosis in man. J Clin Invest 1968;47:188–202.
2. Javaheri S, Shore N, Rose B, Kasemi H. Compensatory hypoventilation in metabolic alkalosis. Chest 1982;81:296–301.
3. Irsigler G, Stafford M, Severinghaus J. Relationship of CSF pH, O_2 and CO_2 responses in metabolic acidosis and alkalosis in humans. J Appl Physiol 1980;48:355–361.
4. Glaser G, Stark L. Excitability in experimental myopathy: potassium deficiency. Neurology 1958;8:708–711.
5. Weller J, Lown B, Hoigne R, et al. Effects of acute removal of potassium from dogs: changes in the electrocardiogram. Circulation 1955;11:44–51.
6. Nordrehaug J, Johannessen K, Von Der Lippe G. Serum potassium concentration as risk factor for ventricular arrhythmias early in acute myocardial infarction. Circulation 1985;71:645–649.
7. Follis R, Orent-Keiles E, McCollum E.: The production of cardiac and renal lesions in rats by a diet extremely deficient in potassium. Am J Pathol 1942; 18:29–35.
8. McAllen P. Myocardial changes occurring in potassium deficiency. Br Heart J 1955;17:5–14.
9. Vanderwinden JM, Mailleux P, Schiftman SN, et al. Nitric oxide synthase activity in infantile hypertrophic pyloric stenosis. New Engl J Med 1992;327:511–515.

Case 35

Joseph R. Tobin
The Johns Hopkins Hospital
Baltimore, Maryland, USA

HISTORY

A 6-year-old boy, scheduled for an elective hypospadias repair had had nothing to eat or drink since midnight prior to the morning of surgery. He had no prior hospitalizations and no prior surgical treatment. The family history was remarkable for a sister with arthrogryposis. With his otherwise good health, general anesthesia was induced first with premedication by midazolam 15 mg per rectum (approximately 1 mg/kg) followed by inhalation of nitrous oxide and halothane via mask. The induction of anesthesia continued uneventfully and the boy had a patent airway throughout. After a few minutes at 4% halothane concentration, he became hypotensive (60/38 mm Hg) while intravenous access attempts continued. The halothane was decreased to 1% concentration, and an oral airway was inserted while intravenous access was obtained. At this time, the boy was given atropine 0.3 mg and succinylcholine 22 mg intravenously. His pulse increased to 200 beats/min, his fingers curled tonically, and he became rigid. His jaw tightened, and his mouth could not be opened beyond the extent of the oral airway previously inserted. Ventilation continued to be performed without difficulty via bag mask apparatus. Pancuronium bromide 1.5 mg was given intravenously. Pulse oximetry demonstrated 98–100% oxygen saturation throughout. Intubation was performed following pancuronium administration, with approximately 90 seconds required for visualization of the vocal cords. The endotracheal tube was immediately connected to an end-tidal carbon dioxide monitor, which measured a carbon dioxide concentration of 90 mm Hg. A rectal thermometer was inserted, and the boy's temperature was 38.5°C. He was hyperventilated and arterial blood gas readings were as follows: pH 7.28, PCO_2 30 mm Hg, PO_2 123 mm Hg, HCO_3 15, with an end-tidal CO_2 reading of 40 mm Hg. Halothane was discontinued and the patient was switched to an alternate airway circuit. A central venous line, arterial line, and urinary catheter were inserted. A few drops of clear urine were obtained. He was brought to the PICU intubated and receiving assisted ventilation.

PHYSICAL EXAMINATION

On arrival at the ICU, his temperature was 38.6°C (peak temperature 38.8°C in the operating room). Other vital signs included: blood pressure 98/60 mm Hg, pulse rate 160 beats/min, respiratory rate 28 breaths/min (artificially ventilated), and arterial oxygen saturation measurement of 99%. His weight was 18.5 kg. The anesthesiologist had sedated and paralyzed him. Eye and ear examination results were normal. Examination of his oropharynynx revealed relaxed muscular tone, and an oral airway and endotracheal tube were in place. His neck was supple without adenopathy or rigidity. Auscultation of the chest revealed equal breath sounds. The precordium was hyperdynamic, and his heart tones were normal, without murmur, rub, or gallop. His abdomen was soft, without palpable masses or organomegaly. Genitourinary examination revealed a penile hypospadias through which the urinary catheter was inserted. His testes were descended bilaterally. His extremities were flushed and pulses were easily palpable and bounding in all extremities. Neurologically, he had equal and briskly reactive pupils. The remainder of his neurologic examination was obscured secondary to neuromuscular blockade.

LABORATORY DATA

Laboratory data are summarized below in Table 35.1.

MANAGEMENT

Immediate management of this patient was initiated in the operating room and included stopping exposure to triggering agents (volatile anesthetics and succinylcholine). The patient was actively cooled, oxygenated, hyperventilated, and received specific pharmacologic therapy to interrupt the vicious cycle of hypermetabolism. Intravenous dantrolene 2–2.5 mg/kg was given. Metabolic acido-

Table 35.1. Laboratory Data

Electrolytes (mEq/l)	
Na$^+$	135
K$^+$	5.3
Cl$^-$	105
HCO$_3$$^-$	15
Blood urea nitrogen (mg/dl)	14
Creatinine (mg/dl)	0.6
Ionized Ca^{++} (mM/l)	0.74 (normal = 1.13–1.32)
Mg^{++} (mEq/l)	1.4 (normal = 1.3–2.0)
Creatine kinase (IU/l)	30,000 (normal = 0–175)
MB fraction (%)	249 (normal = 0–3 of total)
Lactate dehydrogenase (IU/l)	1,380 (normal = 0–220)
Aspartate transaminase(IU/l)	1,492 (normal = 0–35)
Urinalysis results	yellow/amber color, hazy appearance with 1 red blood cell/high power field, and urine dipstick measurement: 4+ positive reaction for hemoglobin (cross-reacts with myoglobin)
Hemoglobin (g/dl)	9.1
Hematocrit (%)	28
Platelets (/mm^3)	331,000
White blood cell count (/mm^3)	9,500
Prothrombin time (sec)	12.7
Activated partial thromboplastin time (sec)	24.5

sis required large doses of sodium bicarbonate (administered in 0.5–1.0 mEq/kg/dose) to titrate the lactic acidemia (from hypermetabolism and inadequate oxygen delivery) and to attempt alkalinization of the urine to combat the renal tubular damage caused by myoglobinemia and myoglobinuria. This child developed rose-colored urine, which continued despite dantrolene and bicarbonate therapy. Forced diuresis was accomplished with the use of large volumes of crystalloid infusion. Therapy was continued to maintain his body temperature at <38°C, to maintain urine output at >1 ml/kg/hr, and assisted respiratory support was provided to clear the excessive CO$_2$ production. The creatine phosphokinase level increased from 30,000–72,000 IU/l over approximately 18 hours. He was extubated 5 hours postadmission, and observed in the PICU for 72 hours demonstrating generalized residual weakness that slowly improved. Dantrolene therapy was continued during the first 36 hours after the incident.

DISCUSSION

This child illustrates a fulminant presentation of malignant hyperthermia (MH), a disease triggered most frequently in the operating room by exposure to volatile anesthetics and succinylcholine. Other rare cases of MH have been reported during severe stress in an MH-susceptible patient without exposure to these agents. It is important that the intensivist be familiar with this disease and be prepared to treat a patient who has had such a hypermetabolic derangement occur, since appropriate therapy has reduced the mortality of this disease from >80% to <10% in 10 years.

Classic malignant hyperthermia is a disorder characterized by hypermetabolism due to excessive release or lack of reuptake of calcium from the sarcoplasmic reticulum. This excessive calcium level is now available to muscular contractile elements and causes excessive sustained muscular contraction. These contractions are responsible for the physical findings of muscle rigidity. However, despite the rigidity of airway musculature (most notably the masseter muscle), most patients can be bag-mask ventilated through this initial crisis. It is important that the child receive assisted ventilation, because hyperventilation will be necessary to manage the excessive CO_2 production. Along with the muscular contraction, there is excessive heat production in the skeletal muscles. This hypermetabolic function increases cardiopulmonary demands. Rhabdomyolysis occurs, which may be extreme, and release of myoglobin may precipitate renal failure. Although not demonstrated in the case of the child we describe, ventricular irritability and dysrhythmias at the onset of malignant hyperthermia are well described. These arrhythmias may be primary and due to cardiac muscle abnormalities or secondary to other metabolic derangements, including hyperkalemia and acidosis, which occur in MH. Dysrhythmias must be aggressively treated, and hyperkalemia must be assumed even if not measured. Treatment with lidocaine is considered appropriate (1 mg/kg), and aggressive therapies to reduce the deleterious effects of hyperkalemia are essential (hyperventilation, sodium bicarbonate, calcium chloride, and glucose and insulin). The excessive demands on cardiopulmonary status during fulminant MH require invasive monitoring in order to optimize preload, measure cardiac performance, and adjust therapy to improve urine output.

The hyperthermia associated in this condition must be aggressively treated with attempts at peripheral/surface cooling, as well as central/core cooling. The patient will be vasodilated at the initiation of surface cooling, but will respond with sympathetic vasoconstriction, making this therapy less effective. Other options are core cooling with the use of gastric and bladder lavage of cold saline or peri-

Table 35.2. Differential Diagnosis of Tachycardia in This Patient

Sepsis
Thyrotoxicosis
Pheochromocytoma
Neuroblastoma
Transfusion reaction
Hyperthermia (environmental)
Intoxication
  Amphetamine
  Cocaine
  Atropine
  Theophylline
  Thyroid hormone
  Ketamine
  Monoamine oxidase inhibitors

toneal irrigation with sterile cold saline. With early aggressive treatment, it should be unnecessary to use an extracorporeal heat exchange circuit.

The differential diagnosis listed in Table 35.2 includes thyrotoxicosis, which can also become apparent at the initiation of anesthesia, as well as pheochromocytoma or neuroblastoma. These diagnoses should not cause muscle rigidity, which places malignant hyperthermia in a classification by itself. However, the goals of treatment of each of these hypermetabolic crises are the same: to reverse the hypermetabolic course and return vital signs to normal before multiorgan failure occurs.

The release of dantrolene sodium in the United States in 1979 by the Food and Drug Administration has offered pharmacologic therapy specific for MH and other muscular metabolic diseases. In a fulminant presentation of malignant hyperthermia, dantrolene therapy is life-saving; however, attention to basic life-support functions are critical in the first few minutes. Comprehensive information regarding the treatment of malignant hyperthermia is available on a 24-hour basis from the Malignant Hyperthermia Association of the United States (MHAUS). The 24-hour hotline number is 1-209-634-4917. It is also imperative that follow-up arrangements for testing of family members (autosomal dominant transmission) be made and that the patient and family members be aware of the need to provide information regarding the patient's diagnosis to anesthesia care providers in the future.

COMMENTARY

I have chosen MH because it is a unique illness that may be seen by the critical care physician. The paradigm of treatment of MH may be useful in other hyperpyrexic or other hypermetabolic syndromes. Early recognition and management of the patient with MH, as well as management of the MH-susceptible patient, have made dramatic advances in the last decade, to provide safe state-of-the-art care for these children.

As pharmacologic research continues, we hope that ultra-short-acting non-depolarizing agents such as mivacurium will supplant the use of succinylcholine. Since the onset of this agent is slower and is also associated with hypotension, it is not an ideal agent for the emergent establishment of an artificial airway. The actions of mivacurium disappear faster than that of vecuronium, but the latter is devoid of cardiovascular effects. Neither of these agents has an onset time as fast as succinylcholine, which is the most rapidly acting neuromuscular-blocking agent. Presently, therefore, succinylcholine remains the neuromuscular-blocking agent of choice for the emergent establishment of an artificial airway. As long as this is the case, anesthesiologists and intensivists must be familiar with the diagnosis and treatment of MH.

Suggested Readings

1. Nelson TE. SR function in malignant hyperthermia. Cell Calcium 1988;9:257.
2. King JD, Denborough MA. Anesthetic-induced malignant hyperpyrexia in children. J Pediatr 1973;83:37.
3. Muldoon SM, Karan S. Hyperthermia and hypothermia. In: Rogers MC, et al. Principles and practice of anesthesiology. St. Louis: Mosby-Year Book, 1992.

Case 36

Thomas V. Ringer,
Jerry J. Zimmerman, and
William H. Perloff
Children's Hospital
Madison, Wisconsin, USA

HISTORY

A previously healthy 3½-year-old boy developed fever to 103°F, diffuse achiness, listlessness, coughing, and mild vomiting. Amoxicillin was started 2 days later for possible otitis media. On day 4 of illness, a periauricular rash developed and the patient was noted to be tachypneic. The next day, he was admitted to his local hospital with lethargy, neck stiffness, and increased respiratory distress. The patient was not confused. His respiratory rate was 32 breaths/min, his heart rate was 120 beats/min, his blood pressure was 94/60 mm Hg, and his temperature was 102.9°F. He had conjunctivitis and a rash on his ears, neck, trunk, buttocks, extremities, and palms. No adenopathy was noted. His white cell count was 26,200 cells/μl with 46% segmented and 24% immature neutrophils, 17% lymphocytes, and 1% monocytes. The creatinine kinase level was 23 U/l. Cerebrospinal fluid examination revealed 8 white cells, 100% lymphocytes, no red cells, protein level of 10 g/dl, glucose level of 70 mg/dl, and no organisms on Gram stain. After blood cultures were obtained, ceftriaxone was instituted for presumed sepsis.

By the next day, the patient had blood pressures as low as 78/52 mm Hg, respiratory rate to 40 breaths/min, grunting, oliguria, and cardiomegaly with prominent pulmonary vasculature seen on chest X-ray. He was transferred to the University of Wisconsin Children's Hospital PICU.

PHYSICAL EXAMINATION

On arrival, the patient was agitated but alert and oriented and in moderately severe respiratory distress. His respiratory rate was 60 breaths/min, his heart rate was 180 beats/min, his blood pressure was 86/38 mm Hg, and his temperature was 39.8°C. A marked, nonpurulent bulbar conjunctivitis was present. The erythematous lips were peeling. The tongue was red and fissured. No adenopathy was palpated. Inspiratory nasal flaring, moderately severe retractions, rales, and expiratory grunting were present. A mitral regurgitation murmur and a gallop were auscultated. The liver was 6 cm below the right midcostal margin. There was no splenomegaly. Erythematous blanching 3- to 4-mm macules were present on the patient's ears, neck, buttocks, distal extremities, and palms. The hands and feet were cool, with delayed capillary refill.

LABORATORY DATA

On arrival at the PICU, a chest X-ray revealed cardiomegaly, markedly increased pulmonary vasculature, and edema. An ECG showed sinus tachycardia and low voltage across all leads. Severely dilatated left-sided chambers, poor left ventricular contractility (fractional shortening 18%), and mitral valvular insufficiency were detected by echocardiography. No coronary aneurysms were noted. The white blood cell count was 11,200 with 40% segmented and 49% immature neutrophils, 5% lymphocytes, and 4% monocytes. Creatinine kinase was 46 U/l with 100% MM pattern. Serum electrolyte and liver studies showed no abnormalities.

MANAGEMENT

Arterial and central venous lines were placed. The initial central venous pressure was 6 mm Hg. The patient received furosemide intravenously, and a dobutamine infusion was begun with only marginal improvement. Mechanical ventilation was instituted following nasotracheal intubation. A balloon flotation pulmonary artery catheter was positioned. Initial pulmonary artery wedge pressure was 23 mm Hg, cardiac index 4.8 l/min/m^2, and systemic vascular resistance index 623 dyne-sec/ cm^5/m^2. Vasoactive infusions including epinephrine, dopamine, dobutamine, amrinone, and, later, nitroprusside resulted in significant improvement in hemodynamics. Daily echocardiograms demonstrated slight but consistent improvements in the patient's poor cardiac contractility.

Complications during the hospital course included pulmonary edema and severe intrapulmonary shunting leading to hypoxemia on F_IO_2 1.0 and poor pulmonary compliance for days despite hemodynamic improvement. Thrombocytopenia was first noted on the second hospital day and did not normalize for $3\frac{1}{2}$ weeks. Severe oliguria necessitated institution of peritoneal dialysis by the third hospital day. After 1 week of hospitalization, the epinephrine infusion was discontinued. On the eighth hospital day, intravenous γ-globulin, 400 mg/kg/d, was started for 4 days because a slightly diffusely dilatated right coronary artery raised the question of atypical Kawasaki's disease. Amphotericin B was begun to treat *Candida albicans* which grew on cultures from a central venous line, peritoneal dialysate, and later from two tracheal aspirates. Subsequent to initiating Amphotericin B, *Candida tropicalis* grew from four different vascular lines, two peripheral blood samples, and a urine specimen.

Oxygen was weaned below F_IO_2 0.7 at 2 weeks after admission and the patient was extubated 2 weeks later. Peritoneal dialysis was stopped the day following extubation. The last parenteral inotrope was discontinued on the 33rd hospital day. A head CT scan demonstrated ventriculomegaly and cerebral atrophy. The patient underwent speech, occupational, and physical therapy and was eventually discharged from the hospital 47 days after admission.

Postdischarge, paired acute and convalescent rubeola complement fixation titers were reported as 1:8 from 10/4 and 1:128 from 11/7. IgG indirect fluorescent antibody for rubeola was positive, with IgM being equivocal. Serology for rubella, herpes simplex, Coxsackie B, influenza A and B, encephalomyocarditis virus, parainfluenza, adenovirus, respiratory syncytial virus, and *Mycoplasma pneumonia* were negative. Subsequent cardiac evaluations have been normal except for a slightly dilatated right coronary artery on echocardiogram and a partial right bundle block on ECG. Serial neurologic examinations have demonstrated the child's complete clinical recovery from his encephalitis.

DISCUSSION

An epidemic resurgence of rubeola has occurred in the United States since 1989 (1). The majority of cases have involved children younger than 5 years of age (2). Rubeola cases precipitously declined after the introduction of the vaccine in 1963. Approximately 80% of patients acquiring the disease in the present epidemic have been unvaccinated (1). Our patient had received a mumps-measles-rubella vaccine 2 years prior to his illness. Typically the vaccine confers protective immunity to 95% of vaccinated subjects (1). Our patient did not have a history of frequent, virulent, or atypical infections. There was no clinical suspicion of cell-mediated or other immunodeficiency.

Rubeola is a highly contagious acute disease characterized by fever, conjunctivitis, photophobia, coryza, cough, and Koplik's spots on buccal mucosa. The characteristic brownish-pink maculopapular rash begins 3–5 days after symptom onset, spreads from the ears, face, and neck to the trunk and limbs, and persists for 4–7 days. Rubeola is usually benign, but uncommon severe manifestations include encephalitis, pneumonia, and thrombocytopenic purpura.

Deaths occur in approximately 0.1% of cases usually due to pneumonia or encephalitis (2). However, severe complications occur in about 80% of immunocompromised patients with a mortality of 40%–70%, primarily because of pneumonia or encephalitis (3).

Relatively few cases of cardiac involvement during rubeola illness have been reported (4–11). The principal type of cardiac pathology has been myocarditis. Acute myocarditis is often characterized by elevated serum creatinine kinase levels and elevated ST segments seen on ECG. The patient we described had unremarkable creatinine kinase levels and ST segments were not elevated. He did however have low QRS voltage diffusely across all leads on ECG and markedly dilated, hypocontractile chambers on echocardiogram, consistent with cardiomyopathy. The patient had no previous symptoms of cardiac dysfunction prior to his illness and had an essentially normal echocardiogram 2 months after his illness. His heart failure was temporally associated with rubeola illness. Perhaps immunoglobulin may have ameliorated the patient's course, although he received this treatment somewhat late in his illness. Some authors have suggested consideration of immunoglobulin therapy in immunocompromised individuals with measles or measles exposure (12,13).

This child exhibited a severe dilated cardiomyopathy associated with rubeola illness requiring very aggressive monitoring and therapy. Clinicians should be aware of this possibly fatal complication of measles and of its potential reversibility with appropriate supportive care.

COMMENTARY

In the past 50 years the focus of general pediatrics has changed. Past generations of pediatricians in the United States spent a great deal of their time making house calls to patients suffering such infectious childhood diseases as mumps, measles, and rubeola. Things have changed. What we are now seeing is a resurgence of these diseases either from a failure of the vaccine, a failure of immunization programs, and/or poor access to health care. As primary care givers see more and more of these diseases, intensivists will see more and more of the rare complicated cases and complications of these diseases. For measles, there is a correlation between vitamin A levels and the severity of the illness. Furthermore, vitamin A supplementation (200,000 IU given orally twice daily with a total dose of 400,000 IU) seems to diminish the morbidity and mortality of the illness (14).

As always in pediatrics, an ounce of prevention is worth a pound of cure. The hope is that immunization programs will again diminish the incidence of these diseases.

References

1. The National Vaccine Advisory Committee. The measles epidemic: the problems, barriers, and recommendations. JAMA 1991;266: 1547–1552.
2. Centers for Disease Control. Measles-United States. MMWR 1991; 40:369–372.
3. Kaplan LJ, Daum RS, Smaron M, McCarthy CA. Severe measles in immunocompromised patients. JAMA 1992;267:1237–1241.
4. Wlodarska EK. The role of viruses in the pathogenesis of myocarditis and dilated cardiomyopathy. Kardiol Pol 1991;34:250–255.
5. Tokuyama T, et al. A case of measles in an adolescent with myocarditis and pneumonia. Kansenshogaku Zasshi 1989;63:530–533.
6. Frustaci A, Abdulla AK, Caldarulo M, Buffon A. Fatal measles myocarditis. Cadiologio 1990;35:347–349.
7. Herdy GV, de Oliveira SA, Lopes VG. Measles myocarditis. Arq Bras Cardiol 1982;38:115–117.
8. Ananko J, Vieth J, Czarski W. Two cases of toxic myocardial injury in the course of measles complicated by lobar pneumonia. Przegl Epidemiol 1976;30:271–273.
9. Provvidenza G, Ciarla MV, DiNardo V. On a case of acute myocarditis during measles. G Malattie Infet Parassist 1971;23:35–36.
10. Cristofani M. Electrographic findings in an epidemic of measles in Milan. Minerva Cardioangiol 1967;115:287–293.
11. Navarro EE, Gonzaga NC, Lucero MG, et al. Clinicopathologic studies of children who die of acute lower respiratory tract infections: mechanisms of death. Rev Infect Dis 12 (suppl 8) 1990;S5: 1065–1073.

12. Kay HEN, Rankin A. Immunoglobulin prophylaxis of measles in acute lymphoblastic leukemia. Lancet 1984;1:901–902.
13. Ross LA, Kim KS, Mason WH, Gomperts C. Successful treatment of disseminated measles in a patient with AIDS: consideration of antiviral and passive immunotherapy. Am J Med 1990;88:313–314.
14. Hussey GD, Klein M. A randomized, controlled trial of vitamin A in children with severe measles. New Engl J Med 1990;323:160–164.

Case 37

**Steven E. Haun,
Donna A. Caniano,
David L. Anglin,
and Linda L. Sell**
*Children's Hospital
Columbus, Ohio, USA*

HISTORY

A 6-year-old girl suffered burns and smoke inhalation in a house fire. Her past medical history was unremarkable except for morbid obesity. She developed stridor shortly after arrival to the PICU and her trachea was intubated. Her burns were estimated to involve 50% of her total body surface area. The burns were second and third degree involving both upper extremities, anterior and posterior trunk, buttocks, posterior and lateral portions of both lower extremities, and the lateral aspect of the left face and neck. The burns of the forearms were circumferential, and emergent escharotomies were performed to restore perfusion to the distal upper extremities. Fluid resuscitation was initiated using the Parkland formula. During the first day of hospitalization, the patient developed increasingly severe respiratory failure and anuria. Escharotomies were performed on the anterior trunk and back without improvement in oxygenation or ventilation. The abdomen became progressively more distended. Approximately 18 hours after admission, the patient could no longer be supported by a mechanical ventilator. Adequate arterial oxygen saturations could be maintained only by ventilating the patient with 100% oxygen by means of a self-inflating manual ventilation bag; peak inflating pressures exceeded 150 cm H_2O. Arterial blood gas values revealed pH 6.88, $PaCO_2$ 109 mm Hg, and PaO_2 55 mm Hg. Chest X-ray per-

239

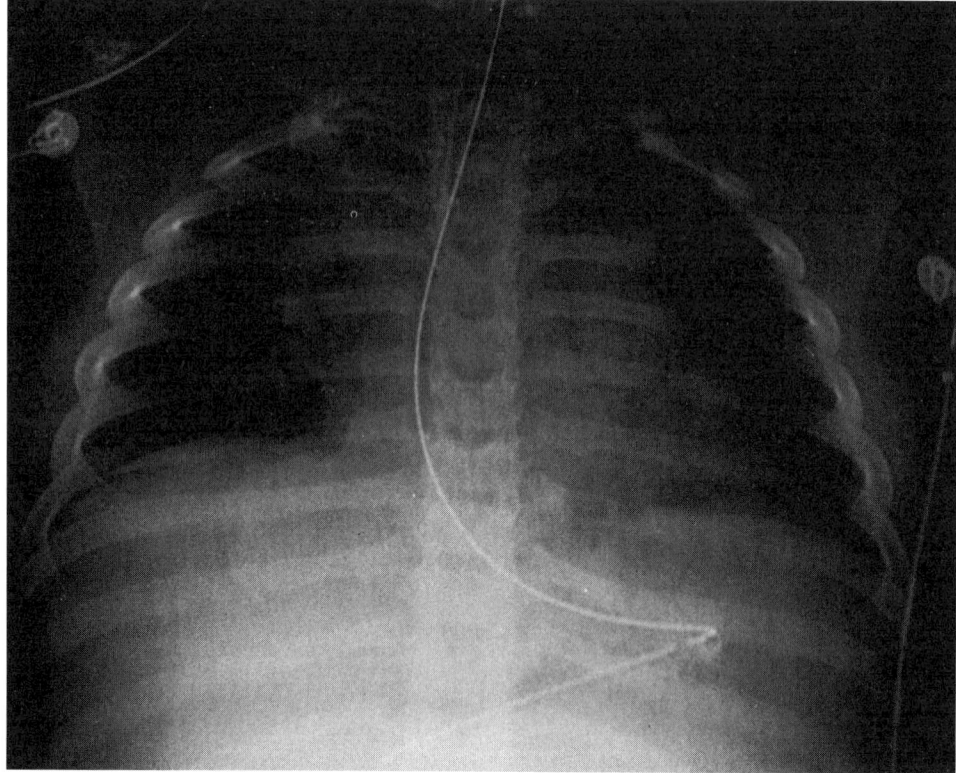

Figure 37.1. Preoperative chest X-ray demonstrating a high diaphragm, small lung volumes, and generalized atelectasis.

formed at this time (Fig. 37.1) demonstrated a high diaphragm, very small lung volumes, and generalized atelectasis.

PHYSICAL EXAMINATION

The girl's temperature was 93.0°F, her heart rate was 115 beats/min, her respiratory rate was approximately 30 breaths/min (with self-inflating manual ventilation bag), her blood pressure was 95/54 mm Hg, her height was 132 cm (>95th percentile for age), and her weight was 45 kg (>95th percentile for age).

The patient was a morbidly obese girl with massive generalized edema. There were second- and third-degree burns involving both upper extremities, anterior and posterior trunk, buttocks, posterior and lateral portions of both lower extremities, and the lateral aspect of the left face and neck. Auscultation of the heart revealed a regular rhythm, distant heart sounds, and no audible murmurs. Capillary refill was delayed, and peripheral pulses of the lower extremities were not palpable. Inspection of the thorax revealed barely perceptible chest excursion with positive pressure inspiration. Breath sounds were diminished in all lung fields. The abdomen was distended and tense. Bowel sounds were absent. The patient was alert and followed commands prior to the administration of morphine sulfate, diazepam, and pancuronium bromide.

LABORATORY DATA

Shortly after arrival at the emergency room, arterial blood gas values obtained while the patient was breathing 100% oxygen via a non-rebreather mask revealed pH 7.31, $PaCO_2$ 43 mm Hg, and PaO_2 345 mm Hg. The carboxyhemoglobin was 7.0%. The initial complete blood count was as follows: hemoglobin 16.6 g/dl, hematocrit 46.8%, white blood count 59,900 cells/mm^3, and platelets 435,000 cells/mm^3.

MANAGEMENT

The patient was transported to the operating room. She was anesthetized with fentanyl and vecuronium. A midline incision was made from the sternum to just above the pubis, and the peritoneal cavity was entered. Immediate evisceration of the intestine resulted in dramatic improvement of the patient's respiratory mechanics. The end-tidal CO_2 fell from 108 to 30 mm Hg. A large ventral hernia was then created. Four 20 × 15-cm patches of 2.0-mm Gortex were sewn together to create the silo. In addition, fasciotomies were performed on both lower extremities, with resultant dramatic improvement in perfusion of the distal lower extremities. At the conclusion of the operation, the arterial oxygen saturation was 100%, the end-tidal CO_2 was 30 mm Hg, and the peak inflating pressure was 45 cm H_2O. Arterial blood gas values obtained immediately after the operative procedure revealed pH 7.40, $PaCO_2$ 17 mm Hg, and PaO_2 338 mm Hg. Chest X-ray performed at this time (Fig. 37.2) demonstrated good lung expansion with resolution of the atelectasis and a right pleural effusion. Urinary output resumed at greater than 1.0 ml/kg/hr. The patient's postoperative course was complicated by severe coagulopathy, septic shock, and respiratory failure. On the eighth day of hospitalization, she was taken to the

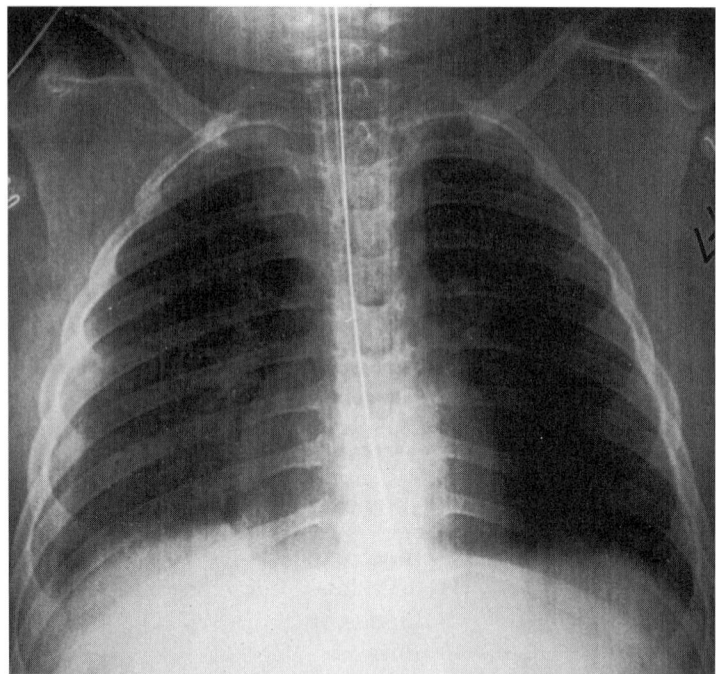

Figure 37.2. Postoperative chest X-ray demonstrating restoration of normal lung volumes, resolution of atelectasis, and a right pleural effusion.

operating room to remove the Gortex silo and partially close the abdominal wall. The patient's septic state and coagulopathy resolved, but she developed chronic respiratory failure. A tracheostomy was performed on the 28th hospital day. She had a protracted ICU course and underwent numerous skin grafting procedures. She remained ventilator-dependent for 6 months and was discharged after a 7-month hospital stay. Pulmonary function tests performed 11 months after her burn injury revealed normal forced vital capacity and forced expiratory volume at 1 second. Maximum voluntary ventilation was 70% of expected, and her arterial oxygen saturations while breathing room air were 98%. During 5 years of follow-up care, she has required only two brief hospitalizations for elective reconstructive procedures and has never been hospitalized for respiratory disease.

DISCUSSION

It is widely recognized that elevated intra-abdominal pressure can result in life-threatening renal (1–9), cardiovascular (1,3,9–17), and pulmonary dysfunction (3,12,16,

18,19). We described a patient whose prominent manifestation of increased intra-abdominal pressure was respiratory failure, although she demonstrated significant renal and cardiovascular dysfunction as well. The only recourse in this situation was to decompress the abdomen, and indeed, the patient's condition improved dramatically following decompression. We deemed the risk of sepsis resulting from the open abdomen to be acceptable in the face of certain death without decompression.

Renal dysfunction secondary to increased intra-abdominal pressure is characterized by decreases in renal blood flow (1,5,9,15), glomerular filtration rate (5,9), and urine output (1,5,9) and increases in renal vascular resistance (5,9). These changes appear to result from the local effects of direct compression rather than from decreases in cardiac output (1,5). Our patient's urinary output resumed following surgical decompression, which is consistent with numerous previously reported cases (2–4,6–8).

The detrimental effects of increased intra-abdominal pressure on the cardiovascular system have been well documented. These include reductions in stroke volume (3,10,15), cardiac output (1,3,5,9–16), venous return (13,16), and splanchnic blood flow (1,5,9,10,15,17) and elevations in cardiac filling pressures (1,3,5,9,11,13, 15,17), systemic vascular resistance (1,5,9,11,13,15), and pulmonary vascular resistance (11).

Elevated intra-abdominal pressure produces dramatic alterations in respiratory mechanics that appear to result from stiffening of the diaphragm/abdomen portion of the chest wall and limitation of lung expansion (19). In a model of increased intra-abdominal pressure in piglets, Mutoh and coworkers (19) demonstrated significant reductions (>40%) in total lung capacity, functional residual capacity, respiratory system compliance, chest wall compliance, and lung compliance after increasing the intra-abdominal pressure to 15 cm H_2O. Elevations in intra-abdominal pressure also lead to impaired oxygenation (3,12,16), presumably because of nonuniformity of ventilation resulting in areas of lung with low ventilation/perfusion ratios, that is, intrapulmonary right-to-left shunting. Oxygenation may be improved by the addition of continuous positive airway pressure or positive end-expiratory pressure; however, this may cause further decrements in cardiac output (11,12) and splanchnic blood flow. In summary, elevated intra-abdominal pressure can produce significant renal, cardiovascular, and pulmonary dysfunction. Surgical decompression may be indicated in situations where supportive care is inadequate to maintain acceptable function of these vital organ systems.

COMMENTARY ▬▬▬▬▬▬▬▬▬▬▬▬▬▬▬▬▬▬▬▬

Surgical decompression as a last resort life-saving maneuver is becoming more common, as in this situation or as in the case of decompressive craniotomy. What is impressive is that this patient survived, given the extent and variety of her pathologies. A working knowledge of the relative compliance of the abdominal and the thoracic cage allows for an understanding and sound management of cases such as this.

References

1. Caldwell CB, Ricotta JJ. Changes in visceral blood flow with elevated intraabdominal pressure. J Surg Res 1987;43:14–20.
2. Celoria G, Steingrub J, Dawson JA, et al. Oliguria from high intra-abdominal pressure secondary to ovarian mass. Crit Care Med 1987; 15:78–79.
3. Cullen DJ, Coyle JP, Teplick R, et al. Cardiovascular, pulmonary, and renal effects of massively increased intra-abdominal pressure in critically ill patients. Crit Care Med 1989;17:118–121.
4. Gehrig JJ, Jr. Oliguria and increased intra-abdominal pressure. JAMA 1985;253:39.
5. Harman PK, Kron IL, McLachlan HD, et al. Elevated intra-abdominal pressure and renal function. Ann Surg 1982;196:594–597.
6. Jacques T, Lee R. Improvement of renal function after relief of raised intra-abdominal pressure due to traumatic retroperitoneal haematoma. Anaesth Intensive Care 1988;16:478–482.
7. Platell C, Hall J, Dobb G. Impaired renal function due to raised intra-abdominal pressure. Intensive Care Med 1990;16:328–329.
8. Richards WO, Scovill W, Shin B, et al. Acute renal failure associated with increased intra-abdominal pressure. Ann Surg 1983;197: 183–187.
9. Shenasky JH, Gillenwater JY. The renal hemodynamic and functional effects of external counterpressure. Surg Gynecol Obstet 1972;134:253–258.
10. Barnes GE, Laine GA, Giam PY, et al. Cardiovascular responses to elevation of intra-abdominal hydrostatic pressure. Am J Physiol 1985;248:R208–R213.
11. Burchard KW, Ciombor DM, McLeod MK, et al. Positive end expiratory pressure with increased intra-abdominal pressure. Surg Gynecol Obstet 1985;161:313–318.
12. Buyukpamukcu N, Hicsonmez A. The effect of C.P.A.P. upon pulmonary reserve and cardiac output under increased abdominal pressure. J Pediatr Surg 1977;12:49–53.
13. Kashtan J, Green JF, Parsons EQ, et al. Hemodynamic effect of increased abdominal pressure. J Surg Res 1981;30:249–255.
14. Lynch FP, Ochi T, Scully JM, et al. Cardiovascular effects of increased intra-abdominal pressure in newborn piglets. J Pediatr Surg 1974;9:621–626.
15. Masey SA, Koehler RC, Buck JR, et al. Effect of abdominal distension on central and regional hemodynamics in neonatal lambs. Pediatr Res 1985;19:1244–1249.

16. Richardson JD, Trinkle JK. Hemodynamic and respiratory alterations with increased intra-abdominal pressure. J Surg Res 1976; 20:401–404.
17. Robotham JL, Wise RA, Bromberger BB. Effects of changes in abdominal pressure on left ventricular performance and regional blood flow. Crit Care Med 1985;13:803–809.
18. Gilroy RJ, Jr, Lavietes MH, Loring SH, et al. Respiratory mechanical effects of abdominal distension. J Appl Physiol 1985;58:1997–2003.
19. Mutoh T, Lamm WJ, Embree LJ, et al. Abdominal distension alters regional pleural pressures and chest wall mechanics in pigs in vivo. J Appl Physiol 1991;70:2611–2618.

Case 38

Robert T. Mansfield and Patrick M. Kochanek

Children's Hospital of Pittsburgh
Pittsburgh, Pennsylvania, USA

HISTORY

A 7-year-old boy fell into a pond while trying to retrieve a toy. He was submerged under 4 feet of water for 10–15 min. The estimated water temperature was 45°–55°F. Emergency medical technicians removed the boy from the pond. He had no spontaneous respirations and was pulseless. Cardiopulmonary resuscitation was initiated, and he was transported to the local hospital. His pupils were fixed and dilated. The cardiac rhythm was ventricular fibrillation, which was electroconverted to asystole and then to a slow sinus rhythm of 30 beats/min. Epinephrine (two doses) and atropine (one dose) were given, and the patient was intubated. By this time, he was having spontaneous respiratory efforts. His vital signs were as follows: temperature 86°F (30°C) rectally, heart rate 82 beats/min, systolic blood pressure 130 mm Hg. Arterial blood gas values were: pH 6.63, pCO_2 156 torr, pO_2 76 torr, HCO_3 15 mmol/l, and base excess − 13 mmol/l. He was placed under warm blankets and received warmed intravenous fluids and sodium bicarbonate. His blood glucose level measured 372 mg%. The next blood gas values showed improvement, with a pH of 7.24, pCO_2 of 30 torr, pO_2 of 111 torr, HCO_3 of 13 mmol/l, and a base excess of − 12 mmol/l. Because there were copious pink frothy secretions from the endotracheal tube, which were consistent with pulmonary edema, positive end-expiratory pressure (PEEP) of 15 cm H_2O was initiated. Before transport to our tertiary-care center, the boy had sluggishly reactive pupils and decorticate posturing. He was assigned a Glasgow coma score of 5, and he required high peak inspiratory airway pressures

(60–80 cm H_2O) with 100% oxygen to maintain adequate arterial saturation by pulse oximetry.

PHYSICAL EXAMINATION

On arrival at the PICU, the child's rectal temperature was 30.4°C (86.7°F), his heart rate was 76 beats/min, and his blood pressure was 96/50 mm Hg. He had very cold extremities with thready pulses and prolonged capillary refill, and diffuse rales throughout all lung fields. Neurologically, he had no eye opening, flexion withdrawal on painful stimuli, and indeterminate verbal response (Glasgow coma score equal to 6). His pupils were sluggishly reactive and symmetric. There was no response to corneal stimulation and only occasional respiratory efforts.

LABORATORY DATA

Arterial blood gas values were as follows: pH 7.53, pO_2 35 torr, and pCO_2 23 torr; serum sodium was 128 mEq/l, potassium was 2.7 mEq/l, and glucose was 512 mg%. The total white blood cell count was $4.7 \times 10^9/l$, and the hemoglobin was 15.7 g/dl. The pO_2 improved rapidly and remained >100 torr.

MANAGEMENT

Management of the patient included external rewarming, and within 3 hours of admission to the PICU (approximately 8 hours after the accident) the boy's rectal temperature was 36.8°C (98.2°F). Because of severe peripheral vasoconstriction and a suspicion of high vascular resistance, infusions of dobutamine (10 µg/kg/min) and sodium nitroprusside (1–2 µg/kg/min) were started. A pulmonary artery catheter was inserted and revealed a cardiac index of 2.3 l/m²/min, pulmonary capillary wedge pressure of 2 mm Hg, high vascular resistance in both the systemic and pulmonary beds, and a mixed venous saturation of 49%. Volume infusion raised the cardiac index to 4.7 l/m²/min and the mixed venous saturation to 70%. Over the initial 36 hours, the vital signs remained in the normal range except for a temperature of 39.5°C once, with the temperature occasionally in the 38°C range. Metabolic abnormalities corrected, perfusion improved, and pulmonary edema resolved. In the first few hours the patient required high airway pressures (peak 44 cm H_2O, PEEP 16 cm H_2O) with a rate of 20 breaths/min and 60% oxygen, but by 48 hours postaccident, as the lung compliance improved, the airway pressures were lowered (peak 38 cm H_2O and PEEP 8 cm H_2O) and only 40% oxygen was needed.

On the first PICU day, painful stimuli produced decorticate posturing and eye opening (Glasgow coma scale 6), and the boy reacted to endotracheal tube suctioning by jerking his body. Corneal reflex was absent, and there was no response to nasopharyngeal irritation. An electroencephalogram revealed the absence of a normal background rhythm, but reaction to stimuli, low-amplitude admixture of slow and fast frequencies primarily in the β and τ range with lack of a well-developed posterior rhythm, and no seizures.

On the third PICU day, the patient had pupils that were 3 mm and not reactive to light, no response to painful stimuli (no motor response, no eye opening, no verbal response (Glasgow coma scale 3), no corneal reflex, and a "weak" oculocephalic reflex. Earlier in the day, the boy reportedly opened his eyes to command. His head CT scan was normal, with no edema, good grey-white differentiation, normal-sized ventricles and sulci, and no evidence of infarct. A stable xenon CT cerebral blood flow (CBF) study revealed hyperemia (CBF 70–112 ml/100 g/min) at an arterial pCO_2 of 40 torr, but the CBF decreased to between 40 and 60 ml/100 g/min when the arterial pCO_2 was lowered to 30 torr (Fig. 38.1) , indicating intact CO_2 reactivity.

On the fourth PICU day, the boy showed extreme hypertonicity and bruxism, and he remained comatose. We considered the prognosis for this child to be very guarded and that the eventual outcome was quite likely to be poor, based on his initial clinical appearance and his neurologic condition 3 days after the accident.

On the fifth hospital day, the patient opened his eyes spontaneously, was thrashing all extremities, withdrew to pain, had reactive pupils and normal corneal reflex. He was successfully extubated. The following day he said, "What are you doing?" to a nurse, and had good visual fixation. This dramatic improvement was astonishing to all.

He was transferred from the ICU to the ward on day 8. He remained combative, agitated, and withdrawn, occasionally making simple requests (such as, "I want water"). On day 19, he was transferred to a rehabilitation facility, where he continued to show gradual improvement. He was diagnosed with hyperactivity and a movement disorder

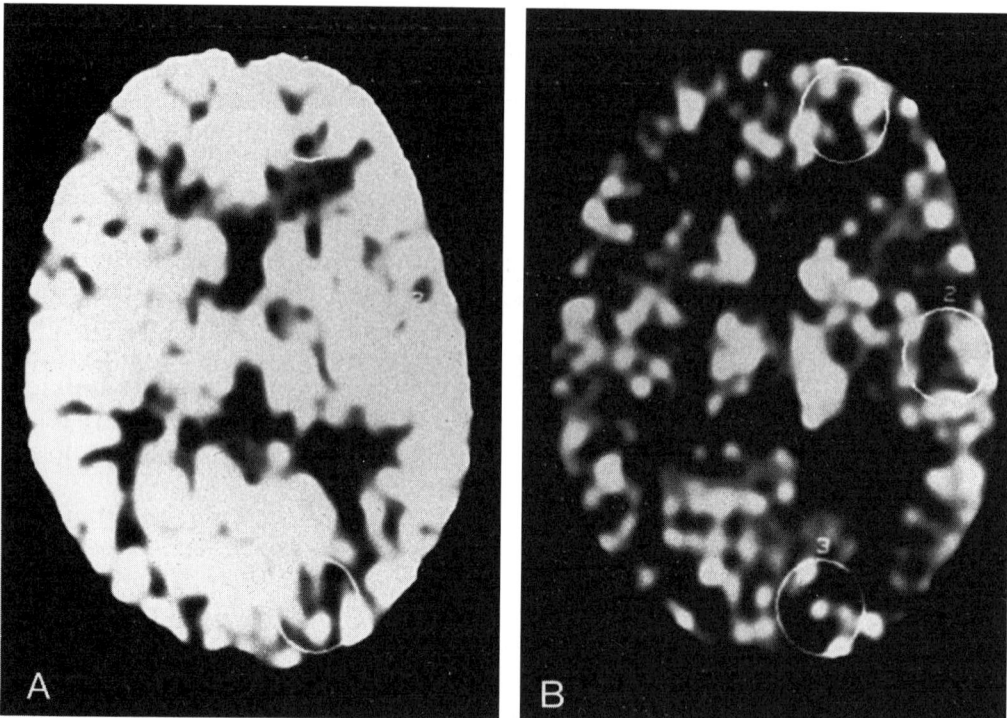

Figure 38.1. Stable xenon CT cerebral blood flow (CBF) scan demonstrating excessive CBF (70–112 ml/100 g tissue/min) at an arterial pCO_2 of 40 torr (*A*). Despite hyperemia, there is intact CBF reactivity to changes in pCO_2 with an appropriate reduction of flow (to 40–60 ml/100 g tissue/min) at pCO_2 of 30 torr (*B*).

characterized by dystonia and choreoathetosis. He was treated with Sinemet and methylphenidate, with marked improvement. On a recent visit to the neurology clinic 2 years after his near-drowning event, he is in the appropriate grade for his age, although he has mild learning disabilities and hyperactivity.

DISCUSSION

We report this case of near-drowning for several reasons. First, it re-emphasizes the difficulty in predicting neurologic outcome in the setting of intra-asphyxial hypothermia. The case also presents an excellent opportunity to discuss current knowledge of the implications of hypothermia and hyperthermia associated with cerebral ischemia. Lastly, the interpretation of the interesting results of the cerebral blood flow study in this patient and cerebral blood flow in the postarrest setting merit discussion.

Predicting Outcome

There are certain features of this child's history that might have led us to be optimistic about his neurologic outcome. Most importantly, he was submerged in cold water and was hypothermic (rectal temperature 30°C) on initial presentation. Biggart and Bohn (1) studied 55 pediatric near-drowning victims, 27 of whom were in cardiopulmonary arrest, as was our patient. Of these 27, 13 had an initial temperature of >33°C and either died or had severe neurologic impairment. However, of 14 patients in cardiopulmonary arrest but with temperature <33°C, 4 survived intact. There are several reports in the literature of dramatic recoveries after cold water drowning (2,3), presumably due to the cerebroprotective effects of hypothermia. Also, our patient had spontaneous respirations after the initial resuscitation. Jacobsen et al. (4) noted that 13 of 26 nearly drowned children who had spontaneous respirations after their initial resuscitation recovered with little or no residual neurologic impairment, whereas the 13 who were apneic either died or suffered severe neurologic impairment. Another piece of data favoring a good outcome was the Glasgow coma score of 6 when the boy was admitted to the PICU. Allman et al. (5) found that of those patients with a Glasgow coma scale of >5 at the time of presentation to the PICU, most are neurologically intact at discharge, but only 50% do well if the Glasgow coma scale is 4 or 5, and all do poorly if it is 3.

In contrast, other factors about our patient predicted a poor outcome. Peterson (6) noted that the need for cardiopulmonary resuscitation in the emergency facility and submersion time >6 minutes are invariably associated with severe anoxic encephalopathy. Similarly, if we were to score our patient according to the method of Orlowski (7), he would receive a 3 (for pH <7.1, submersion time >5 min, and cardiopulmonary resuscitation in the hospital), which was found to predict death or severe neurologic impairment in 89% of cases. Other authors have stated that a low pH by itself is associated with a poor outcome (1,8). Hyperglycemia (our patient's initial blood glucose was 372 mg%) is associated with severe neurologic damage after near-drowning (9). In this study, all children who died or had severe neurologic impairment had an initial blood glucose level >300 mg%, and only one of four who went on to complete recovery had a glucose level >300 mg%. Our patient had an initial Glasgow coma scale of 5, which falls between the good and bad ranges described by Dean and Kaufman (10). They predict a good outcome if the initial Glasgow coma scale is 6 or greater, and a poor outcome if it is 4 or less, but none of the patients in their series had a score of 5. Also, "eyes-closed coma" at 3 days after an arrest is associated with a 96% chance of poor outcome in adults (11). Although there are features in this case consistent with both a good and a bad neurologic outcome, in the absence of hypothermia a negative outcome would be far more likely.

Hypothermia

Hypothermia is protective in the setting of near-drowning (1). The medical literature contains numerous examples of dramatic recoveries after prolonged submersion in cold water (2,3). The everyday use of hypothermia during cardiac surgery is testimony to its protective effects. In the past few years there have been an increasing number of studies regarding the cerebroprotective effects of hypothermia induced before (12) and after (13) ischemic insults to the brain, and there is currently a resurgence of hope for the therapeutic potential of induced hypothermia after a variety of brain insults (14,15). Even small differences of 2°–3°C in the postischemic temperature can improve the neurologic outcome in experimental animal models (16).

To date, the use of hypothermia induced after near-drowning has been controversial and unproven. Conn vigorously recommended induced hypothermia as part of the "HYPER" protocol (17), although prospective data were lacking. In an abstract, Maggi et al. reported improved outcome in comatose near-drowning patients with the use of hypothermia (30 ± 1°C) and pentobarbital (18). In a later study, these authors demonstrated that similar results were obtained using hypothermia with or without pentobarbital, suggesting that hypothermia was the protective factor (19). However, these studies were done at different times and involve other therapies (e.g., hyperventilation, osmotic diuretics) that may have a confounding effect, and in the latter published study there was no control group without hypothermia. Bohn and Biggar retrospectively evaluated the use of hypothermia and barbiturate therapy and found no improvement in the frequency of neurologic salvage, and an increase in infectious complications (20). In summary, accidental hypothermia sustained during a near-drowning event can offer protection against cerebral ischemia, but randomized prospective studies on induced hypothermia as a therapeutic modality are lacking in humans.

The urgency of rewarming depends on the cardiovascular stability of the patient. When he arrived at the PICU, our patient was still poorly perfused with a low mixed venous saturation and was believed to be unstable. Therefore, he was rewarmed in a short time. Unfortunately, perhaps through overwarming or an endogenous febrile response, the boy we treated had mild hyperthermia for some of the first 24 hours postaccident. Studies in animal models of cerebral ischemia suggest that it is important that hyperthermia not occur after an ischemic brain insult, because this has been shown to worsen the degree of insult (21,22). Fever in the postarrest patient should be aggressively treated. Furthermore, in the absence of hemodynamic instability, patients should be allowed to passively rewarm once a temperature of approximately 34°C has been achieved.

Cerebral Blood Flow

Our patient had excessive cerebral blood flow (CBF) 2 days after the insult, with intact CO_2 reactivity (i.e., a 4.5% decrease in CBF per torr decrease in P_aCO_2, with normal being approximately 3% [16]). Patterns of CBF after ischemic insults have been delineated in both animal and human studies. In general, there is a very transient period (0–5 min) of hyperemia followed by a variable period (hours to days) of low flow (23,24). CBF will normalize in those subjects sustaining a milder insult who would be expected to have good recovery, but in those with more severe insults, CBF often becomes excessive in relation to the metabolic needs of the brain (so-called "uncoupling of flow" or "luxury perfusion"). Beckstead studied 25 patients who were comatose after cardiac arrest, and noted low CBF and $CMRO_2$ (cerebral metabolic rate of O_2 consumption) at 2–6 hours postresuscitation (25). By 24–48 hours, both flow and metabolism were increasing, with CBF increasing disproportionately more than $CMRO_2$. Nearly all of these patients died. Cohan et al. found that patients with good neurologic recovery after cardiac arrest had relatively normal CBF, whereas those patients who died without regaining consciousness all had excessive CBF beginning around 15 hours postarrest (26). In some of these patients, the hyperemia eventually progressed to profound hypoperfusion before brain death. These studies suggest that the finding of absolute or relative hyperemia after an ischemic brain insult carries a poor prognosis, as does very low flow.

There are two clinical studies on CBF in pediatric near-drowning. Beyda collected such data on 34 patients (27). Intact survivors had CBF that was slightly low at 12 hours and returned toward normal by 24 hours (there were no normal control subjects in his study). Patients with a vegetative outcome had CBF that became relatively high at 24–48 hours, and then fell. In patients who died, the flows became quite low by 24 hours. Ashwal et al. found low CBF in nonsurvivors after near-drowning (measured at 24–48 hours) and a dichotomy in those with a persistent vegetative state, some having normal flows and some having low flows (9).

A recent study by Connors et al. (28) on near-drowning in children shows that those children with a poor neurologic outcome had a higher ratio of CBF to $CMRO_2$, suggesting uncoupling of flow. There was no information regarding CO_2 reactivity.

In the only study we found that evaluated CO_2 reactivity in the postarrest setting (29), it was noted that patients who eventually regained consciousness had intact CO_2 reactivity. The only other human studies describing CO_2 reactivity concern trauma patients, and the findings are consistent with the little that is known about the postarrest situation. Nordstrom et al. showed a positive correlation between good outcome and preserved CO_2 reactivity (30), and Jaggi et al. found that the loss of CO_2 reactivity is associated with a fatal outcome (31). No information is available regarding the *combination* of delayed postarrest hyperemia with intact CO_2 reactivity—the findings observed in our patient.

COMMENTARY

The case described demonstrates the difficulty in predicting neurologic outcome of a hypothermic near-drowning victim, even with numerous poor prognostic indicators at initial presentation and a poor neurologic examination at 3 days. After a true *cold water* near-drowning episode, attempts at prognostication should be made with great caution, and a longer period of observation than that traditionally applied after normothermic cardiorespiratory arrest may be indicated. While there remains variability and controversy concerning the management of these patients, it is important to remember that hyperthermia can be detrimental after an ischemic brain insult. Therefore one should avoid overwarming (*primum non nocere*), and passive rewarming is recommended when cardiovascular stability is present and a temperature of about 34°C has been reached. The time course and patterns of CBF and cerebral metabolic rate after neurologic insult are still being investigated in humans, although much is known from animal data. Coupled with other diagnostic information, the increasing availability of the noninvasive stable xenon CT scan CBF technology may prove useful in helping to make more accurate predictions of outcome, and also in guiding therapies if these become available in the future.

This patient was treated at a center that has a mandate of interfacing the clinical and basic science realms in the field of resuscitation. Undoubtedly, these clinical observations linked with excellent basic sciences will yield changes that will continue to benefit our patients.

References

1. Biggart MJ, Bohn DJ. Effect of hypothermia and cardiac arrest on outcome of near-drowning accidents in children. J Pediatr 1990; 117:179–183.
2. Young RSK, et al. Neurological outcome in cold water drowning. JAMA 1980;244:1233–1235.
3. Siebke H, Rod T, et al. Survival after 40 minutes submersion without cerebral sequelae. Lancet 1975;1:1275–1277.
4. Jacobsen W, Mason LJ, Briggs BA, Schneider S, Thompson JC. Correlation of spontaneous respiration and neurological damage in near-drowning. Crit Care Med 1983;11:487–489.
5. Allman FD, Nelson WB, Pacentine GA, McComb G. Outcome following cardiopulmonary resuscitation in severe pediatric near-drowning. Am J Dis Child 1986;140:571–575.
6. Peterson B. Morbidity of childhood near-drowning. Pediatrics 1977; 59:364–370.
7. Orlowski JP. Prognostic factors in pediatric cases of drowning and near-drowning. Ann Emerg Med 1979;8:176.
8. Fandel I, Bancalari E. Near-drowning in children: clinical aspects. Pediatrics 1976;58:573–579.
9. Ashwal S, Schneider S, et al. Prognostic implications of hyperglycemia and reduced cerebral blood flow in childhood near-drowning. Neurology 1990;40:820–823.
10. Dean JM, Kaufman ND. Prognostic indicators in pediatric near-drowning: the Glasgow coma scale. Crit Care Med 1981;9:536–539.
11. Levy DE, Caronna JJ, et al. Predicting outcome from hypoxic ischemic coma. JAMA 1985;253:1420.
12. Busto R, Dietrich WD, et al. Small differences in intra-ischemic brain temperature critically determine the extent of ischemic neuronal injury. J Cereb Blood Flow Metab 1987; 7:729–738.
13. Busto R, Dietrich WD, Globus M, Ginsberg MD. Postischemic moderate hypothermia inhibits CA, hippocampal ischemic neuronal injury. Neurosci Let 1989;101;299–304.
14. Dietrich WD. The importance of brain temperature in cerebral injury. J Neurotrauma 1992;9(suppl 2):S475–485.

15. Clifton GL, Allen S, et al. Systemic hypothermia in treatment of brain injury. J Neurotrauma 1992;9(suppl 2):S487–495.
16. Ackerman RH. The relationship of regional cerebrovascular CO_2 reactivity to blood pressure and regional resting flow. Stroke 1973; 4:725–731.
17. Conn AW, Edmonds JE. Near-drowning in cold fresh water: current treatment regimen. Can Anaesth Soc J 1978;25:259.
18. Maggi JC, Allman F, Nussbaum E. Early use of hypothermia and pentobarbital therapy in pediatric near-drowning. CCM 1984;12: 281.
19. Nussbaum E, Maggi JC. Pentobarbital therapy does not improve neurologic outcome in nearly-drowned, flaccid-comatose children. Pediatrics 1988;81:630–634.
20. Bohn DJ, Biggar WD, et al. Influence of hypothermia, barbiturate therapy, and intracranial pressure monitoring on morbidity and mortality after near-drowning. CCM 1986; 14:529.
21. Kuroiwa T, Bonnekoh P, et al. Prevention of postischemic hyperthermia prevents ischemic injury of CA_1 neurons in gerbils. J Cereb Blood Flow Metab 1990;10:550–557.
22. Dietrich WD, Busto R, et al. Effects of normothermic versus mild hyperthermic forebrain ischemia in rats. Stroke 1990; 21: 1318–1325.
23. Hossman KA, Lechtabe-Gruter, Hossman V. The role of cerebral blood flow for the recovery of the brain after prolonged ischemia. Z Neurol 1973;204:281–299.
24. Singh NC, Kochanek PM, et al. Uncoupled cerebral blood flow and metabolism after severe global ischemia in rats. J Cereb Blood Flow Metab 1992;12:802–808.
25. Beckstead JE, Tweed WA, Lee J, MacKeen WL. Cerebral blood flow and metabolism in man following cardiac arrest. Stroke 1978;9: 569–573.
26. Cohan SL, Mun SK, Petite J, Correia J, DaSilva AT, Waldhorn RE. Cerebral blood flow in humans following resuscitation from cardiac arrest. Stroke 1989;20:761–765.
27. Beyda DH. The prognostic value of measuring regional cerebral blood flow in the neuro-compromized paediatric patient. In: Wade J, et al, eds. Current problems in neurology: impact of functional imaging in neurology and psychiatry. London: J Libbey, 1987:145–150.
28. Connors R, Frewen TC, Kissoon N, et al. Relationship of cross-brain oxygen content difference, cerebral blood flow, and metabolic rate to neurologic outcome after near-drowning. J Pediatr 1992;121: 839–844.
29. Love JT, Darby JM, Yonas H, Nemoto EM. CO_2 reactivity and cerebral blood flow in comatose survivors of cardiac arrest [Abstract]. Crit Care Med 1989;S146.
30. Nordstrom C-H, Messeter K, Sundbarg G, Schalen W, Werner M, Ryding E. Cerebral blood flow, vasoreactivity, and oxygen consumption during barbiturate therapy in severe traumatic brain lesions. J Neurosurg 1988;68:424–431.
31. Jaggi JL, Obrist WD, Gennarelli TA, et al. Relationship of early cerebral blood flow and metabolism to outcome in acute head injury. J Neurosurg 1990;72:176–182.

Case 39

Jorge E. Montes and Arno L. Zaritsky

Children's Hospital of the King's Daughters
Norfolk, Virginia, USA

HISTORY

A 5½-month-old infant boy was brought to the pediatrician's office because of fever, poor feeding, and decreased activity. The temperature for the previous 3 days ranged from 38.3°–39.5°C. His parents reported that the infant was not moving as much as usual. While dressing him, his mother noticed a red rash on his trunk and abdomen; there were no other signs or symptoms. The only medication administered was acetaminophen for his fever. The child's pre- and postnatal history were unremarkable, his developmental milestones were appropriate for his age, and his immunizations were current.

PHYSICAL EXAMINATION

At the pediatrician's office, the infant's vital signs were as follows: temperature 39°C, heart rate 160 beats/min, and respiratory rate 30–45 breaths/min. The baby was irritable but consolable, and seemed to be quite alert otherwise. The pediatrician noticed that the boy was not moving all four extremities as much as expected for his age. There was rhinorrhea, an injected oropharynx, and neck flaccidity. The infant was unable to hold his neck up, which represented a marked change according to the parents. Multiple small cervical lymph nodes were palpable. There was a fine red rash over the trunk and abdomen; in some

Table 39.1.

Date	Hb	Hct	10⁶ WBC	% POL	% LYM	Plate 10⁹	ESR	PT	PTT	Na / K	Cl / CO₂	GLUC / BUN	AST / ALT
7/21*	12.5	38	8.6	38	55	425				142 / 4.1	108 / 17	96 / 11	
7/24†	11	34	7.0	20	75	348	5	11.9	24.2	131 / 4.9	100 / 19	180 / 9	40 / 10
8/4	10.5	32	7.3	35	56					140 / 4.8	104 / 19	102 / 2	

	HSV IFA	CMV EIA	ADENO	ECHO	COX	Polio
Admission	<1:16	40	Neg	Neg	Neg	
3rd Hospital week	<1:16	39	Neg	Neg	Neg	
4th Hospital week						

Abbreviations: Hb, hemoglobin; Hct, hematocrit; WBC, white blood cell count; POL, polymorphonuclear lymphocytes; LYM, lym tin time; GLUC, glucose; BUN, blood urea nitrogen; AST, aspartate transaminase; ALT, alanine transaminase; CPK, creatinine antibody test; CMV, cytomegalovirus; EIA, enzyme immunoassay; ADENO, adenovirus; ECHO, echovirus; COX, coxsackie antigen.
* 7/21 community hospital.
† 7/24 children's hospital.

areas the rash was petechial. The chest was clear with good air entry bilaterally, and there was a tachycardia to 160 beats/min, without murmurs. There were symmetric pulses and 2-second capillary refill. The liver was palpable 2 cm below the right costal margin, the spleen was not palpable, and no other masses were noted. The infant was alert, but with generalized hypotonia, and he was areflexic. He had bilateral upgoing toes. There were no focal findings. The office nurse noted that the baby did not react to blood drawing, starting of an intravenous line, a suprapubic tap, and a lumbar puncture.

The boy was admitted to a local community hospital. He was started on intravenous fluids, intravenous antibiotics, and oral acetaminophen. His laboratory data are seen in Table 39.1. Over the subsequent 2 days, his respiratory status continued to deteriorate: his breathing became diaphragmatic, his cry and cough were weak, and he did not have a gag reflex. At this point, the patient was transferred to the Children's Hospital of the King's Daughters for further evaluation and treatment.

| CPK / LDH | Ion CA / PHOS | Mg | Blood Culture | WBC | RBC | CSF | | | | | | Latex Panel | Viral Bacterial Cultures |
						% Pol	% Lym	Gluc	Prot	Gram Stain		
		—	Neg	0	600	0	0	21	78	Neg	Neg	Neg
168 236	5.0 —	1.8	Neg	0	0	0	0	58	39	Neg	Neg	Neg
				1	0	100	0	63	19	Neg	Neg	Neg

Serology

| | | Epstein-Barr Virus | | | |
Rubella	TOXO	Nuc Ag	VCA IgM	VCA IgG	EA IgG
Not IMM	Neg	Neg	Neg	1:640	Neg
Not IMM	Neg	<1:20	Neg	Neg	Neg
		<1:20	Neg	Neg	Neg

phocytes; Plate, platelets; ESR, erythrocyte sedimentation rate; PT, prothrombin time; PTT, partial thromboplas-
phosphokinase; LDH, lactic dehydrogenase; Neg, negative; HSV, herpes simplex virus; IFA, indirect fluorescent
virus; Polio, poliovirus; IMM, immune; VCA, viral capsid antigen; EA, early antigen complex; Nuc Ag, nuclear

Upon arrival at the PICU, his vital signs were as follows: temperature 38.3°C, heart rate 116 beats/min, blood pressure 84/50 mm Hg, respiratory rate 60 breaths/min, and his weight was 7.7 kg. He was noted to be alert but quite anxious and in marked respiratory distress, only using his diaphragm to breathe. There was clear rhinorrhea, facial symmetry, neck flaccidity, and an inability to move his head from side to side. No rashes were noted, his breathing was diaphragmatic, with air entry decreased bilaterally, and the patient had no cough or gag. Normal heart sounds were appreciated without murmurs, pulses were symmetric, and capillary refill was 2 seconds. The abdomen was soft, and the liver was palpable 2 cm below the right costal margin; there were no other masses or visceromegaly. The rectal sphincter was atonic. The infant was flaccid and unable to move any of his extremities to painful stimulation. He was alert, but had generalized hypotonia. Deep tendon reflexes were absent. He had upgoing toes bilaterally. Both sensory and motor levels were thought to be at C5–C6.

MANAGEMENT

It was evident that this infant was in impending respiratory failure; therefore, an endotracheal tube was placed emergently. Neurologic and neurosurgical evaluations were obtained. A spinal tap, myelogram, and enhanced CT scan of the cervical spine were done. The following morning, a magnetic resonance imaging (MRI) of his cervical spine was obtained (Fig. 39.1A).

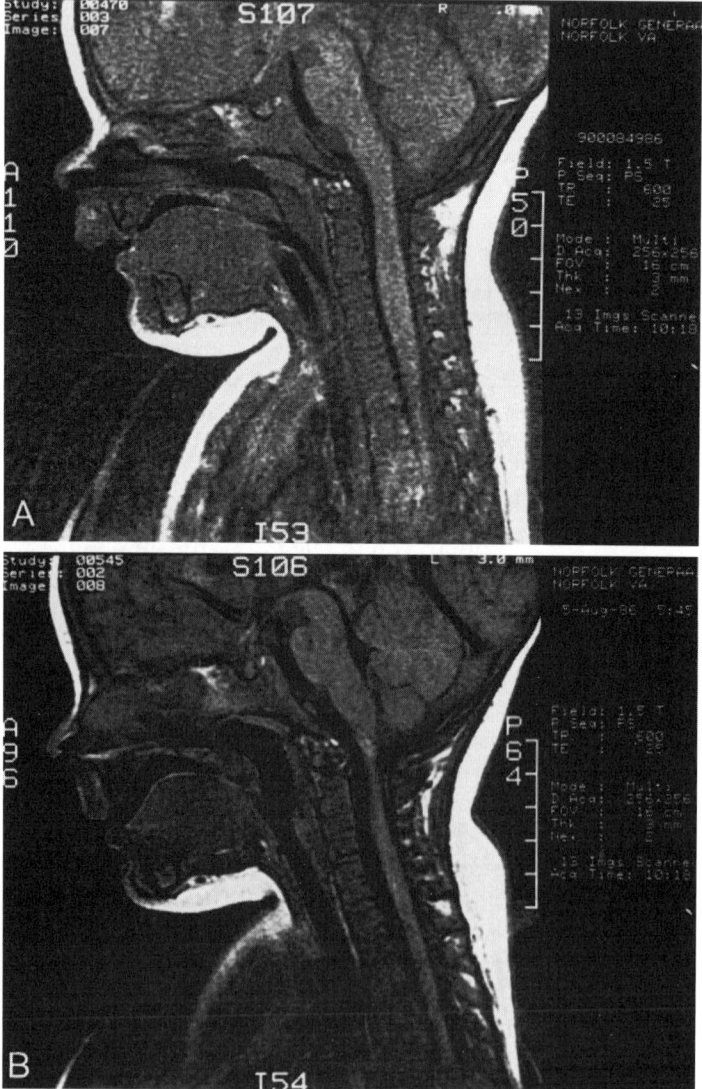

Figure 39.1. *A,* On the day after admission the T1-weighted midsagittal image shows fusiform swelling of the cervical cord, especially at C5–C6 levels. *B,* 10 days later the cervical cord appears normal.

Our patient, like 5 of the 69 other patients with acute transverse myelitis described in the three pediatric series, needed mechanical ventilation for a total of 17 days. He was given corticosteroids, as recommended by several authors (1,2). The rest of his therapy was supportive. There was quick resolution of the edema of his spinal cord as demonstrated on a follow-up MRI done on day 9 of his hospitalization (Fig. 39.1B). The patient never recovered any motor function, and he was eventually discharged home. He has had several hospitalizations for management of recurrent pulmonary infections. At the present time, 6 years later, he is wheelchair bound, has normal intellect, but has marked scoliosis for which a surgical procedure is being considered.

DISCUSSION

This 5½-month-old infant was examined for an acute febrile illness accompanied by rhinorrhea, an injected oropharynx, cervical adenopathy, petechial skin rash, palpable liver, and acute quadriplegia with normal mental status. The level of his neurologic injury was believed to be C5–C6. He required airway protection and mechanical ventilation shortly after PICU admission. The differential diagnosis of acute-onset quadriplegia is outlined in Figure 39.2.

By clinical history and physical examination, we established that this patient had spinal quadriplegia. A number of congenital malformations have a clinical appearance of spinal quadriplegia in this age group.

Arachnoid cysts of the spinal cord are very rare in infancy, and are usually asymptomatic and discovered incidentally. They can be single or multiple and are usually located in the thoracic spine. They rarely cause quadriplegia. This diagnosis was ruled out by MRI of the spine.

Arteriovenous malformations of the spinal cord are also very uncommon in infancy. The youngest patient described in the literature was a 1-yr-old infant (3). Only 14% of the patients described by Scarff and Reigel (3) became symptomatic before 5 years of age. Early paraplegia was the presenting symptom in about one-third of the children. When subarachnoid hemorrhage was the initial manifestation, the malformation was more likely to be located in the cervical region of the spinal cord, in which case MRI is diagnostic (4,5). Although the patient we described had 600 red blood cells in his initial spinal tap, we ruled out that diagnosis with our neuroimaging studies.

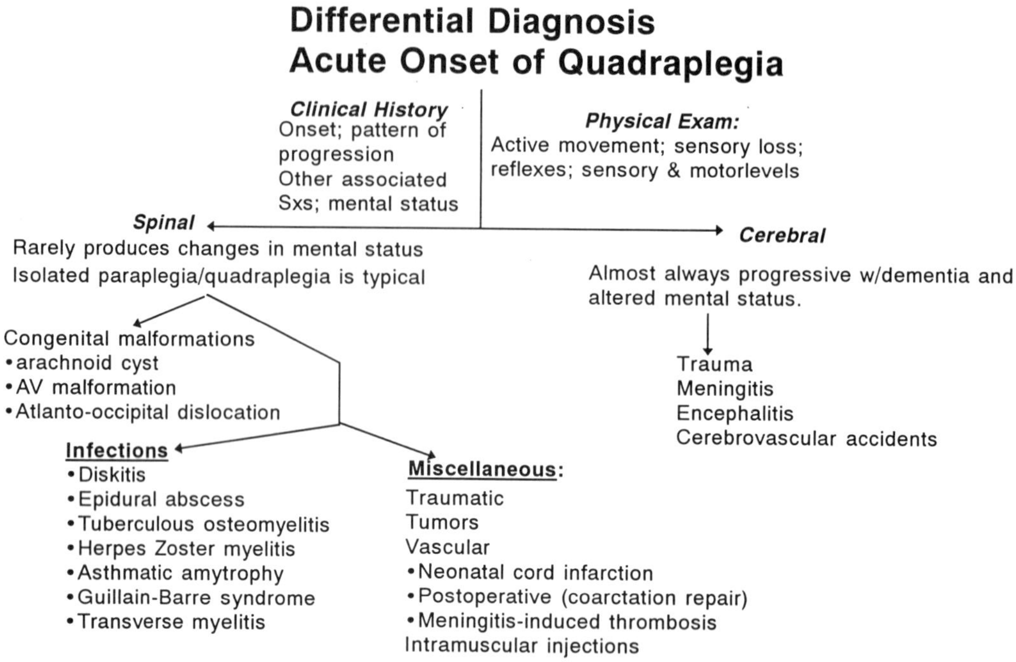

Differential Diagnosis
Acute Onset of Quadraplegia

Clinical History
Onset; pattern of
progression
Other associated
Sxs; mental status

Physical Exam:
Active movement; sensory loss;
reflexes; sensory & motorlevels

Spinal
Rarely produces changes in mental status
Isolated paraplegia/quadraplegia is typical

Cerebral
Almost always progressive w/dementia and
altered mental status.

Congenital malformations
• arachnoid cyst
• AV malformation
• Atlanto-occipital dislocation

Trauma
Meningitis
Encephalitis
Cerebrovascular accidents

Infections
• Diskitis
• Epidural abscess
• Tuberculous osteomyelitis
• Herpes Zoster myelitis
• Asthmatic amytrophy
• Guillain-Barre syndrome
• Transverse myelitis

Miscellaneous:
Traumatic
Tumors
Vascular
• Neonatal cord infarction
• Postoperative (coarctation repair)
• Meningitis-induced thrombosis
Intramuscular injections

Figure 39.2. Flow chart showing the differential diagnosis of acute onset quadriplegia.

Atlantoaxial dislocation can be traumatic or part of a number of congenital syndromes much as Morquio and Klippel-Feil syndromes, mucopolysaccharidoses, and several types of chondrodysplasias. Asymptomatic subluxation is reported in 20% of children with Down's syndrome (6); symptomatic dislocation in these patients is much less common. Clinical history, physical examination, and neuroimaging studies ruled out this diagnosis.

Other miscellaneous conditions such as *trauma, tumors, vascular problems,* and *Transverse myelitis induced by intramuscular injections* (7) can all be ruled out in this patient.

Most likely this patient's quadriplegia is related to an infectious process. *Diskitis* is a relatively common disorder in childhood. It is said to be a benign, self-limited inflammation or infection of the intervertebral disc space. The peak incidence has been reported at 2–3, 5.3, or 7.5 years (8–10) and it is twice as common among girls (8). There are very few cases reported in patients <1 year of age and none <6 months of age. The great majority of cases involve the thoracic and lumbar spine. To our knowledge there are <10 reported cases of cervical spine involvement; none of these patients was <6 months of age and none presented with flaccid quadriplegia as did our patient. The etiology remains obscure and controversial. Some authors proposed an infectious origin; others suggest that the process is more likely traumatic. In one series (10), 50% of cultures from the blood or intervertebral space grew *Staphylococcus aureus*; others have isolated *Haemophilus influenzae* from similar specimens (11). Most authors agree that the infecting organism is blood borne (9).

The clinical presentation of diskitis is quite variable, but patients are not systemically ill. Low-grade temperature, irritability, and pain are common features. Other symptoms vary with age. Refusal to stand and ambulate accompanied by "hip irritability in extension" (positive log roll) are the most common clinical findings in patients <3 years of age. Abdominal pain with reluctance to ambulate are the most common symptoms in patients >3 years of age. The white blood cell count and erythrocyte sedimentation rate are usually elevated, and the diagnosis is confirmed by MRI of the spine. Clinical presentation and diagnostic evaluation excluded this condition in our patient.

Epidural abscess is a relative uncommon condition in infancy; there are less than 60 cases described in the literature. It is known to occur in any age group including infancy, but there are only 8 cases described in children <1 year of age (12). Of these, 4 patients were <2 months of age (13). Children may be seen with fever, malaise, irritability or excessive crying with handling or movement, and reluctance to lie prone. Particularly in younger children, the diagnosis was not made until weakness or paralysis occurred. Most reported series (12–14) document that the majority of the abscesses are located in the dorsal epidural space at the level of the lower thoracic and lumbar spine.

The most common mechanism of spinal epidural abscess in children is by hematogenous spread (13). Reported sites of original infection included upper and lower respiratory tract, skin and soft tissue infections, and upper and lower urinary tract infections. Other cases have been described following blunt trauma that produced a hematoma that became infected. Epidural anesthesia, lumbar puncture, and disk surgery may also result in a local epidural hematoma. Spinal epidural abscess can also be seen from direct extension of a local infection, most commonly vertebral osteomyelitis (12,13).

The organism most frequently seen is *S. aureus*; other organisms include *Streptococcus pneumonia* and Gram-negative organisms when the process is associated with urosepsis. Other laboratory data may include an elevated white blood cell count and erythrocyte sedimentation rate. The cerebral spinal fluid (CSF) findings are usually not specific; there may be an elevated protein concentration with normal glucose and mild leukocytosis. CSF cultures are almost always negative.

The diagnosis can be confirmed by myelography and CT scan of the spine. MRI of the spine is the technique of choice because of its superior resolution and lack of invasiveness (12,15).

Spinal epidural abscess is considered by most to be a surgical emergency, especially in patients with rapidly deteriorating neurologic function (16), as was seen in our patient. The clinical features of our patient were quite compatible with this diagnosis, but this possibility was ruled out by our radiologic findings.

Tuberculous osteomyelitis is a very uncommon condition in infancy and childhood. There are two published series of cervical spine tuberculosis with presenting ages ranging from 2–65 years; 26 were <10 years old, but none were <2 years (17,18). Like epidural abscess, this condition occurs more frequently in the lower thoracic and upper lumbar spine. The organism reaches the vertebral body via hematogenous dissemination. The infection usually starts at one vertebral body and spreads to adjacent vertebrae and surrounding tissues. Based on clinical, radiographic, and operative findings, we observe two different types of disease: that seen in children <10 years old, and that which occurs in patients >10 year old (the "adult" type). The infection in younger children is characterized by more diffuse and extensive involvement, forming large abscesses with a low incidence of paraplegia or quadriplegia. The adult type was more localized and produced less pus, but had a higher incidence of paraplegia (80%). Four patients <4 years of age had stridor and cyanotic spells and two others had dysphagia.

There may be a cord granuloma in the absence of vertebral disease. The clinical symptoms are chronic. In the series we observed, most patients have been symptomatic for at least 1 month before they were seen by a physician. A small but significant number of patients had a second lesion lower on the spine.

Several imaging techniques can be diagnostic, including plain radiographs of the spine, technetium bone scan, and MRI. The clinical picture and radiographic findings ruled out this condition in our patient.

Herpes zoster myelitis usually occurs in persons whose immunity has been compromised. The cord becomes involved within 2–3 weeks after the appearance of the trunk rash (19). The cord involvement is characteristically ipsi-lateral to the rash, with motor disfunction predominating, followed by spinothalamic involvement and, less often, posterior column sensory deficit. The cervical spine may be affected, but myelitis can occur at any level. This diagnosis can be easily ruled out in our patient.

Two other entities, *asthmatic amyotrophy* and *Guillain-Barré* syndrome, were excluded based on the clinical history, physical examination results, and CSF findings.

The diagnosis of acute transverse myelitis was confirmed in the patient we treated by myelogram, enhanced CT cervical myelogram, and MRI of the cervical spine, which showed cervical cord enlargement beginning at the level of C2–C3 and extending down to the T1–T2 level. The maximum enlargement was found at the level of C4–C5. The cord tapered to a normal caliber at the level of T2–T3 (Fig. 39.1A).

Acute transverse myelitis is a relatively uncommon but not rare condition in childhood. Precise incidence figures in children are not available, but one of the three pediatric series (1,2,20) quotes an annual incidence of 1 per 1.34 million population (2). There have been cases reported in patients ranging from 7 months–15 years of age, with the mean age of onset being 9 years. The etiology remains unclear, but the onset has been noted to follow an acute febrile illness in approximately 30–60% of patients described. In some instances, the original illness resolved prior to the development of clinical symptoms, suggesting a postinfectious immune etiology. There also have been a number of patients who developed this syndrome after minor trauma or exercise, suggesting a possible vascular event at the level of the anterior vertebral artery. A multitude of infectious agents have been implicated including measles, varicella, mumps, rubella, herpes simplex and zoster, echovirus, cytomegalovirus (CMV), hepatitis viruses, and *Mycoplasma pneumoniae*. Our patient developed symptomatology during an acute febrile episode. Comprehensive viral cultures from stool, nasopharynx, and CSF were all negative. CMV was grown from his urine, but there was no change in his CMV-specific IgG antibody titers from admission compared with a specimen obtained 3 weeks later. This finding suggests that the presence of a positive CMV culture was just an incidental finding. Studies for Epstein-Barr virus demonstrated that his viral capsid antigen (VCA)-IgG antibodies were elevated at 1/640, but his EBNA-EIA, EA IgM, and VCA-IgM remained negative on a second sample obtained 3 weeks later (Table 39.1). The presence of an acute febrile illness accompanied by rhinorrhea, an injected oropharynx, cervical adenopathy, petechial skin rash, and hepatomegaly with a complete blood count that showed a relative neutropenia with marked lymphocytosis and an elevated VCA IgG titer for Epstein-Barr virus that subsequently became negative (Table 39.1) makes the diagnosis of infectious mononucleosis very provocative, although we did not grow the virus from nasopharyngeal secretions. These clinical and laboratory findings meet the diagnostic criteria of Sumaya and Ench (21,22), who described the clinical and serologic manifestations of Epstein-Barr virus infectious mononucleosis in children. To our knowledge, the patient we treated may represent the first case of Epstein-Barr virus-associated transverse myelitis described in the literature.

Other diagnostic investigations of the infant included multiple sclerosis profile in the CSF that was normal, somatosensory-evoked responses that were consistent with myelopathy at the level of C5–C6, and brainstem visual- and auditory-evoked responses that were considered to be within normal limits.

COMMENTARY

The case of our patient illustrates the diagnostic approach to patients with cervical pathology. I think it is appropriate to amplify one issue that was mentioned, namely, children with Down's syndrome. As pediatricians, we care for a great number of patients with Down's syndrome. Atlantoaxial instability in Down's syndrome is the subject of much literature. Identification of patients at risk for injuries due to that instability is problematic. X-rays of flexion and extension of the neck may identify abnormalities, but the implications for patients is unclear. The most common circumstance under which these issues become germane is when we intubate patients with Down's syndrome. While intubating, the triple maneuver involves not only extension but anterior displacement of the neck. This is theoretically a more disrupting maneuver compared with the simple extension maneuver that the radiologist performs. This disruption can be exaggerated when the stability offered by the musculature is eliminated by neuromuscular blocking agents. Since a specific and sensitive test for children at risk is not readily available, it is important to be cognizant of the problem and sensitive to gentle manipulation of the neck in patients with Down's syndrome.

References

1. Paine RS, Ryers RK. Transverse myelopathy in childhood. Am J Dis Child 1953;85:151–163.
2. Dunne K, Hopkins JJ, Shield LK. Acute transverse myelopathy in childhood. Dev Med Child Neurol 1986;28:198–204.
3. Scarff TB, Reigel DH. Arteriovenous malformations of the spinal cord in children. Child Brain 1979; 5:341–351.
4. Doppman JL, DiChiro G, Dwyer AJ, et al. Magnetic resonance imaging of spinal arteriovenous malformations. J Neurosurg 1987;66: 830–834.
5. DiChiro G, Doppman JL, Dwayer AJ, et al. Tumors and arteriovenous malformations of the spinal cord: assessment using MR. Radiology 1985;156:689–697.
6. Chaudry V, Sturgeon C, Gates AJ, et al. Symptomatic atlantoaxial dislocation in Down's syndrome. Ann Neurol 1987;21:606–609.
7. Weir MR, Fearnow RG. Transverse myelitis and penicillin. Pediatrics 1983;71:98.
8. Magera BE, Klein SG. Radiological case of the month, diskitis. Am J Dis Child 1989; 143:1479–1480.
9. Crawford AH, Kucharzyk DW, Ruda R, et al. Diskitis in children. Clin Orthop 1991;266:70–79.
10. Wenger DR, Bobechko WP, Gilday DL. The spectrum of intervertebral disc-space infection in children. J Bone Joint Surg 1978;60A: 100–108.
11. Amit H, Hurvitz H, Korn-Lubetzki I, et al. Gower's sign in discitis in children. Clin Pediatr 1986;25:459–461.
12. Rockney R, Ryan R, Knuckey N. Spinal epidural abscess: an infectious emergency, case report and review. Clin Pediatr 1989;28: 332–334.
13. Enberg RN, Kaplan RJ. Spinal epidural abscess in children, early diagnosis and immediate surgical drainage is essential to forestall paralysis. Clin Pediatr 1974;13:247–253.
14. Danner RL, Hartman BJ. Update of spinal epidural abscess: 35 cases and review of the literature. Rev Infect Dis 1987;9:265–274.
15. Angtuaco E, McConnell J, Chadduck W, et al. MR imaging of spinal epidural sepsis. AJR 1987;149:1249–1253.
16. Leys D, Petit H. Spinal epidural abscess: surgery or conservative treatment? Clin Neurol Neurosurg 1988;90:181–182.
17. Hsu LC, Leong JC. Tuberculosis in the lower cervical spine (C2–C7): a report of 40 cases. J Bone Joint Surg 1984;66B:1–4.
18. Fang D, Leong JCY, Fang HSY. Tuberculosis of the upper cervical spine. J Bone Joint Surg 1983;65B:47–50.
19. Devinsky O, Wun–Sook C, Petito CK, et al. Herpes zoster myelitis. Brain 1991;114:1181–1196.
20. Adams C, Armstrong D. Acute transverse myelopathy in children. Can J Neurol Sci 1990;17:40–45.
21. Sumaya CV, Ench Y. Epstein-Barr virus infectious mononucleosis in children. I. Clinical and general laboratory findings. Pediatrics 1985;75:1003–1010.
22. Sumaya CV, Ench Y. Epstein-Barr virus infectious mononucleosis in children. II. Clinical and general laboratory findings. Pediatrics 1985;75:1011–1019.

Case 40

**Francis X. McGowan, Jr.,
Linda K. Snelling, and
Howard A. Zucker**
*Yale New Haven Hospital
New Haven, Connecticut, USA*

HISTORY

The patient was a 27-month-old girl with the diagnosis of tricuspid and pulmonic atresia, D-transposition of the great arteries, and ventricular septal defect, who was status post bilateral Blalock-Taussig shunts in the neonatal period. She did fairly well until increasing cyanosis and waning growth necessitated a Fontan procedure and shunt takedown. This situation was complicated by bilateral pleural fluid accumulations that were present from the early postoperative period. The right pleural collection remained despite continuous thoracostomy drainage and a low-fat diet. Because of this persistent and large chylothorax and the possible surgical risk to the child, we decided to attempt chemical pleurodesis 2 months after her Fontan procedure.

In the PICU, we placed a lumbar epidural catheter, using intravenous ketamine (1 mg/kg) sedation in order to provide adequate analgesia over the thoracic dermatomes and minimize possible hypoventilation (from pain, splinting, or systemic narcotics). Initial epidural analgesia was produced with 0.03 mg/kg of preservative-free morphine solution, 1.25 mg/kg bupivicaine, and 2.5 μg/kg epinephrine injected into the epidural space. A sensory level of T6 was obtained without incident. Two and one-half hours later and ½ hour prior to pleurodesis, the epidural analgesia was reinforced with 0.5 mg/kg bupivicaine, and a total of 4 mg/kg lidocaine and 3 μg/kg epinephrine over approximately 20 minutes; a sensory level of T4 was obtained.

Heart rate, blood pressure, and oxygen saturation were unchanged following each of the epidural injections, indicating that this was not an intravenous injection. There were no signs of intrathecal local anesthetic injection.

It was the choice of the surgical team to utilize erythromycin for the pleurodesis. Therefore, 20 ml of a preservative-free saline solution containing 1 g of erythromycin lactobionate was instilled into the right pleural cavity via the indwelling thoracostomy tube, which was then clamped. There was no evidence of respiratory distress, desaturation, or pain following this instillation.

Subsequent events are summarized in Table 40.1. Two hours after the most recent epidural injection of local anesthetic and 1½ hours after the beginning of pleurodesis, the patient experienced two to three brief (10- to 15-second) right focal seizures. The last of these became generalized tonic-clonic and was treated with mask oxygen and 0.05 mg/kg diazepam, with immediate termination of apparent seizure activity. At this point, the sclerosis solution was drained from the pleural cavity. One-half hour later (2 hours after beginning pleurodesis), the patient was noted to have an approximately 10–15% decrease in blood pressure and cool extremities, which responded to 10 ml/kg intravenous saline.

Table 40.1. Toxicity following Intrapleural Erythromycin-Benzyl Alcohol Instillation

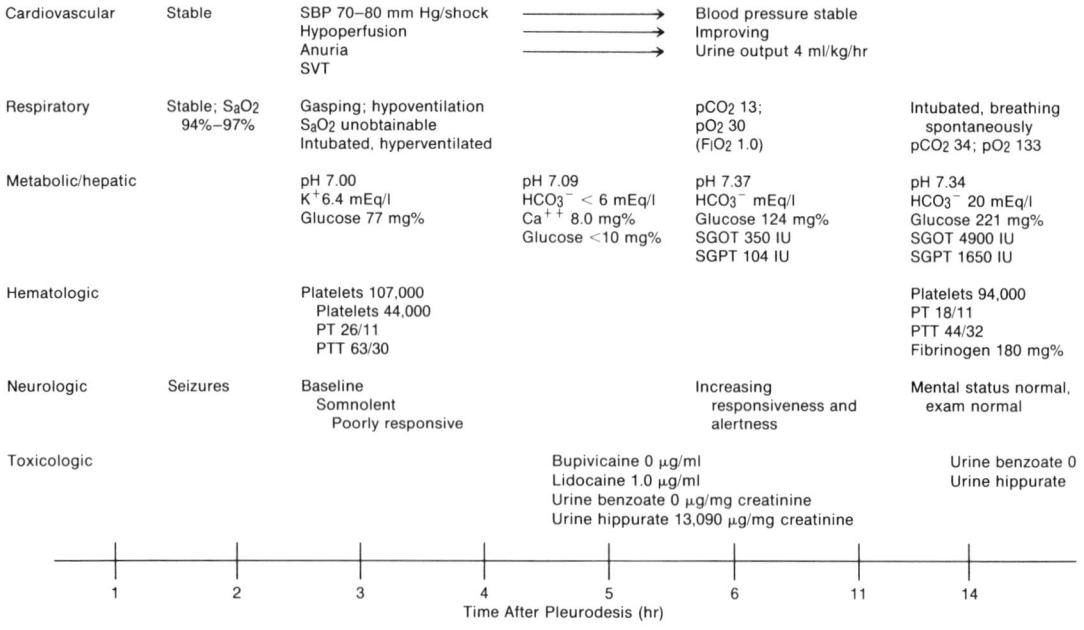

Cardiovascular	Stable	SBP 70–80 mm Hg/shock ———⟶ Hypoperfusion ———⟶ Anuria ———⟶ SVT		Blood pressure stable Improving Urine output 4 ml/kg/hr	
Respiratory	Stable; S_aO_2 94%–97%	Gasping; hypoventilation S_aO_2 unobtainable Intubated, hyperventilated		pCO_2 13; pO_2 30 (F_iO_2 1.0)	Intubated, breathing spontaneously pCO_2 34; pO_2 133
Metabolic/hepatic		pH 7.00 K^+ 6.4 mEq/l Glucose 77 mg%	pH 7.09 HCO_3^- < 6 mEq/l Ca^{++} 8.0 mg% Glucose <10 mg%	pH 7.37 HCO_3^- mEq/l Glucose 124 mg% SGOT 350 IU SGPT 104 IU	pH 7.34 HCO_3^- 20 mEq/l Glucose 221 mg% SGOT 4900 IU SGPT 1650 IU
Hematologic		Platelets 107,000 Platelets 44,000 PT 26/11 PTT 63/30			Platelets 94,000 PT 18/11 PTT 44/32 Fibrinogen 180 mg%
Neurologic	Seizures	Baseline Somnolent Poorly responsive		Increasing responsiveness and alertness	Mental status normal, exam normal
Toxicologic			Bupivicaine 0 µg/ml Lidocaine 1.0 µg/ml Urine benzoate 0 µg/mg creatinine Urine hippurate 13,090 µg/mg creatinine		Urine benzoate 0 Urine hippurate

Time axis (hr): 1 2 3 4 5 6 11 14 — Time After Pleurodesis (hr)

Abbreviations: SBP, systolic blood pressure; SVT, supraventricular tachycardia; SGOT, serum glutamic oxalocetic transaminase; SGPT, serum glutamic pyruvic transaminase; PT, prothrombin time; PTT, partial thromboplastin time.

Her condition remained stable for the next $1\frac{1}{2}$ hours (now $3\frac{1}{2}$ hours after intrapleural erythromycin and 4 hours after the most recent epidural local anesthetic administration). At this point, the child became progressively somnolent, with gasping, labored respirations, and had an unobtainable blood pressure by noninvasive means with extremely poor peripheral perfusion. She had two episodes of a wide complex tachydysrhythmia consistent with supraventricular tachycardia with aberrant conduction that was treated successfully with synchronized cardioversion. Initial blood gas analysis revealed a profound metabolic acidosis (venous pH 7.0; Table 40.1). The patient was immediately treated with intubation and hyperventilation, sodium bicarbonate, dobutamine and epinephrine infusions, as well as approximately 75 ml/kg colloid over the ensuing 90 minutes. Despite these measures, her clinical picture remained one of profound circulatory collapse. Laboratory investigations revealed coagulopathy and elevated hepatic enzymes. An echocardiogram during this interval demonstrated good ventricular filling volume and contractility.

Over the following 4–6 hours (approximately 6–12 hours after pleurodesis), her condition steadily improved, with resolution of the hypoperfusion, metabolic acidosis, and hypoglycemia. Fresh frozen plasma was administered for 18 hours, after which her coagulopathy continued to improve. Abnormal hepatic enzyme levels improved similarly. Blood cultures were negative. The child recovered fully, and her pleural effusion did not recur.

As serum bupivacaine concentration 3 hours after the onset of cardiovascular collapse was undetectable, and a serum lidocaine concentration was 1 μg/ml (therapeutic range 1.5–5.0 μg/ml). Urine assayed for benzoic acid (the oxidation product of benzyl alcohol) and hippuric acid (the glycine conjugate of benzoate) contained 13,090 mg hippurate/mg creatinine (normal 0–500 mg creatinine) Benzoic acid was undetectable. A subsequent urine sample obtained 8 hours later contained 64 mg/mg creatinine hippurate and was likewise free of benzoic acid. A review of the contents of the various medications and their diluents revealed that the child had received 180 mg (18.4 mg/kg) of benzyl alcohol in the erythromycin pleurodesis solution. All other drugs administered for the prior 7 days were free of benzyl alcohol.

DISCUSSION

The potential for toxicity in infants from benzyl alcohol that is used as a preservative in multiple-dose vials of numerous intravenous medications is well established (1,2). The major manifestations of this toxic insult include neurologic decompensation, gasping respirations, severe metabolic acidosis, and cardiovascular collapse. This report describes an apparent episode of benzyl alcohol toxicity in a child who underwent pleurodesis with a benzyl alcohol-containing erythromycin solution.

The metabolic fate of benzyl alcohol involves oxidation to benzoic acid followed by conjugation with glycine to form hippuric acid (both in the liver), with subsequent excretion in the urine. The toxic reactions previously described in infants may be, in part, related to immaturity of their oxidative and conjugative pathways. Animal toxicity studies (3,4) have demonstrated a broad range of effects, including respiratory stimulation and failure, cardiovascular collapse with arterial smooth muscle relaxation, vasodilation, severe hypotension, sedation, seizures, and death. Many of these effects, along with profound acidosis and coagulopathy, were seen in the premature infants previously reported (1) with the "gasping syndrome" due to benzyl alcohol. The mean dose of benzyl alcohol received by these infants was 153 mg/kg/day. A subsequent report has also linked kernicterus and intraventricular hemorrhage to the administration of this agent to neonates (5). Although the patient described in this report received just over 18 mg/kg benzyl alcohol, we speculate that the toxicity in this case was due to rapid absorption and metabolism in the 1- to 2-hour period following injection into the pleural cavity. It is also possible that fragile circulatory status and hepatic congestion associated with Fontan physiology played roles in her course. Local anesthetic toxicity can also cause seizures and cardiac arrest. Toxicity from bupivacaine may be exacerbated by cyanosis. However, local anesthetic doses administered to this patient were well below those associated with toxicity, as were plasma concentrations measured subsequently.

Persistent pleural chyle accumulation may occur following traumatic interruption of the thoracic duct, as a congenital malformation, or in the setting of various malignancies. Unchecked chyle loss can result in dehydration, electrolyte imbalance, and reductions in blood proteins, lipids, and lymphocytes. Treatment in infants and young children is controversial. Many authorities recommend a trial (usually 2–3 weeks) of low-fat diet and continuous thoracostomy tube drainage for congenital chylothorax (6). The use of chemical irritants to sclerose the pleura has been most widely used in patients with malignant pleural effusions; tetracycline, erythromycin, talc, and nitrogen mustard have all been employed for this purpose. However, the possible chemical toxicities of these sclerosing solutions have not been reported. Although successful in our patient, most authors believe that nonsurgical treatment is rarely effective in cases of traumatic thoracic duct leak. Given that mortality has been reported to range from 11–83% in those cases resulting from trauma, early attempt at surgical ligation of the duct is most often recommended (6,7). Surgery was not favored in this patient because of her underlying cardiac dysfunction.

In summary, the case of this patient underscores the toxic potential of the benzyl alcohol commonly found in intravenous solutions. It is the first report of toxicity in an older child, and via a nonintravenous route. Heightened vigilance to the presence of this agent and to its myriad effects is certainly warranted.

COMMENTARY

This case illustrates the vigilance necessary to be aware of exactly what we administer to our patients. Preservatives can wreak havoc when administered intravenously with very high dose epinephrine as cautioned in the new American Heart Association cardiopulmonary resuscitation guidelines. Preservatives also can cause problems in unusual circumstances, as this case shows. Intrapleural administration of drugs will often result in prompt and efficient systemic absorption.

Acknowledgments

The authors would like to thank Piero Rinaldo, M.D., Department of Genetics, Yale University School of Medicine, for measuring benzoic acid and its metabolites, and Laura Dillman for secretarial assistance.

References

1. Gershanik J, Boecler B, Ensley H, Mc Closkey S, George W. The gasping syndrome and benzyl alcohol poisoning. N Engl J Med 1982;307: 1384–1388.
2. American Academy of Pediatrics, Committee on Fetus and Newborn and the Committee on Drugs. Benzyl alcohol: toxic agent in neonatal units. Pediatrics 1983;72:356–357.
3. Kimura ET, Darby TD, Krause RA, Brondyk HD. Parenteral toxicity studies with benzyl alcohol. Toxicol Appl Pharmacol 1971;18:60–68.
4. Gruber CM. The pharmacology of benzyl alcohol and its esters: some of the effects of benzyl alcohol, benzyl benzoate, and benzyl acetate

when injected intravenously upon the respiratory and circulatory systems. J Lab Clin Med 1923;9:92–112.

5. Jardine DS, Rogers K. Relationships of benzyl alcohol to kernicterus, intraventricular hemorrhage, and mortality in preterm infants. Pediatrics 1989;83:153–160.

6. Milsom JW, Kron IL, Rheuban KS, Rodgers BM. Chylothorax: an assessment of current surgical management. J Cardiovasc Surg 1985; 89:221–225.

7. Sele JG, Snyder WH, Schreiber JT. Chlothorax. Indications for surgery. Ann Surg 1973;177:245–249.

Case 41

Curt M. Steinhart, Edward J. Truemper, and Edward M. Burton

Medical College of Georgia Hospital and Clinics
Augusta, Georgia, USA

HISTORY

An 8-day-old infant boy was admitted to a pediatric ward at the Medical College of Georgia Hospital and Clinics after referral from his private physician for evaluation of a cool, pale, left lower extremity. The infant was well for his first 7 days of life, until the evening prior to admission when he was noted to be irritable and vomited once. On the day of admission, he remained irritable and vomited two more times. The pallor of the left lower extremity had been noted by the parents 12 hours prior to admission.

The baby had been delivered by cesarean section at 39 weeks' gestation to a mother with poorly controlled diabetes mellitus. The mother had persistent hyperglycemia throughout the pregnancy. She had been hospitalized 1 week prior to delivery for upper respiratory symptoms and received intravenous antibiotics. After an unremarkable delivery, the baby went home with his mother on the fifth day of life. He was breast-fed without difficulty. The infant was the first child of a married couple who were not related. The father was a chicken farmer. Except for the maternal diabetes mellitus, the family history was noncontributory.

PHYSICAL EXAMINATION

Physical examination revealed a heart rate of 126 beats/min, respiratory rate of 40 breaths/min, and temperature of 38.2°C (rectal). Blood pressures were as follows: right arm 120/82 mm Hg, left arm 128/86 mm Hg, right leg 116/80 mm Hg, left leg 54/40 mm Hg. The infant was well-developed with a pale left lower extremity. His anterior and posterior fontanels were full, and his eyes, ears, nose, and throat showed no abnormalities. The neck was supple without adenopathy. His lungs were clear and the heart was regular without murmurs. His abdomen was soft and nontender. His liver and spleen were not enlarged. The baby's left leg was cool and pale and his right leg was warm and moderately red. Brachial and radial pulses were normal and equal bilaterally. The pulses in the right leg were normal, but the left femoral pulse was decreased and the pulses in the left foot were only intermittently palpable. The infant was lethargic. His tone was normal and all infantile reflexes were intact.

LABORATORY DATA

Initial laboratory values included: hemoglobin 19.2 g/dl, hematocrit 57.6%, white blood cell (WBC) count 21,600/mm^3 with a normal differential, platelets 128,000/mm^3. The blood type was O positive; direct Coombs test was negative. Arterial blood gas values on room air were: PaO$_2$ 89 mm Hg, PaCO$_2$ 31 mm Hg, and pH 7.44. Urinalysis revealed a dipstick positive for blood, glucose, ketones, and protein, with a pH of 7.5 and specific gravity of 1.015.

MANAGEMENT

The infant was initially admitted to the pediatric ward, where he continued to feed poorly. Intravenous fluids were added to supplement breast feedings. Elevated blood pressures were frequently noted, particularly in the upper extremities. Abdominal ultrasound did not reveal any masses. Echocardiogram did not reveal aortic coarctation.

On the evening of admission, the infant became more lethargic. A CT scan was obtained that revealed a large posterior fossa hemorrhage (Fig. 41.1). Shortly after the scan, the baby had a seizure and a brief respiratory arrest. He was assisted with bag valve mask ventilation and intubated. He was then transferred to the PICU.

He was initially treated with intravenous phenobarbital to control seizures and mannitol because his fontanels had become increasingly tense. Clotting studies were not obtained prior to fresh frozen plasma administration. Neu-

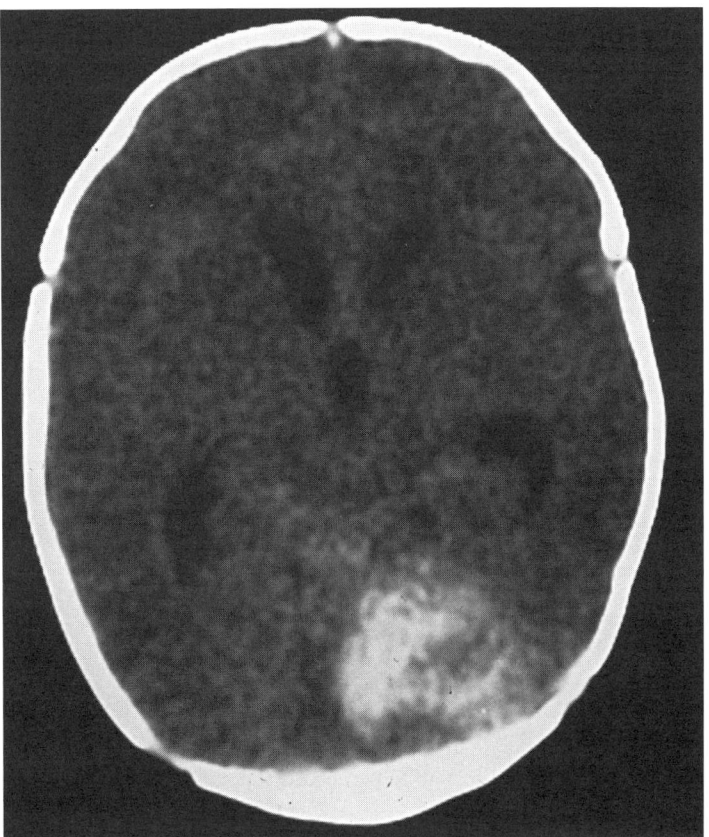

Figure 41.1. Noncontrast CT scan obtained when the infant was admitted demonstrates a large posterior fossa hematoma and subarachnoid hemorrhage. Note the mild ventriculomegaly.

rosurgeons placed a ventriculostomy to monitor intracranial pressure (ICP) and to remove cerebrospinal fluid (CSF) for intracranial pressure control. The initial ICP was 5 torr. CSF studies showed 6 WBC/mm^3, 1810 red blood cells (RBC)/mm^3, protein 480 mg/dl, and glucose 101 mg/dl. During the next 2 days, the patient was stabilized, but hypertension persisted. Sodium nitroprusside by continuous infusion at 1.0–4.0 μg/kg/min effectively controlled blood pressure. Repeat echocardiogram again failed to demonstrate coarctation. Oliguria ensued despite treatment with intravenous furosemide. A repeat abdominal ultrasound showed a thrombus in the abdominal aorta (Fig. 41.2). Surgical consultation was obtained and a consensus was reached that surgical intervention would not be successful. During cardiac catheterization, aortography confirmed the aortic thrombus (Fig. 41.3), and the catheter was placed directly into the thrombus. Intraaortic

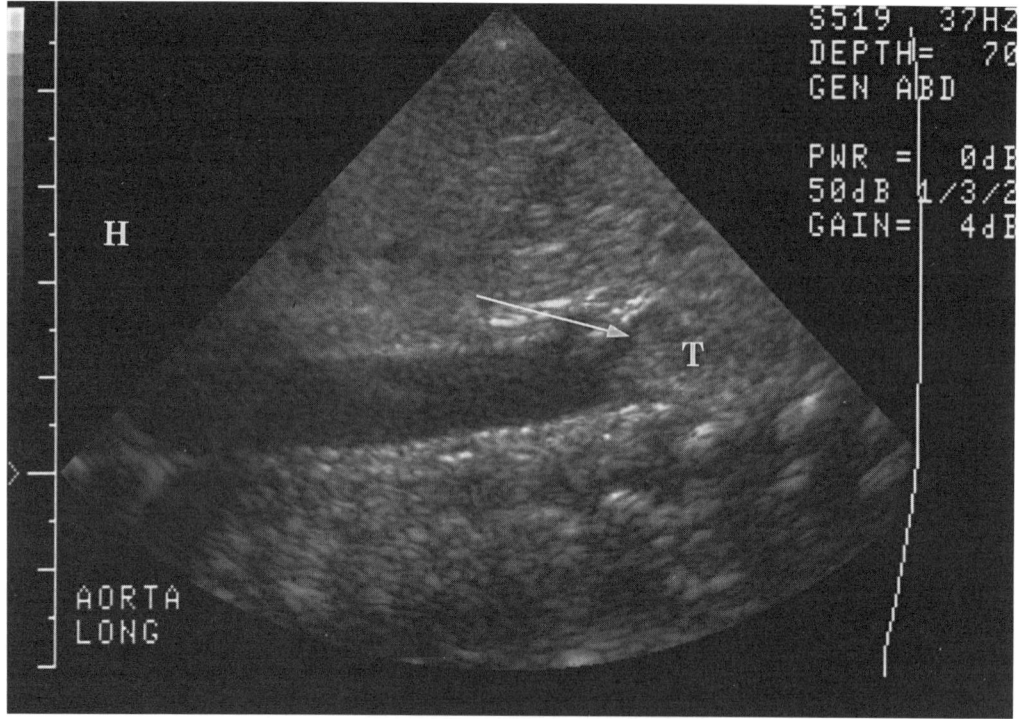

Figure 41.2. Parasagittal abdominal ultrasound shows thrombus (*T*) filling the aorta from the level of the aortic bifurcation to just below the superior mesenteric artery (*arrow*). H = head.

streptokinase was begun at 50 IU/kg/hr, increased to 67 and then 80 IU/kg/hr as urine output and distal pulses did not appear to improve.

Over the next 2 days, oliguria and hypertension persisted despite administration of nitroprusside and hydralazine. On hospital day 7, continuous arteriovenous hemofiltration (CAVH) was begun from the left radial artery to the right femoral vein. On hospital day 9, there was a slight increase in urine output, and by day 10, urine output exceeded 1.0 ml/kg/hr and blood pressure returned to normal. In addition to streptokinase, heparin infusion into the CAVH circuit had been initiated. CAVH was discontinued on hospital day 11.

Intraaortic streptokinase at 80 IU/kg/hr was administered for 9 more days and heparin at 20 U/kg/hr was continued for 14 more days. The baby was extubated on the 16th hospital day. He began to take oral fluids and his neurologic condition gradually improved. The ventriculostomy was maintained for a total of 13 days. There were no periods of increased ICP. Prior to discharge from the ICU, the baby was placed on oral Coumadin (warfarin sodium). Magnetic resonance imaging (MRI) of the brain showed a

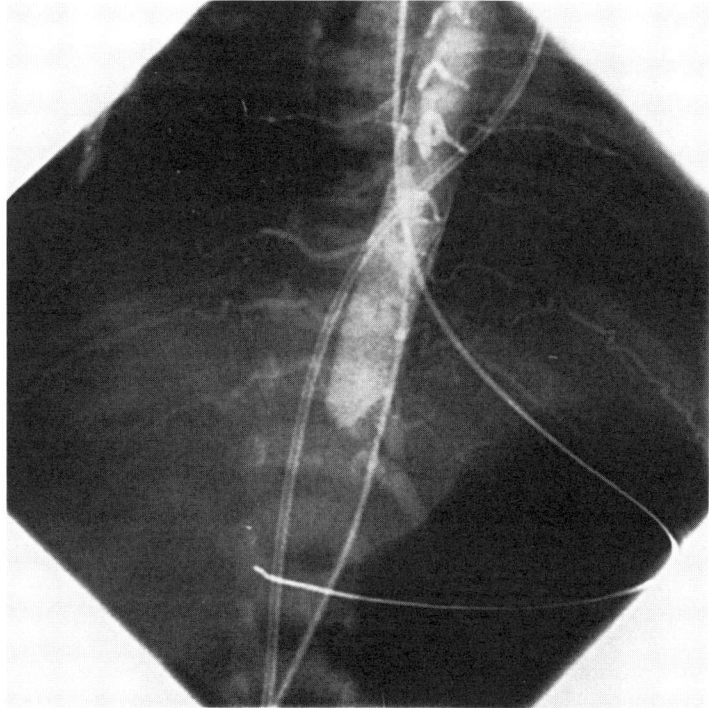

Figure 41.3. Abdominal aortogram demonstrates abrupt discontinuity of the abdominal aorta at the L4 level due to a large thrombus. The aortic catheter is through the thrombus. The adjacent catheter enters the inferior vena cava via the left femoral vein.

subacute subdural hematoma of the tentorium and interhemispheric fissure (Fig. 41.4). The infant was discharged from the hospital on day 34. Follow-up examination at 2 weeks postdischarge and again at 4 months of age revealed a normally growing and developing child.

DISCUSSION

The case of this patient posed a number of diagnostic and therapeutic dilemmas. From the diagnostic standpoint, hypertension and decreased femoral pulses in an 8-day-old infant would usually suggest coarctation of the aorta. Two echocardiograms done several days apart failed to demonstrate coarctation. The initial abdominal ultrasound failed to demonstrate the aortic thrombus, which was readily visible on the repeat study. Intraaortic thrombosis is associated with umbilical artery catheterization, sepsis, dehydration, and coagulation disorders. Maternal diabetes can be associated with a number of these poten-

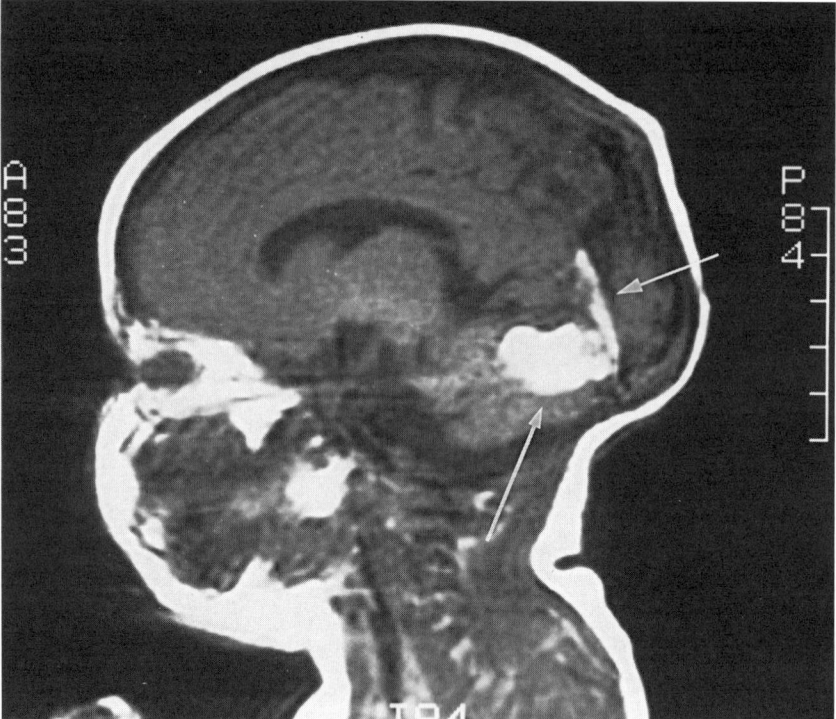

Figure 41.4. Midline sagittal and coronal (not shown) T_1-weighted magnetic resonance images obtained 1 month after hospital admission demonstrate a subacute subdural hematoma of the tentorium (*long arrow*) and interhemispheric fissure (*short arrow*).

tial conditions and also with polycythemia, which could lead to vascular stasis. Poor feeding may have exacerbated the problem with hydration and blood viscosity. Differential flow to the two lower extremities could have "clued" us in to the diagnosis of aortic thrombus earlier, but the initial "normal" abdominal ultrasound proved to be misleading.

The posterior fossa hemorrhage had no obvious etiology. It might have been secondary to hypertension. No coagulopathy was ever uncovered, with a protein C level done while the infant was on Coumadin (2.5 µg/ml; normal 2.7–5.6 µg/ml), which was considered normal for an infant who was receiving an oral anticoagulant and not considered to indicate protein C deficiency. Protein S level was normal at 25 µg/ml (normal 13–32 µg/ml).

Thrombolytic agents were used in the presence of an intracranial hemorrhage with great trepidation. By utilizing direct intraaortic infusion of streptokinase, we sought to limit possible systemic effects that could have resulted in extension of the intracranial bleeding. Support for local intraarterial streptokinase infusion comes from a number of literature citations indicating that successful clot lysis is more often achieved with direct intraarterial infusion than with systemic infusion and that hemorrhagic complications are minimized by avoiding systemic therapy (1–4).

CAVH was utilized to control fluid balance and hypertension. Parenteral nutrition was made possible by our ability to remove fluid extracorporeally.

We were fortunate to have no therapeutic complications. Thrombolytic therapy along with standard anticoagulation resulted in clot dissolution before complications such as bleeding and/or sepsis developed. Concomitant use of systemic anticoagulation continues to be controversial (1,3,4), but prevention of catheter-induced thrombus propagation appears to make heparin therapy a valuable adjunct. When utilized, heparin should be titrated to achieve a partial prothrombin time (PPT) around 1.5 times normal. Monitoring prothrombin time, fibrinogen, fibrin degradation, and antithrombin III levels should be done on an individual basis. Ventriculostomy and repeated CT scanning allowed us to monitor ICP and bleeding. Hydrocephalus did not develop.

This case indicates that careful monitoring for complications of locally infused thrombolytic therapy and anticoagulation may allow successful clot lysis even in the presence of major organ hemorrhage. Intraaortic thrombolysis offers direct, local therapy with less risk of systemic effects. Concomitant use of CAVH allowed improved supportive care, particularly parenteral nutrition for this infant with multiple organ system dysfunction.

COMMENTARY

We seem to be seeing an increase in the number of intravascular clots. These occur either as a presenting illness such as in the case of this patient (and in Case 12) or as a complication of intravascular catheters. The incidence of these clots around catheters is extremely high, but only a small percentage go on to become problematic. Prevention of the catheter-related clots would seem to be the best approach if we are to maintain our intravascular monitoring standards. Heparin-bonded catheters will soon be available and may help. Low-molecular weight heparin shows promise in avoidance of the bleeding complications of anticoagulation. Our (appropriate) aversion to aspirin may need to be reevaluated. Under some circumstances, this or another antiplatelet medication may become a part of our ICU protocol for selected patients who are not at risk for bleeding, but are at risk for intravascular clot formation.

References

1. Becker GJ, Rabe FE, Richmond BD, Holden RW, Yune HY, Dilley RS, Bang NU, Glover JL, Klatte EC. Low-dose fibrinolytic therapy—results and new concepts. Radiology 1983;148:663–670.
2. Ino T, Benson LN, Freedom RM, Barker GA, Aipursky A, Rowe RD. Thrombolytic therapy for femoral artery thrombosis after pediatric cardiac catheterization. Am Heart J 1988;115:633–639.
3. LeBlanc JG, Culham JAG, Chan K, Patterson MW, Tipple M, Sandor GG. Treatment of grafts and major vessel thrombosis with low-dose streptokinase in children. Ann Thorac Surg 1986;41:630–635.
4. Pritchard SL, Culham JAG, Rogers PCJ. Low-dose fibrinolytic therapy in infants. J Pediatr 1985;106:594–598.

Case 42

Barry Gelman,
G. Patricia Cantwell, and
Charles L. Schleien

Jackson Memorial Hospital
Miami, Florida, USA

HISTORY

A 3-week-old baby girl returned to the hospital with fever, generalized seizures, and apnea 1 day after discharge following an uneventful hospitalization for suspected sepsis that was ruled out. This infant was first referred to the emergency room (ER) from a local clinic at 16 days of age with the chief complaints of vomiting and tactile fever. Prenatally, the mother was diagnosed with a urinary tract infection 2 weeks prior to delivery for which she was treated with 7 days of antibiotics. She reported no other intrapartum illnesses and prenatal vitamins with iron were the only other medications taken during pregnancy. Perinatal history was significant for birth at 38 weeks' gestation to a 23-year-old mother, gravida 3, para 0, 0, 2, 0, by vacuum extraction; spontaneous rupture of membranes occurred 15 hours prior to delivery. Apgar scores were 8 at 1 minute, 9 at 5 minutes, and 9 at 10 minutes. Birth weight was 2.66 kg (5 pounds 14 ounces; 10th percentile). Length was 48 cm (25th percentile) and head circumference was 31.5 cm (<5th percentile). The baby received 4 days of phototherapy for indirect hyperbilirubinemia (peak total bilirubin 18.1 mg/dl) and was discharged home on the 10th day of life.

When the infant was admitted to the ER at 21 days of age, her temperature was 101.5°F rectally, her heart rate was 166 beats/min, her respiratory rate was 56 breaths/min, and her blood pressure was 91/40 mm Hg. Her weight was 2.78 kg, with head circumference of 31.5 cm and length of 49 cm. She was alert and active with no distress. Physical examination results were entirely normal. A routine sepsis work-up was performed with laboratory results as follows: white blood cell count 11,600/mm³ with 34% granulocytes, 4% bands, and 57% lymphocytes; hemoglobin 12.1 g/dl; hematocrit 35%; and platelets 566,000/mm³. Lumbar puncture was traumatic, revealing 21,750/mm³ red blood cells and 580/mm³ white blood cells with 92% monocytes and 8% polymorphocytes. The following cerebrospinal fluid (CSF) levels were obtained: protein 165 mg/dl, glucose 39.2 mg/dl, and plasma glucose 100 mg/dl. The CSF Gram stain showed rare white blood cells but no bacteria were seen. Serum electrolytes, urinalysis, and chest X-ray were normal. The infant was admitted to the ward and begun on intravenous ampicillin and cefotaxime. She had no further fever and fed very well throughout the hospitalization. After 72 hours, blood, urine, and CSF bacterial cultures were all negative, and antibiotics were stopped. She continued to do well; however, on hospital day 4, a vesicular lesion was discovered on her back midway between the scapulae, which was thought to be varicella. The infant's mother thought she recalled having had varicella as a young girl; there was no known nosocomial exposure. After 36 hours in isolation, the patient continued to do well and remained afebrile with no new lesions appearing. She was discharged on hospital day 6 with a follow-up appointment scheduled 3 days later.

She returned to the ER the following morning with her mother describing an episode of the baby stiffening with her eyes rolling back, pallor, and apnea. She had fed poorly the night before and had a fever of 101°F at that time. In the morning when she was readmitted, her temperature was 102°F. While in the ER, she had another episode of apnea and a short, nonfocal, generalized seizure lasting less than 1 minute.

PHYSICAL EXAMINATION

Her vital signs at the time of admission were as follows: temperature 101.4°F rectally, heart rate 185 beats/min, respiratory rate 60 breaths/min, and blood pressure 90/52 mm Hg.

She appeared ill, pale, and mottled with mild respiratory distress. Her head circumference was 32 cm, her length was 50 cm, and her weight was 2.7 kg. Her anterior fontanel was open and flat. The pupils were equal and reactive. Her neck was supple and she exhibited opisthotonic posturing. Cardiorespiratory examination results were normal except for mild intercostal retractions. Her abdomen appeared normal. The pulses were normal throughout and capillary refill was 2.5 seconds. Neurologic examination revealed an irritable and lethargic baby who was easily arouseable. There were no focal neurologic findings. The lower extremities were hypertonic but without clonus. There were two vesicular lesions on her midback that appeared scabbed; no other lesions were noted. The remainder of her physical examination results were normal.

LABORATORY DATA

At the time of admission, laboratory data were as follows: arterial blood gas: pH 7.46, pCO_2 31 mm Hg, pO_2 100 mm Hg; HCO_{3-} 22 mEq/l, base excess -0.3, O_2 saturation 98% on room air; white blood cells 11,600/mm^3 with 53% granulocytes, 36% lymphocytes, and 10% monocytes. Hemoglobin was 8.6 g/dl; hematocrit 25%; reticulocyte count 0.7%; platelets 419,000/mm^3; CSF red blood cells 30/mm^3; CSF white blood cells 250/mm^3 with 99% monocytes and 1% polymorphocytes. CSF glucose level was 43 mg/dl, plasma glucose was 80 mg/dl, and CSF protein was 173 mg/dl. Gram stain of CSF was negative for organisms or cells. Electrolytes were: sodium 135 mEq/l, potassium 5.6 mEq/l, chloride 102 mEq/l, and bicarbonate 19 mEq/l. Blood urea nitrogen was 13 mg/dl, creatinine was 0.4 mg/dl, calcium (total) was 9.7 mg/dl, and magnesium was 2.0 mg/dl. Aspartate aminotransferase (AST) was 59 U/l, alanine aminotransferase (ALT) was 41 U/l, and alkaline phosphatase was 136 mU/ml. Urinalysis results were as follows: pH 7.0 specific gravity 1.010, 1–5 white blood cells per high-power field, and 1–5 red blood cells per high-power field. Results were negative for protein, blood, glucose, and urobilinogen.

MANAGEMENT

The infant was stabilized with oxygen delivered by face mask and intravenous hydration. She was loaded with phenytoin 15 mg/kg soon after arrival at the ICU. She was begun on ampicillin 200 mg/kg/d, cefotaxime 150 mg/kg/d, and acyclovir 30 mg/kg/d with the presumptive diagnosis of herpes simplex encephalitis. The following day she had several episodes of rapid blinking and lip smacking; her electroencephalograph (EEG) revealed multiple epileptogenic foci (left more than right) consistent with multifocal status epilepticus. A very attenuated δ frequency background was noted between ictal events. A CT scan of the brain showed diffuse low density in cortical white matter bilaterally, probably representing an immature central nervous system, but was otherwise normal. There were no enhancing lesions with intravenous contrast. With the addition of phenobarbital to her regimen, the seizures improved clinically; however, the EEG still showed a burst suppression pattern with left temporal seizures superimposed upon very slow background activity. She continued to have occasional episodes of lip smacking with a very depressed level of consciousness over the next 5 days. A repeat EEG with therapeutic serum levels of phenytoin and phenobarbital showed improvement without seizure activity; however, electrical activity remained very slow. Magnetic resonance imaging (MRI) of the brain done on the 8th hospital day was significant for an abnormally low signal in the anterior portion of the left temporal lobe on the T1-weighted image. This was believed to represent an acute vascular or infectious event. A Tzanck preparation of the skin lesion was positive for multinucleated giant cells, and herpes simplex virus (HSV) type II was isolated in cell culture from scrapings of the lesion. In addition, CSF anti-HSV IgG had increased as measured by enzyme-linked immunosorbent assay (ELISA) index from the time of admission (2.87) to 14 days later (3.57).

During the second week of hospitalization, the patient improved slowly, with increasing wakefulness and improved feeding. There were no focal neurologic deficits. She did, however, manifest intermittent hypothermia (temperatures 94.7°–95.5°F), generalized hypotonia, and ongoing facial and eye movements that were considered to be myoclonic jerking. The EEG remained slowed without epileptiform activity. After 14 days of intravenous acyclovir, she was discharged to home on phenytoin with follow-up examination scheduled for 2 weeks later.

Ten days later, the infant again returned to the ER with a history of increasing frequency of seizures, vomiting, and blisters on her back. These lesions had been present for 1 or 2 days and were again Tzanck positive. Intravenous acyclovir was restarted and carbamazepine (40 mg/kg/d) was added for seizure control; phenytoin was tapered off over a several-day period. After 21 days of intravenous acyclovir administration, the baby's clinical condition improved somewhat. She was more interactive and began nippling again; however, developmental milestones were severely delayed. A brain CT scan at that time showed diffuse low-density areas throughout both cortices and discrete hypodense lesions in the basal ganglia, thalami, and pons. She was discharged with a regimen of carbamazepine and oral acyclovir (50 mg/d) to continue for another 3 weeks.

DISCUSSION

The PICU physician commonly faces the clinical scenario of an infant or child with fever, seizures, and CSF pleocytosis. It is important to consider HSV encephalitis at the time of admission of such a patient, because the prognosis is poor without early initiation of appropriate treatment. Suspicion should be especially high for newborns, because most mothers may be unaware of their genital infection at the time of delivery. Neonates with HSV encephalitis are seen most often in the second or third week of life with fever, an altered level of consciousness, and sudden onset of seizure activity. These seizures are often focal and difficult to control. An asymmetric neurologic examination, common in older children, may be difficult to appreciate in a neonate. CSF from these patients, classically described as hemorrhagic, may not contain red blood cells early in the course of disease. Only in a minority of patients are skin lesions or other evidence of localized infection present.

Unfortunately, other diagnostic tests are limited in their ability to confirm the presence of HSV encephalitis. The virus is very difficult to isolate from CSF. CT scan of the brain often appears normal in the early stages of illness. MRI may be more sensitive; however, this modality may not be available to all patients. EEG may show focal epileptiform activity, most commonly arising in the temporal lobe. Such findings are only suggestive of the diagnosis, however. Measurement of IgM and IgG anti-HSV in CSF may allow an early diagnosis. Single photon emission computerized tomography (SPECT) may lead to a more rapid diagnosis by identifying regional cerebral perfusion abnormalities. The most reliable method for diagnosis of HSV encephalitis remains a brain biopsy, but because of its invasive nature, its use may not always be desirable. A brain biopsy can help in the diagnosis of other diseases, such as other herpes viruses (cytomegalovirus, Epstein-Barr virus), fungal infections, tuberculosis, toxoplasmosis, and other viral encephalitides (St. Louis, eastern equine, California).

Management principles in caring for a patient with HSV

encephalitis are supportive in nature and can be applied to most acute central nervous system (CNS) infections. Airway management and cardiorespiratory support may be indicated, especially if the level of consciousness is severely depressed. Focal or generalized seizures may be a prominent clinical feature. Aggressive therapy with multiple anticonvulsants may be required for seizure control. Continuous EEG monitoring can be helpful in patients with refractory seizures and is an essential tool if a patient is paralyzed pharmacologically to facilitate mechanical ventilation. The patient with severe encephalitis is at risk for intracranial hypertension due to perivascular infiltration, venous congestion, and diffuse cerebral edema; therefore meticulous attention should be paid to the neurologic examination. Intracranial pressure monitoring may prove useful in extreme cases. Fluid therapy should be closely tailored to the patient's clinical state. The presence of cerebral edema, inappropriate antidiuretic hormone, diabetes insipidus, or cerebral salt wasting can complicate fluid management.

The treatment of choice for suspected or proven HSV encephalitis is administration of intravenous acyclovir, 30 mg/kg/day, in three divided doses for 10–14 days. The drug is well tolerated by pediatric patients and has relatively few, minor side effects including rash, gastrointestinal discomfort, thrombophlebitis, and mild azotemia. Anticipated mortality is 10–15% despite adequate treatment. Between 50% and 70% of patients treated with acyclovir may be expected to experience some morbidity, usually manifested as transient or permanent neurologic impairment. Morbidity is often associated with a delay in diagnosis and treatment. Some patients may have an early relapse or evidence of persistent "low-grade" CNS infection. Several isolated case reports exist describing modest results with prolonged acyclovir therapy (14–21 days) in cases of relapse. Neonates with HSV infection appear to be at significant risk for relapse; 46% of infants will have recurrent skin lesions by 6 months after appropriate therapy. Eight percent of those with encephalitis or disseminated disease will have a CNS relapse within 1 month. The exact pathophysiology of CNS relapse is unknown, although an abnormal neonatal immune response to HSV infection most likely plays a significant role. Investigations are underway to evaluate the efficacy of acyclovir prophylaxis for recurrent HSV infections. Finally, despite state-of-the-art intensive care, the outcome from HSV encephalitis may be devastating, even with timely and appropriate therapy. The potentially poor outcome from this disease should be stressed to parents and family members. Some children will not recover; many children will recover without return to their neurologic baseline.

In summary, HSV may be seen as a nonspecific febrile encephalitis in a healthy infant or child. Focal seizures or focal neurologic findings should raise suspicion of a diagnosis of HSV encephalitis. It is a devastating illness that results in severe neurologic sequelae if left untreated. ICU management should include general supportive measures as well as vigilant neurointensive care. Special attention should be paid to issues of seizure control, intracranial hypertension, and level of neurologic functioning. Because rapid confirmation of the diagnosis is difficult, the clinician should strongly consider early empiric therapy with acyclovir. Treatment with acyclovir has little risk and thus may significantly improve the course of disease and outcome.

COMMENTARY

HSV is a ubiquitous agent. It is unclear why some neonates develop fulminant disease, but most do not. By understanding the differences in immune responses to this pathogen, we will better be able to prevent, diagnose, and treat the disease more effectively. Certainly early recognition and treatment of herpes simplex disease will improve the outlook for symptomatic children.

Suggested Readings

1. Ackerman AD. Meningitis, infectious encephalopathies, and other central nervous system infections. In: Rogers MC, ed. Textbook of pediatric intensive care. Baltimore: Williams & Wilkins, 1992: 1040–1083.
2. Ackerman ES, Tumeh SS, Charron M, English R, Deresiewicv R. Viral encephalitis: imaging with SPECT. Clin Nucl Med 1988;13(9): 640–643.
3. Arvin AM, Prober CG. Herpes simplex virus infections: the genital tract and the newborn. Pediatr Rev 1992;13(3):107–112.
4. Bergstrom T, Alestig K. Treatment of primary and recurrent herpes simplex virus type 2 induced meningitis with acyclovir. Scand J Infect Dis 1990;22:239–240.
5. Bergstrom T, Trollfors B. Recurrent herpes simplex virus type 2 in a preterm neonate: favourable outcome after prolonged acyclovir treatment. Acta Paediatr Scand 1992;80:878–881.
6. Gutman LT, Wilfert CM, Eppes S. Herpes simplex virus encephalitis in children: analysis of cerebrospinal fluid and progressive neurodevelopmental deterioration. J Infect Dis 1986;154:415–421.
7. Hanada N, Kido S, Terashima M, Nishikawa K, Morishima T. Noninvasive method for early diagnosis of herpes simplex encephalitis. Arch Dis Child 1988;63(12):1470–1473.

8. Knezevic W, Carroll WM. Relapse of herpes simplex encephalitis after acyclovir therapy. Aust NZ J Med 1983;13:625–626.

9. Kohl S. Herpes simplex virus encephalitis in children. Pediatr Clin North Am 1988;35(3):465–483.

10. Kohl S. The neonatal human's immune response to herpes simplex virus infection: a critical review. Pediatr Infect Dis J 1989;8:67–74.

11. Pike MG, Kennedy CR, Neville BGR, Levin M. Herpes simplex encephalitis with relapse. Arch Dis Child 1991;66:1242–1244.

12. Schroth G, Gawehn J, Thron A, et al. Early diagnosis of herpes simplex encephalitis in MRI. Neurology 1987;37:179–183.

13. VanLandingham KE, Marsteller HB, Ross GW, Hayden FG. Relapse of herpes simplex encephalitis after conventional acyclovir therapy. JAMA 1988;259(7):1051–1053.

14. Wasiewski WW, Lee RT, Armstrong DL, et al. Brain biopsy for herpes simplex encephalitis (HSE): Is it valid? Pediatr Res 1986;20:468A.

15. Whitley RJ. Herpes simplex virus infections of the central nervous system—encephalitis and neonatal herpes. Drugs 1991;42(3):406–427.

16. Whitley R, Arvin A, Prober C, et al. A controlled trial comparing vidarabine with acyclovir in neonatal herpes simplex virus infection. N Engl J Med 1991;324:444–449.

17. Whitley R, Arvin A, Prober C, et al. Predictors of morbidity and mortality in neonates with herpes simplex virus infections. N Engl J Med 1991;324:450–454.

18. Whitley RJ, Cobbs CG, Alford CA Jr, et al. Diseases that mimic herpes simplex encephalitis: diagnosis, presentation, and outcome. JAMA 1989;262(2):234–239.

Case 43

Eric L. Gunnoe
and Gary A. Bellus
The Johns Hopkins Hospital
Baltimore, Maryland, USA

HISTORY

A 19-day-old male infant was admitted to the PICU for cyanosis and dehydration. This child was the 3570-g full-term product of a 17-year-old gravida 1, para 1 female with a benign prenatal course. The child was delivered by spontaneous vaginal delivery and had apparently normal Apgar scores. His newborn nursery course was uneventful, and the child was sent home on cow's milk-base formula with iron. He tolerated this well until 2 days prior to admission, when he developed watery nonbloody stools totaling 8 times per day. His mother denied any history of fever or vomiting, although she had noted that he had been somewhat lethargic. The baby was initially taken to another hospital but subsequently referred to the Johns Hopkins Hospital.

The infant was receiving no medications and there was no apparent history of toxin exposure. He had no known allergies and had yet to receive his first immunization. The family history was unremarkable with the exception of maternal sickle-cell carrier status. The father's carrier status was unknown.

PHYSICAL EXAMINATION

When we first examined him, the infant appeared lethargic but became irritable when disturbed. His temperature was 37°C, his pulse was 160 beats/min, his respiratory rate was 40 breaths/min without respiratory distress, and his blood pressure was 90/50 mm Hg. The infant's

291

weight was 2880 g. Examination of his head revealed a soft and slightly sunken anterior fontanel. There were no apparent eye or ear abnormalities. Mucous membranes of the mouth were mildly tacky. The neck was supple without adenopathy. On lung examination, breath sounds were equal and clear bilaterally. Examination of the heart revealed tachycardia without murmurs or gallops. The abdomen was supple with normal bowel sounds and no organomegaly. Genitally, the infant had normal male anatomy, and there was no blood rectally. Examination of the skin revealed both central and peripheral cyanosis, along with coolness distal to ankles and wrists and a capillary refill of 4–5 seconds. Neurologically, the baby's pupils were symmetrically reactive. He had a strong suck and moved all extremities spontaneously.

LABORATORY EXAMINATION

Laboratory examination revealed a hematocrit of 43%, platelets 619,000/ml, and white blood cell count 290,000/ml (44% bands, 7% polymorphocytes, 24% lymphocytes, and 14% monocytes). Electrolytes were as follows: sodium 143 mEq/l, potassium 4.2 mEq/l, chloride 112 mEq/l, bicarbonate 10 mEq/l, blood urea nitrogen (BUN) 18 mg/dl, creatinine 0.9 mg/dl, and glucose 162 mg/dl. The infant's cerebral spinal fluid (CSF) had 22 red blood cells/ml and 1 white blood cell/ml (a monocyte) with a glucose level of 85 mg/dl and a protein level of 74 mg/dl. Arterial blood gas values on 40% face mask oxygen revealed a pH of 7.23, CO_2 of 16 mm Hg, and a PO_2 of 200 mm Hg, along with concurrent pulse oximetry reading 87%. In spite of the high PO_2, the blood drawn for this was noted to be unusually dark colored.

MANAGEMENT

The infant was placed immediately under 100% oxygen, and after establishment of peripheral intravenous access, he received a 20 ml/kg-bolus of lactated Ringer's solution. This resulted in significant improvement in the perfusion, but no change in the cyanosis. Follow-up arterial blood gas was drawn on 100% oxygen, which revealed a pH of 7.23, PCO_2 of 18 mm Hg, PO_2 of 216 mm Hg, base deficit of 19, and an O_2 saturation of 61%. Following this, the infant received an additional bolus of normal saline (10 ml/kg) as well as sodium bicarbonate 1 mEq/kg. Follow-up arterial blood gas values revealed a pH of 7.45, PCO_2 of 16 mm Hg, PO_2 of 420 mm Hg, and -11 base deficit. The color of this repeat blood sample was noted to be chocolate brown when placed on filter paper. A methemoglobin level performed on this sample was found to be 37%. The infant subsequently received methylene blue 1 mg/kg of a 1% solution intravenously over a 5-minute period. Within 10 minutes, he had a clinical resolution of the cyanosis, along with an improvement of the pulse oximetry saturation from 87% to 100% on 100% hood oxygen. A follow-up methemoglobin level was 2%. The infant subsequently remained acyanotic after being weaned to room air. His diarrhea continued until day 5 postadmission. He received both ampicillin and cefotaxime while awaiting culture results, which remained negative at 72 hours. On day 2 of his hospital stay, the infant's methemoglobin level was found to be 8%. He was subsequently started on oral methylene blue at 1 mg/kg/day. A follow-up methemoglobin level 24 hours after starting the oral methylene blue revealed an increase to 11%, and the infant's dose of methylene blue was doubled. By day 5 of the hospital stay, the diarrhea had resolved and the infant was gradually weaned off the methylene blue over the next 2 days without reoccurrence of methemoglobinemia. The patient continued to do well and was discharged home, where he tolerated his original formula well.

DISCUSSION

The case of this patient illustrates the initial stabilization and management of hypovolemic shock and cyanosis. Hypovolemic shock is seen at the PICU relatively frequently and will not be discussed here. Although cyanosis is a common presenting sign at the PICU, methemoglobinemia is not and thus warrants further discussion.

Cyanosis in the neonate invokes a wide differential diagnosis, including lung disease, congenital heart disease, and various metabolic abnormalities. In this infant, lung disease was unlikely, given the absence of respiratory distress, normal chest X-ray, and the PaO_2 >400 mm Hg on 100% oxygen. Likewise, cyanotic congenital heart disease is unlikely, given the high PaO_2 on 100% oxygen. Both hypoglycemia and hypothermia are known to cause cyanosis in neonates; however, this infant was mildly hyperglycemic and normothermic.

Methemoglobinemia is a rare but important cause of cyanosis in both children and adults. Methemoglobinemia is hemoglobin in its oxidized or ferric form, which cannot bind reversibly to oxygen. Thus, high concentrations of methemoglobin can result in hypoxemia in spite of normal or even high levels of dissolved oxygen (PaO_2). Although methemoglobinemia is rare, it deserves discussion because of the severity of its presentation, which often necessitates admission to PICU.

In normal individuals, methemoglobin is constantly formed, but its concentration is maintained at <2% by nicotinamide adenine dinucleotide phosphate (NADPH) and NADPH-dependent methemoglobin reductase. These enzymes reduce ferric to ferrous hemoglobin which is capable of reversibly binding oxygen. An accumulation of methemoglobin results in clinical cyanosis when methemoglobin exceeds 1.5 g/dl. As would be expected, a defect in the hemoglobin-reducing enzymes would result in methemoglobinemia. Numerous toxins and oxidized hemoglobin overwhelm the normal hemoglobin reductase capacities, resulting in methemoglobinemia. These toxins include aniline dyes, some sulfur drugs, bismuth-containing antidiarrheal compounds, benzine compounds, some local anesthetics such as lidocaine and benzocaine, and nitrites. It should be noted that both nitroglycerin and sodium nitroprusside are capable of producing methemoglobinemia. A congenital defect in hemoglobin results in the formation of methemoglobin (hemoglobin M), which cannot be reduced to ferrous hemoglobin (1).

In young infants, transient methemoglobinemia has been reported to occur in association with vomiting, diarrhea, and metabolic acidosis (2). Although this methemoglobinemia is transient and resolves along with the diarrhea, it occasionally necessitates the acute administration of methylene blue. It has been postulated that increased bacterial colonization of the small bowel leads to the conversion of nitrites from nitrates. The patient had a history of diarrhea, as well as a negative history of toxin exposure, normal hemoglobin reductase capacity, and a positive response to methylene blue (thus ruling out congenital abnormal hemoglobin). All this would suggest the etiology of this case of methemoglobinemia to be bacterial overgrowth in the gut, leading to nitrite formation.

The effect of methemoglobin on pulse oximetry bears further discussion here. Methemoglobin has absorption coefficient similar to hemoglobin and oxyhemoglobin at wavelengths of 660 and 940 nanometers commonly measured by pulse oximetry. Pulse oximetry confuses methemoglobin with both hemoglobin and oxyhemoglobin and the ratio of oxyhemoglobin to all hemoglobins approaches 1. This is read as 85% saturation by the microprocessors in the pulse oximeter. Thus, a valuable clue for methemoglobinemia (or carboxyhemoglobinemia) is the discrepancy between PaO_2 and SaO_2 as measured by pulse oximetry (3).

Treatment of methemoglobinemia begins with removal of the toxin (i.e., clothing removal, skin decontamination). Further treatment may not be required since toxin-induced methemoglobinemia will be reduced to normal hemoglobin level over the next 20 hours. Methylene blue administration is required in the presence of hypoxic symptoms (i.e., metabolic acidosis or mental status changes) or methemoglobin levels >30%. The dosage of methylene blue is 1–2 mg/kg of the 1% solution administered intravenously over a 5-minute period. Methylene blue may then be given either intravenously or orally for the reoccurrence of methemoglobinemia (1).

In summary, methemoglobinemia is a rare but significant cause of cyanosis in childhood. The appearance of the disease frequently necessitates admission to the PICU. Thus, the intensivist must be familiar not only with the broad differential diagnosis of cyanosis, but also with the specific etiologies of methemoglobinemia, as well as the treatment of this disorder.

COMMENTARY

This is another example of the huge impact of pulse oximetry in critical care and in the care of anesthetized patients. Not only is pulse oximetry an early indicator of subtle problems, it offers invaluable diagnostic information. In this case, the discrepancy between pulse oximetry and partial pressure of oxygen makes the likelihood of abnormal hemoglobins most likely. The accuracy of this methodology may be manufacturer dependent. Some companies use a different algorithm to calculate oxygen saturation, making detection of abnormal hemoglobin levels less reliable. Obviously, early recognition and treatment of abnormal hemoglobin levels can lead to a positive outcome, whereas failure to do so will lead to a poor outcome in such a straightforward case of diarrhea, dehydration, and hypovolemic shock.

References

1. Rogers MC. Textbook of pediatric intensive care. 2nd ed. Baltimore: Williams & Wilkins 1992:452–460.
2. Yano SS, Danish EH, Hsia YE. Transient methemoglobinemia with acidosis in infants. J Pediatr 1982;100:415–418.
3. Alexander CM, Teller LE, Gross JB. Principles of pulse oximetry: theoretical and practical considerations. Anesth Analg 1989;68:368–376.

Case 44

Vinay M. Nadkarni
Medical Center of Delaware,
Christiana Hospital
Newark, Delaware, USA

HISTORY

A 7-year-old boy was diagnosed with acute lymphoblastic leukemia 3 years prior to admission and was in good health while receiving maintenance chemotherapy (daily 6-mercaptopurine, weekly methotrexate, monthly vincristine and prednisone). Two days prior to admission, he developed back pain and a papular skin rash on his face, oral mucosa, hands, and feet without fever. The rash became vesicular, and progressed over his trunk and extremities. He had no known varicella exposure, no tick bites, and had been exposed to a child with hand, foot, and mouth disease (coxsackie). He had no known drug allergies and his immunizations were up to date. During the 48 hours prior to admission, fever and dyspnea developed.

PHYSICAL EXAMINATION

At the time of admission, we saw a pale, arousable, 7-year-old boy in moderate respiratory distress with tachypnea, grunting, and alopecia. His temperature was 39°C orally, his heart rate was 125 beats/min (sinus tachycardia), his respiratory rate was 50–70 breaths/min with intercostal retractions and grunting, his blood pressure was 140/94 mm Hg, and his weight was 28.6 kg. He was alert with reactive pupils and a normal fundus examination, had a supple neck without meningismus, and had full pulses with a capillary refill <2 seconds. His lung examination revealed diffuse rales bilaterally with decreased breath sounds at the left base and no wheezing. His heart was regular in rate and rhythm with a 2/6 systolic ejection murmur. His abdomen was distended with a liver edge tender and palpable 4 cm below the costal margin in the midclavicular line. No spleen was palpable. His skin showed a diffuse papular to vesicular rash over the scalp, face, oropharynx, trunk, and extremities with scattered petechiae and easy bruising.

LABORATORY DATA

On admission, his hemoglobin was 13.6 g/dl, white blood cell count was 17,000 with 74% segments, 10% bands, 4% lymphocytes, 1% monocyte, and 1% eosinophil. His platelet count was 83,000, and the following levels were seen: sodium 130 mEq/l, potassium 4.1 mEq/l, chloride 97 mEq/l, bicarbonate 19 mEq/l, blood urea nitrogen (BUN) 15 mg/dl, creatinine 0.3 mg/dl, glucose 145 mg/dl, alanine aminotransferase (ALT) 12 U/l, aspartate aminotransferase (AST) 688 U/l, lactic dehydrogenase (LDH) 124 U/l, amylase 65 U/l, prothrombin time (PT) 15.4 seconds, partial thromboplastin time (PTT) 35.5 seconds, fibrinogen 74 mg/dl, and fibrin degregation products >40. Arterial blood gas values on room air showed pH 7.42, pCO_2 30 mm Hg, pO_2 72 mm Hg, and 96% oxygen saturation. Direct florescent antibody staining of skin lesions was positive for varicella-zoster virus and negative for herpes simplex.

MANAGEMENT

The boy was admitted to the PICU for management of impending respiratory failure, possible sepsis, and early disseminated intravascular coagulopathy. He was treated with oxygen, fluids, cryoprecipitate, acyclovir, and broad-spectrum antibiotics consisting of ceftazidime, oxacillin, and Bactrim. His clinical course progressively worsened to adult respiratory distress syndrome (ARDS), hypotension, and severe oliguria, progressing to anuria with azotemia. The disseminated intravascular coagulopathy (DIC) progressed and upper gastrointestinal bleeding occurred that necessitated transfusion. Endoscopy revealed diffuse excoriations with vesicles consistent with varicella throughout the upper gastrointestinal tract. The patient required intubation, mechanical ventilation, paralysis, and high ventilator settings including peak-inspiratory pressure (PIP) of 60 cm, positive end-expiratory pressure (PEEP) of 15 cm, and vasopressor therapy including dopamine, dobutamine, epinephrine, and ultimately norepinephrine guided by Swan-Ganz catheterization data. Hyperdynamic hemodynamic profiles were demonstrated cardiac index (CI) 7.1 l/min/m^2, pulmonary capillary wedge pressure 15–18 mm Hg, systemic vascular resistance index 400–500, oxygen delivery index (DO$_2$I) 1200–1500 ml/min/m^2, oxygen consumption index (VO$_2$I) 150–180 ml/min/m^2). Bacterial cultures remained negative.

By day 4, the boy developed a persistent metabolic acidosis requiring bicarbonate infusion, hepatopathy (AST >9000 U/l, ALT >3400 U/l, bilirubin 5.2 mg/dl) and progressive anuric renal failure (BUN 41 mg/dl, creatinine 3.7 mg/dl) requiring institution of continuous venovenous hemofiltration (CVVH). An Amicon D20 polysulfone filter was used with a 9-French double-lumen femoral venous catheter, blood flow rate 150 ml/min/M^2, crystalloid predilution of 3.3 ml/min/M^2, and an ultrafiltrate rate of 5 ml/min/M^2. No heparin was required. Following institution of CVVH, a marked improvement in pulmonary gas exchange, decreased PEEP requirement, improved pulmonary compliance and improved PaO$_2$/F$_I$O$_2$ ratio were noted despite continued net positive fluid balance (+ 2.8 l/24 hr) and weight gain (+ 4.5 kg/3 d). In the first 24 hours of CVVH therapy, PEEP was weaned from 12 to 8 cm, the PIP from 60 to 48 cm, and pressors were significantly weaned as follows: dopamine from 20 to 4 µg/kg/min, dobutamine from 24 to 0 µg/kg/min, epinephrine from 1.2 to 0.6 µg/kg/min, and norepinephrine from 1.4 to 0.5 µg/kg/min while maintaining a stable mean arterial pressure and hemodynamic profile (Figs. 44.1 and 44.2). Stroke volume index (SVI) markedly improved after CVVH and pulmonary capillary wedge pressure (PCWP) decreased despite weight gain and positive net fluid balance. Oxygen delivery (DO$_2$) doubled without a change in oxygen consumption during this time period. Intrapulmonary shunt fraction (37%) did not significantly change, but the pulmonary and cardiac compliances improved.

Serial middle molecular weight mediator concentrations were measured in serum and ultrafiltrate (TNF, IL-1α by enzyme-linked immunosorbent assay (ELISA), ENDOGEN, Boston; IL-1β by ELISA, CISTRON, Pinebrook, NJ). Clearance rates and sieving coefficients for these mediators are given in Table 44.1.

Despite maximal medical management, the patient sustained a large pneumothorax and subsequent hemothorax and had persistent multiple organ system failure without evidence of recovery. The patient died after 78 hours on CVVH, which was unrelated to the treatment. Autopsy specimens of skin, spleen, lung, and liver revealed dissemi-

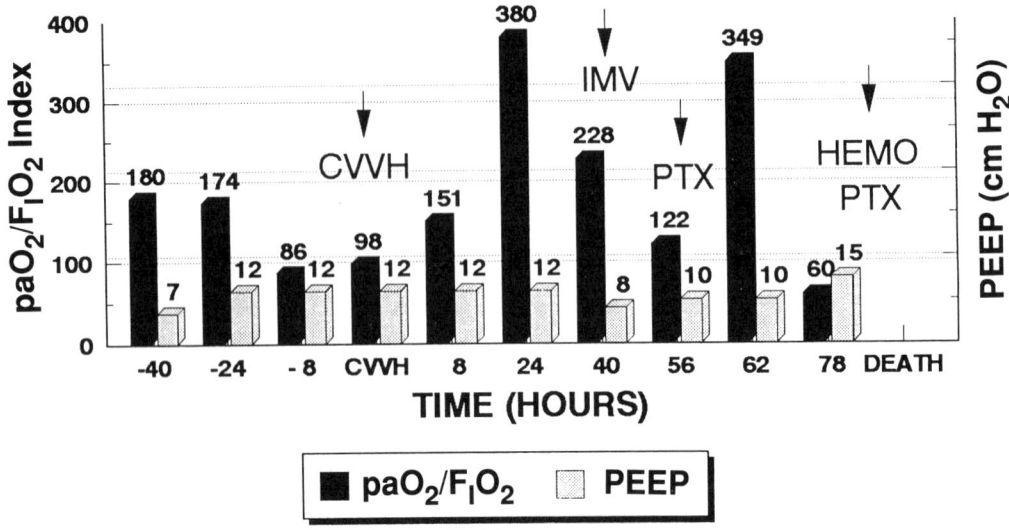

Figure 44.1. Oxygenation index (OI) and peak end-expiratory pressure (PEEP) as a function of time. Marked improvement in OI despite less PEEP was documented after continuous venovenous hemofiltration (CVVH). *CVVH*, institution of CVVH; *IMV* (intermittent mandatory ventilation), change from pressure-limited to volume-limited ventilation; *PTX*, pneumothorax; *HEMO PTX*, hemopneumothorax.

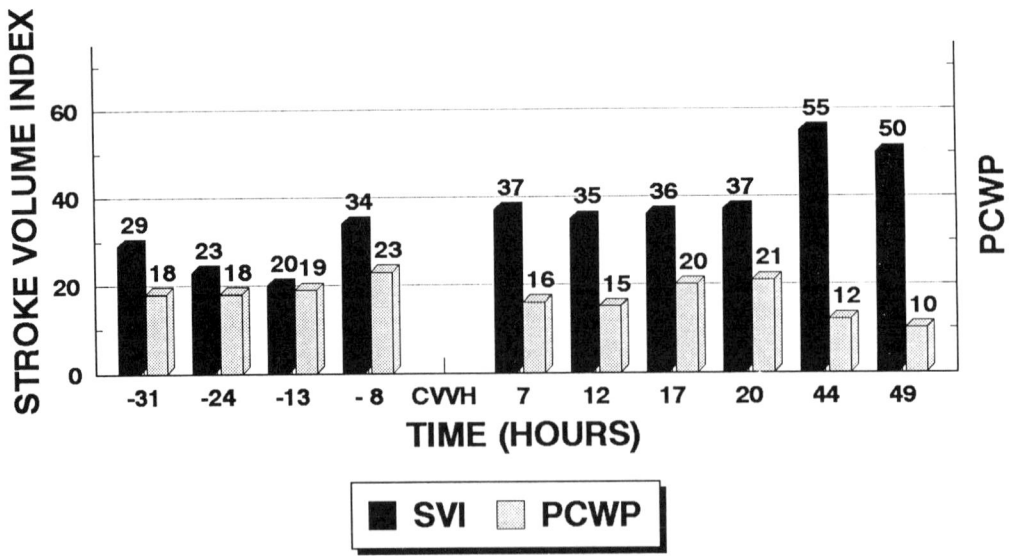

Figure 44.2. Stroke volume index (*SVI*) and pulmonary capillary wedge pressure (*PCWP*) as functions of time. SVI markedly improved after continuous venovenous hemofiltration (CVVH) despite equivalent or lower PCWP. Net fluid gain (+4.9 l) and weight gain (+3.8 kg) were noted during this time period.

Table 44.1   Clearance Rates, Sieving Coefficients, and Serum Levels of TNF, IL-1α, and IL-1β during 72 Hours of CVVH

	Tumor Necrosis Factor	IL-1α	IL-1β
Clearance (hr)			
0–24	75	0	13
25–48	45	0	40
49–72	28	6	56
Sieving coefficients (%)	33	0	33
Serum level (hr)			
0–24	90	160	16
25–48	145	168	17
49–72	223	252	24

Note: Clearance values are given as milliliters per minute per meter squared; serum levels are given as picograms per milliliter.

nated varicella, and necrosis was observed in multiple organs including the heart, brain, and adrenal glands. Focal ulcerations of the distal esophagus were noted. There was no evidence of recurrent leukemia or bacterial superinfection.

DISCUSSION

Hemofiltration is an extracorporeal technique that can easily be applied in the ICU setting for filtrative removal of substances ≤25,000 kD molecular weight via convection. This filtration is not dependent on concentration gradients or diffusion (1–3). Polysulfone material used in CVVH cartridges is less immunogenic than dialysis membranes and requires no large dialytic bath. Although hemofiltration differs from hemodialysis, the factors determining dialyzability still include molecular weight, water solubility, protein binding, volume of distribution, and elimination half-life. Tumor necrosis factor (TNF), Interleukin-1α, and Interleukin-1β are polypeptides that have a broad spectrum of physiologic actions in response to inflammatory stimuli. The mature forms of these molecules are approximately 17,000 kD molecular weight, are synthesized as larger precursor molecules, and may travel in the bloodstream as multimers. Plasma concentrations of these septic mediators are usually below the limit of detection, as have been noted to be elevated in various septic syndromes (4–9). Drapkin and Wisch observed that plasmapheresis could decrease circulating TNF and IL-1 levels in a pediatric patient with severe meningococcemia (10). Decreased mediator levels correlated with improved clinical outcome in this patient. Barzilay et al., in a series of case reports with retrospective or historic control subjects, observed that various extracorporeal filtration techniques may be associated with increased survival in septic acute organ system failure (11,12). They noted no change in pulmonary shunt fraction, low cardiac index, and PaO_2/F_IO_2 ratio, and did not measure peptide clearance. Gotloib et al. described a 21-year-old patient with systemic varicella and streptococcal superinfection who showed a dramatic decrease in intrapulmonary shunt and clinical improvement of multiple organ system failure when hemofiltration was performed (13). This was attributed to clearance of low-molecular weight mediators <5,000 kD including leukotrienes, prostaglandins, and endorphins. DiCarlo et al. described a series of eight children with multiple organ system failure and fluid overload who showed marked improvement in pulmonary gas exchange and increased tolerance of parenteral nutrition and fluids in response to continuous arteriovenous hemofiltration/dialysis (CAVH/D) (14). They postulated that the combination of a decrease in lung and body water and mediator clearance was the mechanism for the pulmonary improvement. Gomez et al. reported reversal of left ventricular systolic dysfunction in hemofiltered septic dogs experimentally (15). Furthermore, when ultrafiltrate was used to perfuse isolated papillary muscles in vitro, papillary muscle contraction was diminished. They concluded that a "myocardial depressant factor" of <30,000 kD molecular weight must be responsible. Byrick et al found that increased plasma tumor necrosis factor concentrations in severe rhabdomyolysis were not reduced by continuous arteriovenous hemodialysis (16).

The case we report documents viral sepsis without bacterial infection developing into ARDS, multiple organ system failure, and typical hyperdynamic septic profiles with associated high levels of plasma septic mediators. The clinical course of this patient with fatal disseminated varicella is consistent with that of previously reported cases (17–20). We noted significant clinical, hemodynamic, and oxygenation improvement after CVVH despite a net positive fluid balance. Related phenomena have been observed in animal models of sepsis (20–23). Clearance rates of middle molecular weight septic mediators (TNF, IL-1α, IL-1β) were low. Sieving coefficients for the mediators involved were low, and serum levels of all three mediators did not decrease over the 78-hour filtration period. Possible explanations for low-mediator clearances may include mediators bound to proteins circulating as multimers too large to filter or induction of inflammatory mediators by the filtration process.

In summary, the case of this patient demonstrates that viral sepsis may hemodynamically mimic bacterial sepsis. Septic hemodynamics may be altered by hemofiltration, independent of water removal or water retention. Middle molecular weight septic mediators may be partially cleared by hemofiltration, but do not appear to alter total serum levels. More efficient or complete mediator removal may be required to affect multiple organ system failure. Hemofiltration may allow adjunctive and supportive treatments such as parenteral nutrition, pressors, and fluids to be administered in the setting of multiple organ system failure. As our understanding of septic mediator patterns improves and the use of extracorporeal means of regulating plasma constituents becomes more common, a role may emerge for extracorporeal manipulation of septic mediators.

COMMENTARY

Adult respiratory distress syndrome as the pulmonary manifestation of multiple organ system failure can occur in many settings. Whether bacterial or viral in etiology, sepsis sets off the cascade, the pieces of which we are just beginning to identify. What is becoming clear is that to make a significant difference we must intervene early and specifically. We can intervene in at least three ways. We can immunologically neutralize some of the mediators with monoclonal antibodies. The modest success of these clinical trials suggests the ability to accomplish this rather than to have identified a present cure. The second approach is to clear the mediators through an extracorporeal circuit. In this case venovenous support allowed more cardiovascular stability. The third method, selective gastrointestinal decontamination, has been reported with variable efficacy. Viewing the intestine as the reservoir of mediators and substrate for mediator proliferation, decontamination makes sense. The liver then becomes a gatekeeper for these processes that becomes overwhelmed.

The mixed results of each of these three modalities may imply that early intervention with all three may offer a synergistic approach to the patient with ARDS or multiple organ system failure.

References

1. Bishof NA, Welch TR, Strife CF, Ryckman FC. Continuous hemodiafiltration in children. Pediatrics 1990;85:819.
2. Cutler RE, Forland SC, Hammond PGS, Evans JR. Extracorporeal

removal of drugs and poisons by hemodialysis and hemoperfusion. Ann Rev Pharmacol Toxicol 1987;27:169.

3. Zobel G, Trop M, Ring E, Grubbauer HM. Arteriovenous hemofiltration in children with multiple organ system failure. Int J Artif Org 1987;10:233.

4. Cannon JG, Tompkins RG, Gelfand J, Michie HR, Stanford G, van der Meer JWM, Endres S, Lonnemann G, Corsetti J, Chernow B, Wilmore DW, Wolff SM, Burke JF, Dinarello CA. Circulating Interleukin-1 and tumor necrosis factor in septic shock and experimental endotoxin fever. J Infect Dis 1990;161:79.

5. Damas P, Reuter A, Gysen P, Demonty J, Lamy M, Franchimont P. Tumor necrosis factor and interleukin-1 serum levels during severe sepsis in humans. Crit Care Med 1989;17:975.

6. Debets JM, Kampmeijer R, Van der Linden M, Buurman MA, Van der Linden CJ. Plasma tumor necrosis factor and mortality in critically ill septic patients. Crit Care Med 1989;17: 489.

7. Michie HR, Manogue KR, Spriggs DR, Revhaug A, O'Dwyer S, Dinarello CA, Cerami A, Wolff SM, Wilmore DW. Detection of circulating tumor necrosis factor after endotoxin administration. N Engl J Med 1988;318:1481.

8. Ohlsson K, Bjork P, Bergenfeldt M, Hageman R, Thompson RC. Interleukin-1 receptor antagonist reduces mortality from endotoxin shock. Nature 1990;348:550.

9. Ziegler EJ, Fisher CJ, Sprung CL, Straube RC, Sadoff JC, Foulke GE, Wortel CH, Fink MP, Dellinger RP, Teng NNH, Allen IE, Berger HJ, Knatterud GL, LoBuglio AF, Smith CR, and the HA-1A Sepsis Study Group. Treatment of Gram-negative bacteremia and septic shock with HA-1A human monoclonal antibody against endotoxin. N Engl J Med 1991;324:429.

10. Drapkin MS, Wisch JS. Plasmapheresis for fulminant meningococcemia. Pediatr Infect Dis 1989;18:399.

11. Barzilay E, Kessler D, Berlot G, Gullo A, Geber D, Zeev IB. Use of extracorporeal supportive techniques as additional treatment for septic-induced multiple organ failure patients. Crit Care Med 1989; 17:634.

12. Barzilay E, Kessler D, Lesmes C, Lev A, Weksler N, Berlot G. Sequential plasmafilter-dialysis with slow continuous hemofiltration: additional treatment for sepsis-induced AOSF patients. J Crit Care 1988; 3:163.

13. Gotloib L, Barzilay E, Shustak A, Waiss Z, Lev A. Hemofiltration in severe septic adult respiratory distress syndrome associated with varicella. Intensive Care Med 1985;11:319.

14. DiCarlo JV, Dudley TE, Sherbotie JR, Kaplan BS, Costarino AT. Continuous arteriovenous hemofiltration/dialysis improves pulmonary gas exchange in children with multiple organ system failure. Crit Care Med 1990;18:822.

15. Gomez A, Unruh H, Light RB, Bose D, Chau T, Eng J, Mink S. Hemofiltration reverses left ventricular systolic dysfunction during E. coli bacteremia in dogs [Abstract]. Am Rev Respir Dis 1988;137:114.

16. Byrick RJ, Goldstein MB, Wong PY. Increased plasma tumor necrosis factor concentration in severe rhabdomyolysisis not reduced by continuous arteriovenous hemodialysis. Crit Care Med 1992;20:1483.

17. Fleisher G, Henry W, McSorley M, Arbeter A, Plotkin S. Life-threatening complications of varicella. Am J Dis Child 1981;135:896.

18. Miliauskas JR, Webber BL. Disseminated varicella at autopsy in children with cancer. Cancer 1984;53:1518.

19. Schlossberg D, Littman M. Varicella pneumonia. Arch Intern Med 1988;148:1630.

20. Scully RE, Mark EJ, McNeely WF, McNeely BU. Case 25-1988: Case records of the Massachusetts General Hospital. N Engl J Med 1988; 318:1669.

21. Lee PA, Matson JR. Continuous arteriovenous hemofiltration (CAVH) as therapy for sepsis-induced acute lung injury in immature swine [Abstract]. Physiologist 1989;32:217.

22. Natanson C, Hoffman WD, Danner RL, Koev LL, Banks SM, Walker LD, Heyman P, Parillo JE. A controlled trial of plasmapheresis fails to improve outcome in an antibiotic treated canine model of human septic shock [Abstract]. Crit Care Med 1989;17:S57.

23. Paschall JA, Nadkarni VM, Hermiller JB, Eckstein JM, Hoban LD, Nevola JJ, Williams TJ. Effects of continuous arteriovenous hemofiltration in porcine intraperitoneal sepsis [Abstract]. Crit Care Med 1990;18:S241.

Case 45

Andrew C. Oken, Steven D. Barnes, Peter Rock, and Lynne G. Maxwell
The Johns Hopkins Hospital
Baltimore, Maryland, USA

HISTORY

A previously healthy 5-month-old boy with no significant past medical or surgical history was seen at the emergency room (ER) with lethargy, drooling, increased irritability, and decreased oral intake of 3 days' duration. He had been treated at another hospital for presumed otitis media and tonsillitis with intramuscular ceftriaxone and oral amoxicillin. At the time of arrival, he was listless and had severe respiratory distress.

PHYSICAL EXAMINATION

His vital signs were as follows: arterial blood pressure 117/59 mm Hg, heart rate 133 beats/min, respiratory rate 36 breaths/min, temperature 37.4°C, and oxygen saturation 90% (O_2 at 5 l/min by face mask). He weighed 5.7 kg (10th–25th percentile for age). In the ER, a jaw thrust maneuver was required to maintain a patent airway. Physical examination results demonstrated upper airway rhonchi, intermittent inspiratory stridor, and sinus tachycardia without significant murmur. Initial white blood cell count was 6000/mm^3 with 50% lymphocytes and 46% bands. A lateral neck roentgenogram showed supraglottic edema and an increase in the size of the epiglottis, with narrowing of the airway.

Reprinted with permission from the International Anesthesia Research Society (Anesthesia and Analgesia, 1992;275:136–138).

HOSPITAL MANAGEMENT

A decision was made to transport the infant to the operating room by physicians expert in airway management for treatment of presumed epiglottitis. This was accomplished uneventfully with the patient breathing supplemental oxygen and with electrocardiographic and pulse oximeter monitoring. Anesthesia was induced by slow incremental mask inhalation of halothane in oxygen (up to 3.5% inspired concentration). Direct laryngoscopy demonstrated supraglottitis with bilateral arytenoid edema, mild erythema, and a white exudate. Orotracheal intubation was performed. Blood and airway mucosa cultures were obtained and the infant was transported to the ICU.

He remained lethargic and hypotonic and required mechanical ventilation. Culture material obtained intraoperatively revealed heavy normal upper respiratory flora and Gram-negative diplococci. *Haemophilus influenzae* was not grown from the culture material. All other culture material (blood, cerebrospinal fluid, and urine) was negative for pathogenic organisms. The patient remained on mechanical ventilation and ceftriaxone but subsequently developed minimally reactive pupils and became progressively weaker by the 5th hospital day. His limbs became floppy, and he had only slight movement in his extremities in reaction to deep painful stimuli. Electrical studies using repetitive nerve stimulation at rates of 20 Hz showed an incremental response of approximately 100%, consistent with botulism (1).

Based on the above clinical features and the baby's response to the nerve stimulation studies, we considered a diagnosis of infant botulism. Stool cultures grew *Clostridium botulinum* type B (Maryland State Health Department). Three days after his first airway examination in the operating room the baby was again examined by direct laryngoscopy and found to have near-resolution of the supraglottic and arytenoid edema. Because of weakness, the patient required ventilatory assistance. He regained his strength over a period of several weeks, and his trachea was subsequently extubated without difficulty.

DISCUSSION

The clinical presentation and neck radiographic findings in this patient strongly suggested acute epiglottitis.

The classic findings of acute epiglottitis, including high fever, irritability, lethargy, and severe sore throat, which progress to dysphagia, dysphonia, dyspnea, and drooling, are usually seen in older children. These children usually assume a characteristic upright posture with forward flexion at the waist, forward chin thrust, and slight cervical flexion, and resist attempts to place them supine. These presentations are seldom missed. Other causes of upper airway obstruction (UAO) such as supraglottitis, laryngotracheobronchitis, and presence of a foreign body must be considered.

Infant epiglottitis (<2 years old) may be very insidious in its clinical appearance, with only mild fever and no characteristic positioning or drooling. A prodromal illness may be present of several days' duration. The diagnosis of acute epiglottitis in this population of patients may be delayed until severe airway obstruction has occurred (2). Lateral neck films have been suggested to aid in the diagnosis; however, the dangers associated with delay in securing the airway, moving the patient, and the necessity for accompaniment by a skilled laryngoscopist must be kept in mind (3).

A definitive diagnosis of epiglottitis may be made in infants by direct laryngoscopy, which should be performed under general anesthesia in a controlled operating room setting where capabilities for tracheal intubation, cricothyroidotomy, or tracheostomy are at hand (4). These procedures were carried out in our patient, and findings in the operating room of supraglottic swelling, inflammation, and exudate supported a diagnosis of UAO of an infectious nature. Subsequent clinical follow-up and evaluation led to the ultimate diagnosis of infant botulism.

Infant botulism has been described as a cause of respiratory distress (5), which is almost always due to progressive weakness culminating in respiratory failure (5,6). As the diaphragm is relatively resistant to neuromuscular block, of which botulism is a type (7), usually the disease is recognized before respiratory failure develops. Our patient was unique, however, in that he had UAO that was associated with supraglottic inflammation and arytenoid edema. It is important to note that in the approximately 600 cases of infant botulism reported in the literature, periglottic inflammation has not been described (8,9). While the issue of whether the botulism caused the glottic inflammation or merely occurred in temporal association with it is important, the association of these two entities must now be kept in mind when managing patients with either of these two diseases. Moreover, this case clearly demonstrates the ability of infant botulism to *mimic* other types of acute UAO.

We can only speculate on the possible association of supraglottic swelling and inflammation with botulism. Weakness may result in either (a) supraglottic pooling of secretions with secondary irritation and/or superinfection, or (b) collapse of supraglottic structures on inspiration and subsequent swelling and inflammation. The case of this patient supports the importance of systematic management of acute UAO (3) and suggests that the differential diagnosis of a hypotonic infant with respiratory distress, drooling, and feeding difficulties should now include botulism.

C. botulinum produces a potent neurotoxin that causes progressive muscle paralysis. *C. botulinum* spores can survive a temperature 100°C for several hours and moist heat at 120°C for 30 minutes. The toxin, however, is destroyed by boiling for 10 minutes. Botulism can occur after ingestion of preformed toxin or after ingestion of *C. botulinum* spores that germinate, proliferate, and then generate toxin in the gastrointestinal tract.

Botulin toxin affects cholinergic synapses peripherally by interfering with presynaptic release of acetylcholine from preganglionic and neuromuscular junction nerve endings. Weakness appears symmetrically and progresses from facial muscles to the distal extremities. Patients are seen with blurred vision, dysphonia, dysphagia, and dysarthria. Subsequent symmetric paralysis of the extremities progresses rapidly to involve the diaphragm. Impaired cholinergic autonomic transmission results in constipation, urinary retention, and nausea and vomiting. In an infant, signs and symptoms include poor feeding and failure to thrive followed by progressive weakness and impaired respirations (5).

When examined, patients are alert and afebrile, with ptosis and failure of accommodation. Pupils are normal in size and react sluggishly. There is weakness of the tongue, larynx, and respiratory muscles. Pooling of oral secretions occurs and may explain the supraglottitis found in this child. Reflexes are diminished or absent but are not pathologic, and sensory examination results usually appear normal.

Infant botulism is a relatively "new" disease first described in 1976 (1). Approximately 90% of recognized cases occur in patients <6 months of age. The intestinal tract is colonized with *C. botulinum* and toxin is gradually produced, leading to slower onset of weakness than when preformed toxin is ingested. The diagnosis of infant botulism requires confirmation of botulinal toxin in stool or isolation of *C. botulinum* from stool culture as was found in our patient. Treatment involves aggressive supportive care. Deaths are uncommon and occur principally when the disease progressed rapidly before supportive treatments could be instituted. Infants with mild hypotonia, poor feeding, and failure to thrive have been found to have botulism, and there is evidence that 5% of cases of sudden infant death syndrome may actually have been severe cases of infant botulism (6).

The increased duration of non-depolarizing muscle relaxants associated with the synaptic blockade must be kept in mind. Depolarizing muscle relaxants should be used with caution because of potential denervation hypersensitivity of postsynaptic receptors and the risk of hyperkalemia. Patients presenting to the operating room may also have a "full" stomach, and appropriate precautions should be taken to prevent aspiration. The most important anesthetic considerations relate to airway management. Some very weak patients with botulism will need tracheal intubation to protect the airway and to allow mechanical ventilation. Moreover, the case of this patient illustrates that patients with botulism are at risk for airway obstruction.

Many questions remain unanswered regarding the relatively new disease of infant botulism. Nevertheless, we recommend that it should be considered in the differential diagnosis of the hypotonic infant with airway obstruction. In the rush to evaluate the obstructed airway, significant weakness may be overlooked. Hypotonia in an infant with airway obstruction should immediately prompt investigation for botulism.

COMMENTARY

The diagnosis of the etiology of acute upper airway obstruction (UAO) presents difficulties in infants. It is critical to treat UAO because any coexisting disease may itself be fatal. While urgently ensuring airway patency, the intensivist must consider the broad differential diagnosis of UAO. Sometimes botulism can come to the attention of the intensivists as a chief complaint of an exaggerated response to agents with neuromuscular blocking properties such as pancuronium and gentamicin.

References

1. Pickett J, Berg B, Chaplin E, Brunstetter-Shafer M. Syndrome of botulism in infancy: clinical and electrophysiologic study. N Engl J Med 1976;14:770–772.
2. Blackstock D, Adderley RJ, Steward DJ. Epiglottitis in young infants. Anesthesiology 1987;67:97–100.
3. Davis HW, Gartner JC, Galvis AG, Michaels RH, Mestad PH. Acute UAO: croup and epiglottitis. Pediatric Clin North Am 1981;28(4): 859–880.
4. Diaz JH. Croup and epiglottitis in children: the anesthesiologist as diagnostician. Anesth Analg 1985;64:621–633.
5. Smith GE, Hinde F, Westmoreland D, Berry PR, Gilbert RJ. Infantile botulism. Arch Dis Child 1989;64:871–872.
6. Long SS. Botulism in infancy. Pediatr Infect Dis 1984;3:266–271.
7. L'Hommedieu C, Polin RA. Progression of clinical signs in severe infant botulism. Clin Pediat 1981;20(2):90–95.
8. Spika JS, Shaffer N, Hargrett-Bean N, Collin S, MacDonald KL, Blake PA. Risk factors for infant botulism in the United States. Am J Dis Child 1989;143:828–832.
9. Thompson JA, Glasgow LA, Warpinski JR, Olson C. Infant botulism: Clinical spectrum and epidemiology. Pediatrics 1980;66(6): 936–942.

Case 46

Mohan R. Mysore,
Linda R. Margraf,
and Daniel L. Levin
Children's Medical Center of Dallas
Dallas, Texas, USA

HISTORY

A 10-year-old boy was brought to the outpatient clinic with a 4 day history of ill-defined chest pain, difficulty in breathing, and nausea. Past medical history was significant only for pneumonia at 13 months of age. He lived at home with his mother and a 7-year-old sister. The pets at home were two dogs and a parrot. The patient's immunizations were up to date.

PHYSICAL EXAMINATION

The patient was afebrile, with a heart rate of 100 beats/min, blood pressure of 127/75 mm Hg, and a respiratory rate of 24 breaths/min with mild intercostal retractions. There was decreased air entry on the left side of his chest and a chest radiograph showed a massive left pleural effusion (Fig. 46.1).

MANAGEMENT

At the time of admission, we evacuated 1250 ml of blood-tinged fluid from the left pleural cavity with an immediate improvement of symptoms. We considered a provisional diagnosis of *Mycoplasma* versus psittacosis pneumonia and began a regimen of clindamycin and erythromycin after we obtained blood and pleural fluid cultures.

313

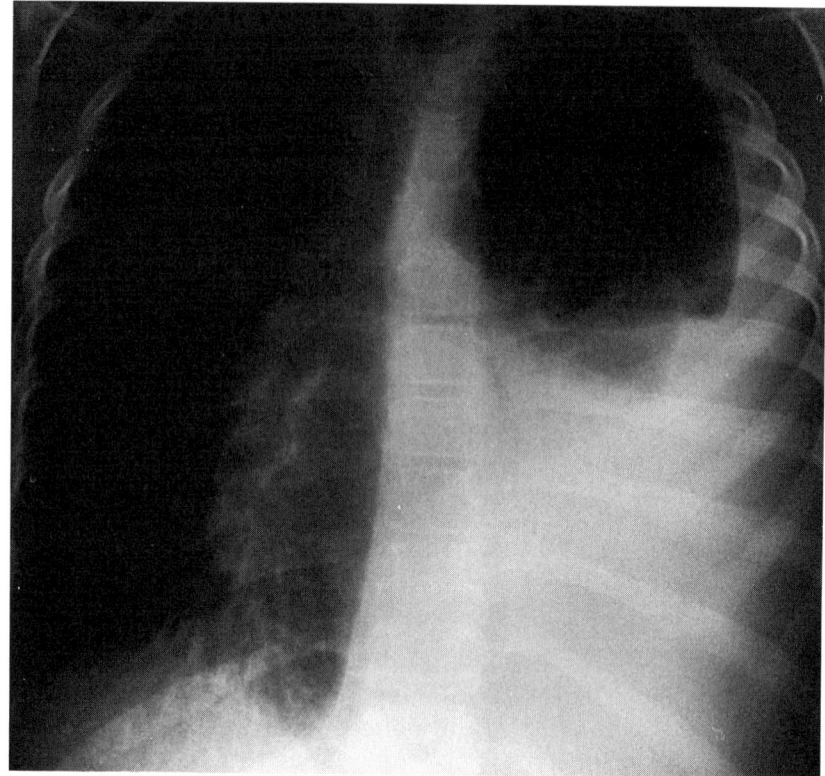

Figure 46.1. Chest radiograph at time of admission showing a large pleural effusion on the left side.

Table 46.1. Laboratory Data: Blood

	Day 1	Day 12	Day 18	Day 19	Day 20
WBC count (/ml)[a]	12,300	12,900	11,700	37,200	32,900
Serum IgG (mg/dl)			163		372
Creatinine (mg/dl)	0.6	0.5	0.7	1.9	1.9
Glucose (mg/dl)	93	86	112	214	176
Platelets (/ml)	250,000	238,000	216,000	34,000	45,000

[a] WBC, white blood cell.

Laboratory results of blood and pleural fluid are shown in Tables 46.1 and 46.2. The Gram stain and stain for acid-fast bacilli on the pleural fluid showed no organisms and the lipid stain was positive for the presence of fat. A magnetic resonance imaging (MRI) of the chest was performed to rule out intrathoracic malignancy. It showed defects in the C7, T1, and T9 vertebral bodies and possibly a left hilar mass.

A bone marrow aspirate and biopsy done on the day of admission were subsequently reported to be normal.

Table 46.2.   Pleural Fluid Volume and Composition[a]

	Day 1	Day 6	Day 11	Day 12	Day 14
Volume (ml)	1,250	2,100	2,500	4,000	1,288
WBC count (/ml)[b]	13,500	6,680		1,750	
RBC count (/ml)[b]	231,000	213,000		61,750	
Triglycerides (mg/dl)		275		87	
Protein (mg/dl)	5.2	4.2		3.2	
LDH (U/l)[b]	547	451			

[a] A chest tube was first placed for continuous drainage on day 11.
[b] Abbreviations: WBC, white blood cell; RBC, red blood cell; LDH, lactic dehydrogenase.

Over the course of the next 5 days, the patient remained afebrile and his appetite improved. Blood and pleural fluid bacterial cultures taken at the time of admission were negative, and the clindamycin was discontinued on the third day. A nuclear medicine bone scan was performed, which showed reduced uptake in the region of the T9 vertebral body. A skeletal survey, however, showed no abnormal bone densities.

Purified protein derivative (PPD) and *Candida* skin tests were negative. Cell mediated immunity and mumps skin tests were placed and showed normal responses. Since the initial pleural fluid was positive for lipids, the boy was started on a low-fat diet because of the possibility of a chylothorax. (Triglyceride levels had not been obtained.)

On the 6th day of hospitalization a thoracentesis was performed for respiratory compromise and 2100 ml of rust-colored fluid was drained. An MRI of the chest performed soon after showed no mediastinal masses or adenopathy.

During the next 4 days, the patient remained afebrile but somewhat tired. The diagnostic evaluation continued and blood cultures remained negative despite a doubling of his total white blood cell count to 24,600/mm^3. Both the C-reactive protein and the erythrocyte sedimentation rate were normal. Cytomegalovirus, Epstein-Barr virus, and *Mycoplasma* infections were ruled out based on cultures and serology, and the erythromycin was discontinued. Urinary catecholamines and vanillylmandelic acid were within normal limits, and since the serum amylase and lipase were both normal, pancreatitis was ruled out as a possible cause of the recurrent pleural effusions.

On the 11th day following admission, chest radiographs revealed a reaccumulation of the pleural effusion on the left, and since the patient was in moderate discomfort, an

18-Fr chest tube was placed in the left pleural space and 2500 ml of blood-tinged fluid was drained at the time of tube placement. The chest tube drained 4 l of fluid in the first 24 hours and fluid boluses (normal saline and 5% albumin) were required to maintain hemodynamic stability. Chest tube output replacement with 5% albumin was begun the following day, and over the next 3 days the chest tube output decreased (Table 46.2). The patient was more comfortable, afebrile, and hemodynamically stable. An abdominal sonogram showed diffuse enlargement of the liver and spleen without any focal (cystic) abnormalities. A moderate amount of ascitic fluid was seen within the pelvis and flanks.

On the 17th day of hospitalization, the patient was febrile (39.8°C) and appeared pale and anxious. Blood cultures were drawn and he was started on intravenous cefotaxime and vancomycin, and a single 5-g dose of intravenous IgG was administered. The following day, his temperature was 40°C and he had chills. Laboratory studies at the time showed hyperglycemia, leukocytosis, thrombocytopenia, and a coagulopathy. In view of the increasing respiratory distress and the rapidly evolving picture of septic shock, he was transferred to the PICU for further management.

Shortly after transfer, his trachea was intubated and mechanical ventilation was begun. He was started on dopamine and epinephrine infusions and needed repeated colloid infusions to correct the coagulopathy and to sustain an adequate blood volume and blood pressure. His weight increased overnight by 2.7 kg (8%) and there was a decrease in urine output to 0.8 ml/kg/hr. He continued to require inotropic support with epinephrine at 0.3 $\mu g/kg/min$, dobutamine at 15 $\mu g/kg/min$, and dopamine at 3 $\mu g/kg/min$. He needed increased ventilatory support with a positive end-expiratory pressure (PEEP) of 6–8 cm H_2O, mean airway pressure of 15.8 cm H_2O, and FiO_2 of 0.8 to maintain the PaO_2 >60 mm Hg. The chest radiographs showed diffuse interstitial involvement consistent with adult respiratory distress syndrome (ARDS). The blood culture from the previous day showed the growth of Gram-negative rods (final report: *Escherichia coli*).

On hospital day 19, the hemodynamic data (Table 46.3) showed a decrease in the blood pressure, cardiac index, and stroke index associated with an elevation of the central venous pressure (CVP). Chest radiograph showed no increase in the heart size. An echocardiogram showed a significant collection of fluid in the pericardium causing a diastolic collapse of the right atrium. A 20-Fr pericardial

Table 46.3. Hemodynamic Data

	3 p.m.	9 a.m.	1 p.m.
Heart rate (beats/min)	154	166	163
Systemic BP	76/37	69/36	136/51
Mean arterial pressure	50	46	76
Central venous pressure	14	18	12
PA wedge pressure	15	16	16
Systolic PA pressure	34	35	32
Diastolic PA pressure	19	23	24
Mean PA pressure	24	28	19
Cardiac output	5.3	2.6	6.8
Cardiac index	4.6	2.2	5.9
Stroke index	29.9	13.6	36.2
SVRI	625.3	989.9	865.2
PVRI	156.3	424.2	40.5

Hemodynamic data was obtained on day 19 using a Swan-Ganz thermodilution catheter. A pericardiostomy was performed between 9 a.m. and 1 p.m. Abbreviations: BP, blood pressure; PA, pulmonary artery; SVRI, systemic vascular resistance index; and PVRI, pulmonary vascular resistance index. Body surface area is 1.15 m^2.

catheter was placed and 225 ml of bloody fluid was drained with an immediate improvement in the hemodynamic status (Table 46.3). Urine output improved and the patient required less inotropic support. The patient gradually recovered from the episode of septic shock, and on the 24th hospital day, pleural, pericardial, and lung biopsies from two sites were obtained (see below).

The following week, an elective tracheostomy was performed because of the need for prolonged ventilatory support. On hospital day 30, the patient was started on daily subcutaneous α-interferon therapy in an effort to halt the progress of the disease process. This therapy was discontinued after 25 days at the mother's request because there had been no improvement in the patient's respiratory status. In addition to the diffuse lung involvement by the disease process (Fig. 46.2), the massive hepatosplenomegaly further compromised his lung compliance. The boy had a gradual decline over the course of the next 4 weeks and he died on the 63rd hospital day despite full supportive care.

HISTOPATHOLOGY

The biopsies of left upper and lower lung lobes and the pericardium demonstrated the same pathologic process. There was extensive expansion of the visceral pleura and pulmonary interlobular septa by a proliferation of anastomosing lymphatic channels (Fig. 46.3). The vascular chan-

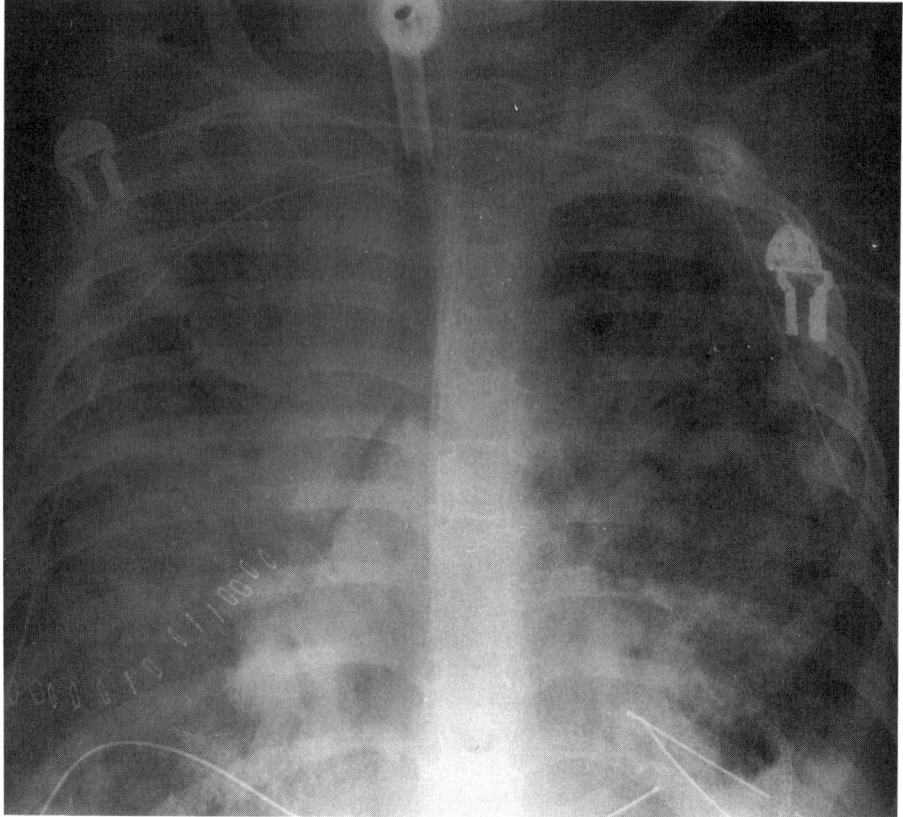

Figure 46.2.   Chest radiograph taken in the 6th week of hospitalization showing diffuse involvement of both lung fields.

nels were lined by bland endothelium with no suggestion of malignancy. This lymphatic proliferation greatly encroached upon the lung parenchyma; however, there was no evidence of obstructive pneumonia or diffuse alveolar damage. The pericardium was similarly expanded from diffuse infiltration by lymphatic channels (Fig. 46.4). An immunocytochemical stain for factor VIII antigen confirmed the vascular origin of this process.

DISCUSSION

Based on the finding of recurrent pleural effusions, the differential diagnosis at the time of presentation was as follows: pulmonary tuberculosis, psittacosis, *Mycoplasma*, Epstein-Barr virus infection, Gorham's syndrome, malignancy (probably lymphoma), trauma (disruption of the thoracic duct), or lymphangiomatosis.

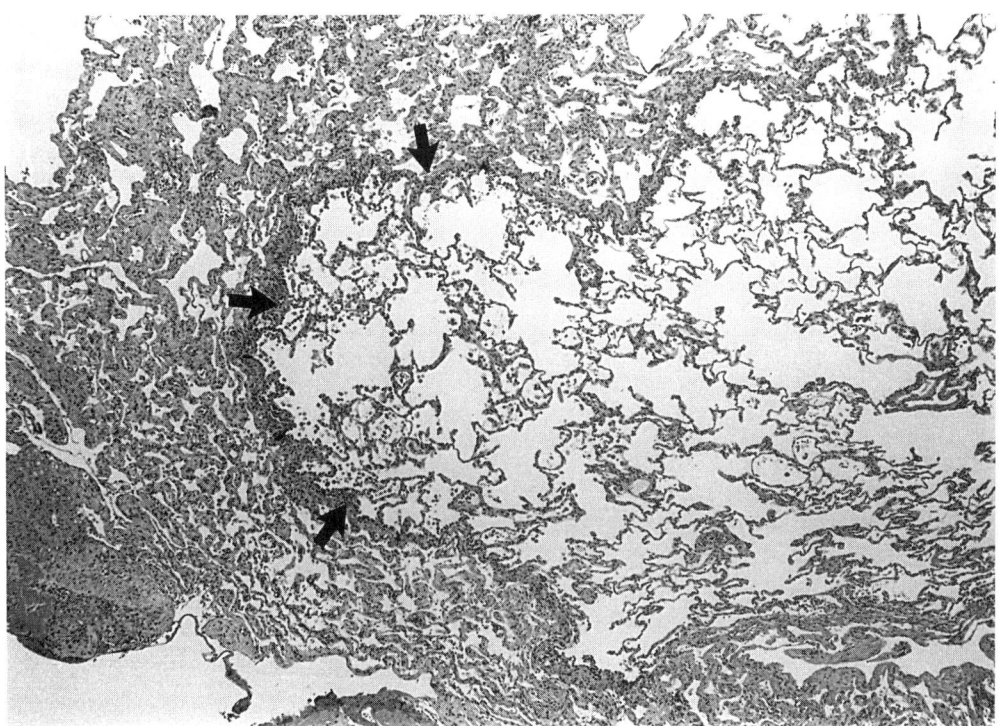

Figure 46.3. Photomicrograph of the biopsy from the left upper lobe demonstrates tremendous expansion of the visceral pleura by numerous anastomosing lymphatic channels. The entrapped lung parenchyma was essentially unremarkable (*arrows*). (Hematoxylin-eosin stain; magnification × 49)

Pulmonary tuberculosis is associated with a history of low-grade fever, weight loss, and loss of appetite. The erythrocyte sedimentation rate is elevated and, except in fulminant tuberculosis (with anergy), the PPD is positive. Psittacosis was considered because of the presence of a parrot at home, but the lack of systemic symptoms did not support this etiology. *Mycoplasma* titer was 1:8, which is not characteristic of an acute infection. Cytomegalovirus and Epstein-Barr virus were excluded on the basis of low or absent titers of antibody. Gorham's disease is a systemic lymphangiomatosis associated with lytic lesions in bones. This diagnosis was considered because of the lesions in the thoracic vertebrae on MRI and the bone scan which were thought to represent lymphangioma or cavernous hemangioma of the bone. Given the presence of these lesions, Gorham's disease could not be entirely ruled out. Disruption of the thoracic duct can occur after direct chest trauma and could explain the ongoing drainage of chylous fluid from the left pleural cavity, but there was no history of trauma. Lymphoma was excluded by the normal bone marrow studies and chest MRI scans showing no evidence

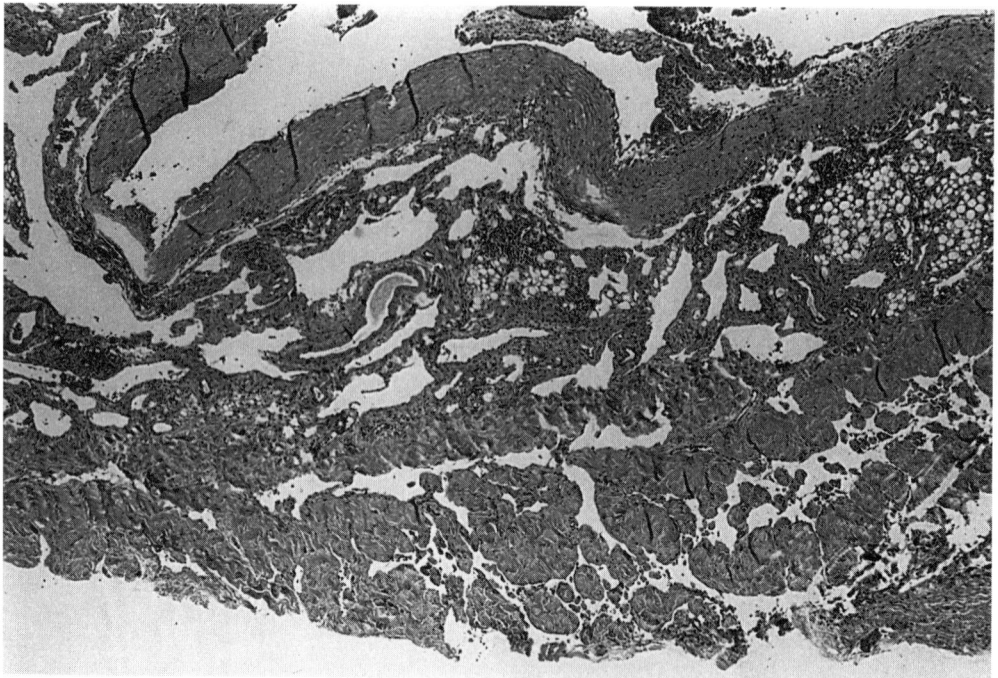

Figure 46.4. Photomicrograph of the pericardial biopsy shows extensive infiltration of the connective tissue by numerous lymphatic channels. (Hematoxylin-eosin; magnification × 48)

of an intrathoracic mass. The diagnosis of lymphangiomatosis fits the clinical picture and the subsequent hospital course.

Clinically, lymphangiomatosis can be diffuse with gradual involvement of the complete lung. There may be areas of lymphatic proliferation within the liver and spleen giving rise to cystic fluid-filled areas within these organs. This patient did not show evidence of splenic involvement initially, but later in the hospital course, there was marked hepatosplenomegaly consistent with lymphatic proliferation in these organs. Since interferon has been shown to be effective in inhibiting angiogenesis in hemangiomas, it was attempted as a rescue therapy to possibly prevent further lymphatic proliferation.

The boy presented to the PICU in septic shock and had two episodes of Gram-negative sepsis. This was most likely due to an altered immune status, including significantly reduced IgG levels (Table 46.2), probably as a result of the ongoing losses of protein-rich fluid from the pleural cavity. IgG was administered to boost these levels.

He developed pericardial tamponade with shock despite there being no change in the cardiac silhouette on chest radiographs. The echocardiogram, however, demonstrated the presence of a significant pericardial effusion causing diastolic collapse of the right atrium. The absence of cardiac enlargement on chest radiographs does not exclude the presence of an effusion or cardiac tamponade.

COMMENTARY

This is an unusual disease, but the pathologic processes are the challenging routine of ICU work. I find it most interesting that pericardial diseases are so difficult to identify, yet can cause such significant disease. Identification and correction (draining the fluid in this case) can cause dramatic improvement.

Suggested Readings

1. Berberich FR, Bernstein ID, Ochs HD, Schaller RT. Lymphangiomatosis with chylothorax. J Pediatr 1975;87[87(Pt 1)]:941–943.
2. Carlson KC, Parnassus WN, Klatt EC. Thoracic lymphangiomatosis. Arch Pathol Lab Med 1987;111:475–477.
3. Ducharme JC, Belanger R, Simard P, Bazinet HP. Chylothorax, chylopericardium with multiple lymphangioma of bone. J Pediatr Surg 1982;17:365–367.
4. Dunkelman H, Sharief N, Berman L, Ninan T. Generalized lymphangiomatosis with chylothorax. Arch Dis Child 1989;64:1058–1060.
5. Folkman J. Successful treatment of an angiogenic disease [Editorial]. N Engl J Med 1989;320:1211–121.
6. Hancock BJ, St-Vil D, Luks FI, Lorenzo MD, Blanchard H. Complications of lymphangiomas in children. J Pediatr Surg 1992;27:220–226.
7. Hellmann JR, Myer CM III, Prenger EC. Therapeutic alternatives in the treatment of life-threatening vasoformative tumors. Am J Otolaryngol 1992;13:48–53.
8. Scully RF, Galdabini JJ, McNeely BU. Case records of the Massachusetts General Hospital: case 30-1980. N Engl J Med 1980;303:270–276.
9. Shah AR, Dinwiddie R, Woolf D, Ramani R, Higgins JNP, Matthew DJ. Generalized lymphangiomatosis and chylothorax in the pediatric age group. Pediatr Pulmonol 1992;14:126–130.
10. Swank DW, Hepper NG, Folkert KE, Colby TV. Intrathoracic lymphangiomatosis mimicking lymphangioleiomyomatosis in a young woman. Mayo Clin Proc 1989;64:1264–1268.
11. White CW, Sondheimer HM, Crouch EC, Wilson H, Fan LL. Treatment of pulmonary hemangiomatosis with recombinant interferon alfa-2a. N Engl J Med 1989;320:1197–1200.
12. Zuckerman E, Shahar J, Lieberman Y, Boss YH, Yeshurun D. Diffuse lymphangioma with intrathoracic involvement. Respiration 1990;57:62–64.

Case 47

Darryl R. Gwyn
The Johns Hopkins Hospital
Baltimore, Maryland, USA

HISTORY

A 7-week-old boy was admitted to the PICU with seizures and depressed mental status. He was the 8-lb 4-oz product of an uncomplicated 42-week gestation and was delivered vaginally. The infant was in good health until 1 week prior to admission. At that time, he was seen by his private medical doctor and diagnosed with a "red throat." He continued to be irritable with some vomiting over the next 3 days, which was attributed to a questionable gastroenteritis at a subsequent physical examination with no other abnormalities apparent. Over the next 3–4 days, the patient's irritability decreased, as did his appetite and playfulness. Concurrently, his mother noticed an increase in his head size and the infant's irritability when she put on his hat.

The baby's social history was unremarkable. He lived at home with his mother, his father, a 10-year-old sister and a male friend of the family. On week days, he was taken care of by a baby-sitter. When the infant was brought to the emergency room by his parents, he was weak, unresponsive, limp, and lethargic, with leftward eye deviation and a questionable swollen head.

PHYSICAL EXAMINATION

At presentation, the patient was unresponsive to stimuli with a positive right eye deviation. His temperature was 38.3°C, his blood pressure was 115/69 mm Hg, his pulse rate was 159 beats/min and regular, and his respirations were regular and unlabored. The physical examination was significant for soft spots noted on his occiput, with questionable swelling. In addition, his fontanel was open and soft, his eyes were opened with pupils equal and reactive to light, and he had a positive corneal reflex and a positive gag reflex. The neurologic examination showed that he was spontaneously moving all extremities bilaterally and his deep tendon reflexes were 2+ and equal throughout. His capillary filling time was markedly decreased >4 seconds, his cardiac, respiratory, abdominal, and genitourinary examination results were all normal, and no further bruising or tenderness was noted physically.

LABORATORY DATA

Laboratory data was as follows: hematocrit 17.7%, hemoglobin 6 g%, platelets 527,000/mm^3, white blood cell count 13.2 × 10^3/mm^3 (57% polymorphonuclears, 10% bands, 25% lymphocytes, 4% monocytes, 2% myelocytes, 2% metamyelocytes), sodium 140 mEq/l, potassium 4.7 mEq/l, chloride 111 mEq/l, bicarbonate 19 mEq/l, blood urea nitrogen (BUN) 7 mg/dl, creatinine 0.4 mg/dl, glucose 135 mg/dl, calcium 7.4 mg/dl, phosphate 4.2 mg/dl, total protein 5 g/dl, albumin 2.9 g/dl, prothrombin time (PT) and partial thromboplastin time (PTT) were 1.1 and 0.9 times control, respectively. Nontraumatic xanthochromic fluid was obtained from the lumbar puncture, which showed 3,862 white blood cells (58% polymorphonuclear, 42% mononuclear) with too numerous to count red blood cells, glucose level of 106 mg/dl, and protein of 1,990, with a negative latex antigen for H-flu and *N. meningitidis* and no organisms seen in the cerebrospinal fluid (CSF). The venous blood gas obtained showed pH 7.31, PCO$_2$ 45 mm Hg, PO$_2$ 38 mm Hg, and bicarbonate 23 mEq/l. Cultures of blood, urine, CSF, and stool were sent.

MANAGEMENT

The child was placed on 100% non-rebreather O$_2$ and an intraosseous line was started with two 15 ml/kg boluses of normal saline given. Decadron 0.15 mg/kg and ceftriaxone 50 mg/kg were given subsequently. After the fluid boluses, the patient was noted to have greatly increased responsiveness and activity. Intravenous access was obtained and fluid was run at 1¼ maintenance. The intraosseous line was discontinued. Arterial blood gas values showed pH 7.37, PCO$_2$ 37 mm Hg, PaO$_2$ 374 mm Hg, and bicarbonate 22 mEq/l. A repeat check of the hemoglobin and hematocrit showed a hemoglobin of 7.2 g% and a hematocrit of 21.7%. At this point, a chest X-ray was obtained and the baby was sent to the CT scanner, which showed acute versus chronic subdural/subarachnoid blood, with blood in the posterior ventricular horns, normal size ventricles, no mass effect or shift, nondepressed biparietal skull fractures, and areas in the right parietal region consistent with contusions. The chest X-ray was significant for positive rib fractures with normal lung fields. Skull films showed parietal and occipital stellate fractures. The child was admitted to the PICU for monitoring while child protective services and social services were contacted. The next several days were significant for increasing frequency of seizures that were unresponsive to anticonvulsants and the infant's decreasing mental status (Glasgow coma scale initially 12–13 decreased to 6–8). His seizures were associated with increasing frequency of desaturations and hypoventilation. Therefore he was electively intubated. Neurosurgical assessment was obtained and bilateral subdural drains were placed. The patient was continued on dilantin and phenobarbital to control his seizures and placed on maintenance 5% dextrose, ½ normal saline with potassium chloride (10 mEq/l). On the third postoperative day, the child was found to be free of seizures, with therapeutic dilantin and phenobarbital levels, and was extubated to room air without incident. His Glasgow coma score continued to improve to 9–10 and the baby showed increasing alertness and activity.

After this brief period of stability, the patient was noted to have increased urine output. Table 47.1 shows the various electrolyte and fluid balances during the next 6 days.

After this period, the patient was started on complete enteral feeds without any problems and transferred to the pediatric ward service.

DISCUSSION

Fluid and electrolyte management is a common concern associated with intracranial trauma and intracranial postoperative care. In Table 47.1, over a 2½-day period, there is an increasing urine output with a decreasing serum sodium concentration. The attendant decrease in urine osmolarity prompted the starting of urine replacements on the third day. The resultant increase in serum sodium

Table 47.1.

Day and Time	Urine Output (ml/hr)	Blood Urea Nitrogen/ Creatinine (mg/dl)	Urine Sodium (mmol/L)	Serum Sodium (mEq/l)	Serum Osmolarity (mOsm/l)	Urine Osmolarity/ Urine Specific Gravity	Sodium Intake (kg/d)	Replacement + Sodium in Urine Output Replacement
11/20								
a.m.	1.5	7/0.5		133–138	284	1.015	9.4	
p.m.								
11/21								
a.m.	3.6	3/0.5		133	272	1.011	5.6	
p.m.	3.3		86–147	128		272–505 1.010	3.4	
late evening	10							
11/22								
a.m.	9.9	1/0.4	25–74	128–135	262	199 1.005–1.000	5.0	7.6
p.m.	7.9			147–150	307	1.005	2.7	
11/23								
a.m.	4.6			148–154	314	1.003	2.9	3.2
p.m.	5.2			149–151		1.002	2.9	4.4
11/24								
a.m.	7.9	1/0.5		148–151	306	1.002	2.2	4.8
p.m.	6.4			145		1.005	a	
11/25								
a.m.	5.4	1/0.5		146–151		1.004	b	
p.m.	3.6			145–146		1.008	b	

[a] Ad lib feeding and keep vein open for intravenous fluids.
[b] Total ad lib.

and urine output prompted discontinuation of urine replacements on the fifth day. For the next 2 days, the infant's urine output continued to decrease, his serum sodium concentration remained stable, and he was advanced to a regular diet.

Throughout this period, the baby was given no diuretics and had normal renal function (potassium, bicarbonate, creatinine). The differential diagnosis considered in this 36- to 48-hour period included: sodium imbalance, fluid overload, diabetes insipidus (DI), syndrome of inappropriate ADH secretion (SIADH), and cerebral salt-wasting syndrome (CSWS). Patients with intracranial trauma or intracranial surgery have fluids administered typically at 2/3 maintenance to avoid complications of cerebral edema and SIADH. Relative hypersthenuria with hyponatremia is the typical clinical situation indicative of SIADH (1). With the decreased sodium concentration, the urine output increased dramatically and the urine osmolarity and specific gravity decreased. Therefore, the decrease in sodium concentration was attributed to something else.

Fluid overload in this situation is not expected, but if

during surgery there is hemodynamic instability or inadvertent perioperative fluid boluses are administered, then the clinical picture seen here may develop. Review of the fluid and electrolyte management of this patient perioperatively showed no such fluid administration.

DI is typically abrupt in onset with a three-stage appearance of initially 3–7 days of diuresis, followed by 2–3 days of antidiuresis, with either a resolution or return to increased diuresis. Clinically, a urine osmolarity ≤300 mOsm/l with a plasma osmolarity of >295 mOsm/l suggests a patient with DI (2). The patient we describe met these criteria except for the dramatic decrease in serum sodium concentration, which is usually noted to be increasing during the initial phase of diuresis.

The syndrome of cerebral salt wasting has an unknown etiology, but is associated with subarachnoid hemorrhage, suprasellar intraventricular blood, or ventricular enlargement, and can be recognized by hyponatremia associated with increased urine output and volume contraction. The etiology has been questioned with no direct correlation seen between atrial natriuretic factor, arginine vasopressin, aldosterone, or renin, although all have been suspected. Most of the evidence initially pointed to atrial natriuretic factor, but subsequent studies have found no correlation between the concentration of atrial natriuretic factor and the occurrence of this syndrome (3–5). The current concept leans toward a nonregulatory hormone or hypothalamic response in which the increased concentration of atrial natriuretic factor may be an indication of the syndrome's presence without being a direct cause of the syndrome. Some other "unknown protein" that may affect renal salt regulation has not been ruled out, however. Review of the chart at the time of increased urine output shows a relatively increased urine sodium compared with the serum sodium. The setting is also correct for the syndrome of cerebral salt wasting.

Intensive care patients may present with drastic changes in organ function, fluid balance, or other "system" failure, prompting quick response. Even expected complications such as increased diuresis after intracranial procedures may be seen in an uncharacteristic fashion. The case of this infant is such an example of an expected complication (increased urine output) presenting with an uncharacteristic finding (decreasing serum sodium concentration). In the intensive care setting, at times of drastic changes, it is important to have an anticipated differential diagnosis generated, appropriate laboratory evidence gathered, and a steady response to correction that must allow for unexpected changes or findings.

COMMENTARY ▬▬▬▬▬▬▬▬▬▬▬▬▬▬▬▬▬▬▬▬▬▬▬

After head trauma or head surgery, unusual fluid and electrolyte abnormalities are seen. Very rarely do we see classic DI or SIADH nor do we see the "classic" cerebral salt wasting syndrome. More commonly, we see a combination of abnormalities that diagnostically do not fit into a single category. Theoretically, management requires maintenance of euvolemia with repletion of the appropriate electrolytes. Child abuse as a cause for head trauma is an increasingly common reason for admission to the PICU. The prevention of this problem through social and educational programs should be a priority.

References

1. Weigle CGM, Tobin JR. Metabolic and endocrine disease in pediatric intensive care. In: Rogers MC, ed. Textbook of pediatric intensive care. 2nd ed. Baltimore: Williams & Wilkins, 1992:1552–1253.
2. Weigle CGM, Tobin JR. Metabolic and endocrine disease in pediatric intensive care. In: Rogers MC, ed. Textbook of pediatric intensive care. 2nd ed. Baltimore: Williams & Wilkins, 1992:1250–1252.
3. Wijdicks EFM, Ropper AH, Hunnicutt EJ, Richardson GS, Nathanson JA. Atrial natriuretic factor and salt wasting after aneurysmal subarachnoid hemorrhage. Stroke 1991;22:1519–1524.
4. Diringer MN, Wu KC, Verbalis JG, Hanley DF. Hypervolemic therapy prevents volume contraction but not hyponatremia following subarachnoid hemorrhage. Ann Neurol 1992;31:543–550.
5. Diringer MN, Lim JS, Kirsch JR, Hanley DF. Suprasellar and intraventricular blood predict elevated plasma atrial natriuretic factor in subarachnoid hemorrhage. Stroke 1991;22:577–581.

Case 48

D. Roddy O'Donnell, Robert C. Tasker, Anthony J. Slater, and Kathy Wilkinson

Hospital for Sick Children
London, United Kingdom

Although head injury, central nervous system (CNS) infection, hypoxic/ischemic insult, or acute toxic encephalopathy are the commonest primary causes of coma in children (1,2), in the critically ill patient referred for intensive care, many and often multiple secondary complicating factors could contribute to cerebral injury and neurologic morbidity (3,4). These potentially interacting factors could include seizures, raised intracranial pressure, acidosis, hypo- or hyperglycemia, hypo- or hypertension, and hypoxia. Furthermore, even in the case of systemic derangements with seemingly uniform cerebral effects, there may be multifocal and not uniform changes in cerebral function (4–6) and neuropathology. We describe the cases of two patients exemplifying the difficulty of such multifactorial insult and multifocal cerebral injury in the pediatric intensive care patient.

HISTORY— PATIENT 1

A 3-year-old boy with high-grade malignant B cell non-Hodgkin's lymphoma was admitted for intensive care during his second course of cyclophosphamide, prednisolone, and vincristine chemotherapy because of uncontrolled seizures. Nine days prior to admission he had a low-grade fever, mild hypertension, and episodes of twitching on the right side of his face. A lumbar puncture for cerebrospinal fluid (CSF) examination had revealed normal CSF pressure, no organisms, blasts, or white blood cells, and CSF

329

biochemistry of glucose 2.8 mmol/l and protein 0.19 g/dl. He was started on broad-spectrum antibiotics, acyclovir, and phenobarbitone. On the day of admission he had intermittent focal seizures and grand mal episodes, and he became very hypertensive with a blood pressure of 170/120 mm Hg. He was intubated, mechanically ventilated, and then transferred for further medical care.

MANAGEMENT

On arrival this boy continued to have repeated grand mal episodes. Examination of the boy revealed consistently low serum magnesium levels (<0.7 mmol/l), mildly low serum calcium (2.15 mmol/l), and a slight elevation in serum creatinine (72 μmol/l). His electroencephalogram (EEG) revealed a marked abnormality, with fluctuating slow activity over the right frontocentral region, and also independently over the left midtemporal and posterotemporal region. His cranial computed tomography (CT) scan (Fig. 48.1) showed extensive low density in the white matter of the cerebral hemisphere that extended into the cortex at some points on the frontal convexity. There was also a small region of low density in the left internal capsule. Over the next 4 days treatment included mechanical ventilation, administration of intravenous antihypertensives, acyclovir, intravenous magnesium, and anticonvulsants. The clinical endpoint used for management was the normalization of biochemical and systemic parameters, and the pharmacologic control of clinically discernable seizures and their electroencephalographic correlates. The latter necessitated the use of phenytoin and the short-acting barbiturate thiopentone with the appropriate monitor-

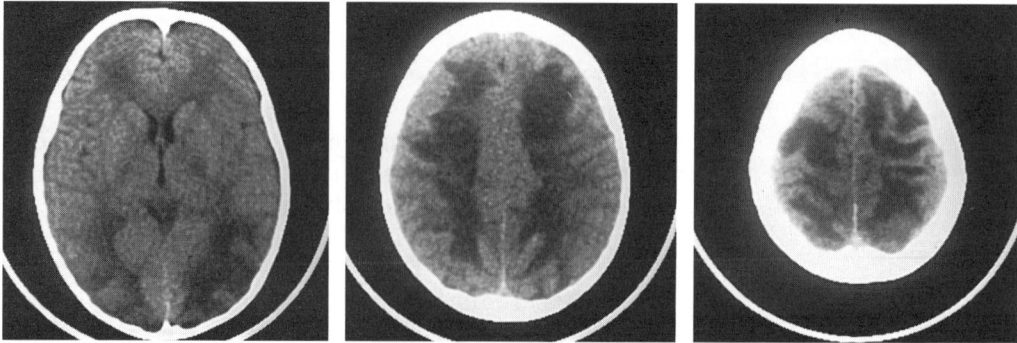

Figure 48.1. Patient 1. Cranial CT scan showing extensive low density in multiple regions of the white matter of the cerebral hemisphere which extends into the cortex at some point on the frontal convexity.

ing (6). By the fourth day postadmission, intravenous anticonvulsant therapy had been weaned and enteral phenobarbitone was started. All investigations for an underlying viral, fungal, or bacterial infective etiology were negative.

After 7 days in the ICU this child was well enough to be transferred back to the referring oncology unit. Six months later he had no detectable neuropsychiatric or neurologic deficits.

HISTORY— PATIENT 2

A 6-year-old boy was admitted for intensive care, having been resuscitated following a fall from a hotel fourth-floor window. At the scene of the accident he was unconscious and initially not breathing. In the emergency room he was hemodynamically stable (pulse 95 beats/min, blood pressure 110/80 mm Hg), he was breathing spontaneously (22 breaths/min), and his initial arterial blood gas in supplementary facial oxygen was: pH 7.2, PaO_2 65 torr (8.6 kPa), and $PaCO_2$ 37 torr (4.96 kPa). His coma scale assessment revealed no spontaneous or stimulated eye opening, incomprehensible sounds as the best verbal response, and flexion to pain as the best motor response. His eye examination showed unequal pupils with the right dilated and nonreactive to bright light. After appropriated airway management, intubation, and hyperventilation, full trauma review revealed right frontal bone and basal skull fractures, as well as a pelvic fracture. His initial cranial CT scan did not show any surgically remediable cause for the raised intracranial pressure (ICP) with mainly diffuse parenchymal changes (Fig. 48.2).

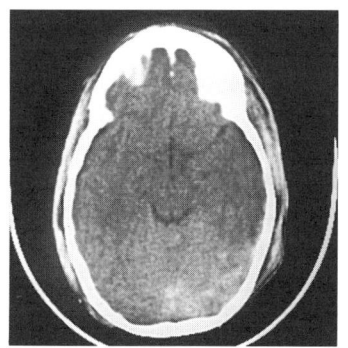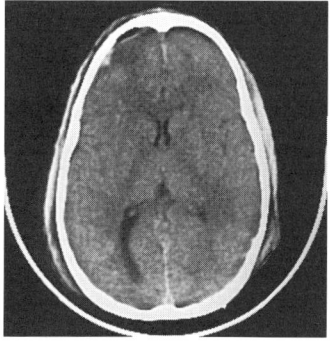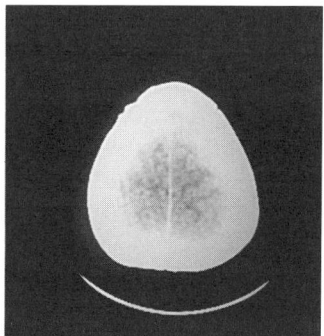

Figure 48.2. Patient 2. Cranial CT scan showing low density in the white matter of the right frontal region extending into the cortex on the frontal convexity, as well as a small amount of subdural air and blood. A not untypical scan for a moderately severe head-injured child.

MANAGEMENT

Following initial stabilization and transfer to the unit, ICP monitoring with a fiberoptic cerebral intraparenchymal device (7) was initiated and a standard active head injury management protocol was followed (8). During the first 24 hours of intensive care, the serum sodium swung between 130 mmol/l and 150 mmol/l, and the maximum ICP was 30 mm Hg. Between the second and the fifth day of ICP monitoring, baseline pressures became more consistently <15 mm Hg, with only intermittently raised levels >20 mm Hg. On the sixth day monitoring was discontinued. On day 7 a technetium-99m hexamethylpropylene amine oxime (HMPAO) brain scan showed at least three focal areas of decreased perfusion (Fig. 48.3).

Three weeks after the accident the boy had no sensory deficits, normal tone, normal motor movement, but a somewhat ataxic gait. Cranial nerve examination results were normal apart from a complete right third nerve palsy. On day 24 he started to speak and subsequently exhibited fair cognitive function.

DISCUSSION

These two patients presenting with an acute cause of coma, one traumatic and the other nontraumatic, had multiple factors that potentially were secondary contributors to the primary cerebral insult—although, of course, there remains the possibility that some of these factors were merely symptomatic of the underlying primary brain injury. In both cases the CNS was not uniformly affected. In the trauma patient this was not an unexpected finding, though the HMPAO scan revealed multifocal abnormalities that are not fully apparent with viewing by conventional imaging.

In the case of the patient 1 there were a number of possible causes that might have precipitated or complicated the encephalopathy. These included tumor lysis with acute renal dysfunction, uncontrolled hypertension, idiosyncratic drug reaction to the antibiotics or chemotherapy, drug toxicities, biochemical derangement, seizures, and possible infection. In patient 2 the additional factors besides trauma included acidosis, hypoxia, hypo- and hypernatremia, and raised ICP. Much of what we now accept and use as standard pediatric neurointensive care practice

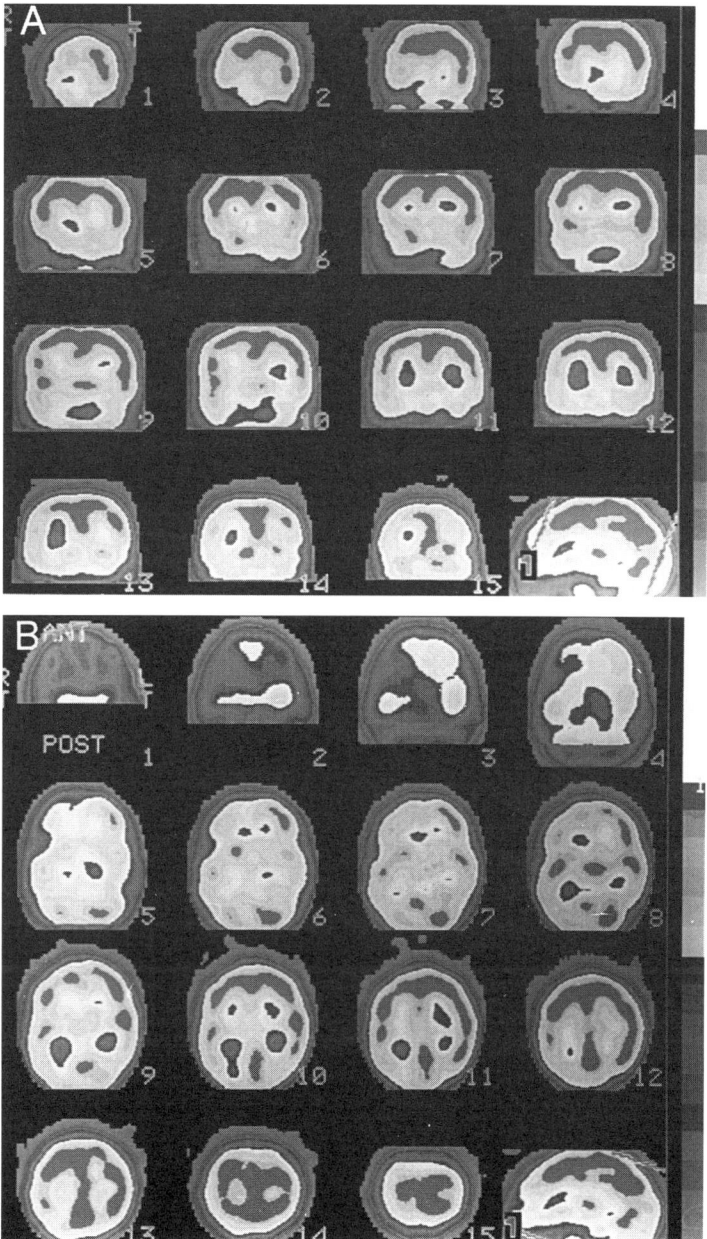

Figure 48.3. Patient 2. Technetium-99m hexamethylpropylene amine oxime (HMPAO) brain scan (*A*, coronal sections; *B*, transverse sections) with increased gray scale indicating increased perfusion or blood flow. In contrast to the CT scan (Fig. 48.2), there are multifocal changes in perfusion, with at least three areas of focal decreased perfusion on the right-hand side (frontal: A 1–3, B 6–8; parietal: A 9–10, B 6–9; occipital: A 13–14, b 11–12).

Table 48.1.   Potential Therapies Based on Experimental Observation

Cellular Mechanism	Potential Therapy
Inadequate perfusion	Calcium antagonists
microvascular circulation	Hypertension
	Hypervolemia
	Hemodilution
Energy failure	Hypothermia
	Barbiturates
Acidosis	Acid-base buffering
Ionic derangement	Diuresis
Cerebral edema	Hyperventilation
Increased intracranial pressure	Temperature control, steroids (?)
Phospholipase activation	Phospholipase inhibitors
Lipolysis	Prostanoid agonists or
Prostaglandin production	antagonists
Leukotriene production	
Neurotransmitter-mediated	Receptor antagonist
Glutamatergic	Inhibition of release
Nonglutamatergic	
Oxygen-radical generation	Scavengers
membrane peroxidation	Antioxidants
Seizure activity	Anticonvulsants
Other	Inhibition of protein synthesis

has evolved from the adult head injury and Reye's syndrome experience of the 1980s (9). The two patients we described had good outcomes despite the severity and complexity of their underlying disease, and what can best be described as the "crudeness" of the medical interventions offered. There are many examples of similar patients in our experience whose outcomes were sadly unfavorable.

Experimental models of such complex insults with multifocal pathologies do not exist. However, extensive study over the past decade into the mechanisms leading to neuronal injury in well-defined focal or global insults such as ischemia and hypoglycemia has revealed a number of separate but interrelated pathophysiological processes that may participate in neurotoxicity (10–12). Each of these potentially have therapeutic agents that could prevent or arrest the injurious process (Table 48.1). It was perhaps fortuitous that the two patients we described received agents which may act on many of the mechanisms indicated in Table 48.1.

COMMENTARY

Clinical trials in such a heterogenous population with injury in potentially multiple brain regions would be impossible to conduct—either because of differential regional vulnerability or differential regional insult. Given that many of the patients with acute encephalopathies admitted for intensive care support fall into this category even when we do not suspect it, a multicenter epidemiologic approach is the only way of identifying and investigating future specific therapeutic strategies or combined therapies.

References

1. Seshia SS, Seshia MMK, Sachdeva RK. Coma in childhood. Dev Med Child Neurol 1977;19:614–628.
2. Brown JK, Habel AH. Toxic encephalopathy and acute brain-swelling in children. Dev Med Child Neurol 1975;17:659–679.
3. Tasker RC, Matthew DJ, Helms P, Dinwiddie R, Boyd S. Monitoring in non-traumatic coma. I: invasive intracranial measurements. Arch Dis Child 1988;63:888–894.
4. Tasker RC, Boyd SG, Harden A, Kendall B, Harding BN, Matthew DJ. The clinical significance of seizures in critically ill young infants requiring intensive care. Neuropediatrics 1991;22:129–138.
5. Tasker RC, Boyd S, Harden A, Matthew DJ. Monitoring in non-traumatic coma. II: electroencephalopathy. Arch Dis Child 1988;63:895–899.
6. Tasker RC, Boyd SG, Harden A, Matthew DJ. EEG monitoring of prolonged thiopentone administration for intractable seizures and status epilepticus in infants and young children. Neuropediatrics 1989;20:147–153.
7. Tasker RC, Matthew DJ. Evaluation of cerebral intraparenchymal pressure monitoring in young children. Neuropediatrics 1991;22:47–49.
8. Davis RJ, Tate VF, Dean JM, Goldberg AL, Rogers MC. Head and spinal cord injury. In: MC Rogers. Textbook of pediatric intensive care. 2nd ed. Baltimore: Williams & Wilkins, 1992.
9. Swedlow DB, Schreiner MS. Management of Reye's syndrome. Crit Care Clin 1985;1:285–311.
10. Wieloch T. Neurochemical correlates to selective neuronal vulnerability. Prog Brain Res 1985;63:69–85.
11. Hoff JT. Cerebral protection. J Neurosurg 1986;65:579–591.
12. Ginsberg MD, Globus MY-T, Busto R, Dietrich WD. The potential of combination pharmacotherapy in cerebral ischemia. In: J Krieglstein, H Oberpichler, eds. Pharmacology of cerebral ischemia 1990. Stuttgart: Wissenchaftliche Verlagsgesellschaft, 1990.

Case 49

D. Lyn Davidson and Donald H. Shaffner

The Johns Hopkins Hospital
Baltimore, Maryland, USA

HISTORY

A 9-year-old boy was admitted to the hospital with a history of lethargy, dizziness, vomiting, and headache of 1 week's duration. On arrival at the emergency room, he had a generalized tonic-clonic seizure while he was receiving inhaled bronchodilators for his reactive airway disease. The seizure spontaneously remitted without administration of anticonvulsant and the patient was hospitalized for observation. No further seizures occurred during the next 3 days. Blood cultures did not demonstrate bacteremia. A urinary toxicology screen was negative. Sinus radiographs appeared normal. An electroencephalogram (EEG) showed diffuse slowing in the left parietal region. A contrast CT scan of the brain showed an enhancing mass lesion obstructing the foramen of Monroe with a marked midline shift and massive hydrocephalus (Fig. 49.1). The patient was transferred to Johns Hopkins University Hospital.

The patient had a 1-year history of episodic afebrile "flu-like" symptoms, with headache, vomiting, and lethargy. These symptoms lasted for several days and responded to bed rest and oral analgesics. These episodes had occurred approximately eight times in the previous 12 months. The remainder of the boy's medical history revealed three prior hospitalizations for exacerbations of asthma and one hospitalization in infancy for hemorrhagic cystitis following circumcision. He had never had any seizures before the presenting event. There was no history of anemia, change in appetite, weight loss, recent additional medications, or

337

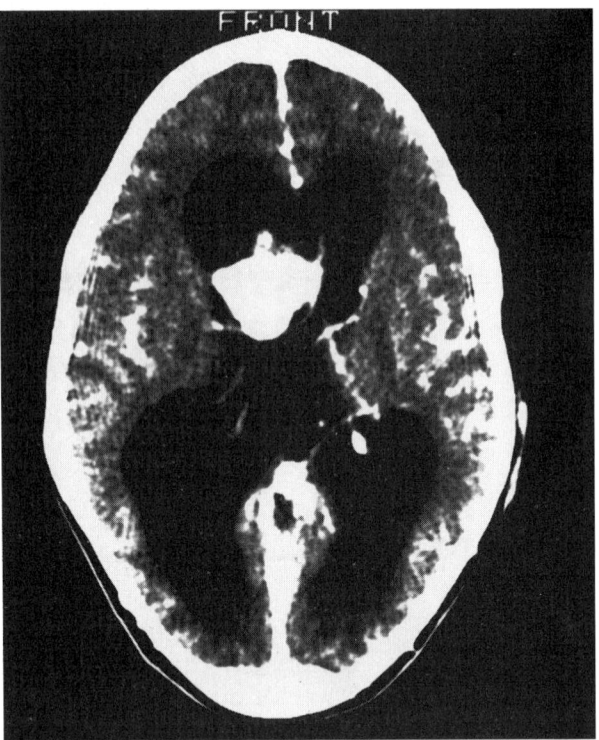

Figure 49.1. Contrast-enhanced brain CT showing massive hydrocephalus and a contrast-enhancing midline mass.

ingestion of unusual materials. Family history was negative for neurologic symptoms.

PHYSICAL EXAMINATION

Physically, we saw an obese child who appeared to be his stated age. He had no enlarged lymph nodes and results of cutaneous examination were normal except for two pigmented papular lesions, each measuring approximately 2 mm, on the right nasolabial fold. The boy's head was normal in shape and size. No retinal hemorrhages could be found but bilateral papilledema was present. His neck was supple, his lungs were clear, and his heart was normal. His abdomen was relaxed and nontender. His liver and spleen were not palpable and no masses were present.

Neurologic examination was significant for arousal only to pain, inconsistent localization of motor responses, and confused verbal utterances. Deep tendon reflexes were symmetrically increased. A brief focal tonic-clonic seizure involving the left arm and leg occurred during the examination.

The boy's temperature was 36.5°C, and his respiratory rate was 15–20 breaths/min. His pulse rate was 50–60 beats/min and regular and his blood pressure was 120/80 mm Hg with the patient supine.

LABORATORY DATA

Pulse oximetry on room air demonstrated an arterial saturation of 100%. Hemoglobin was 12.0 g/dl with a packed cell volume of 35.7%, a mean corpuscular volume of 80.3 μm^3/cell, and a mean corpuscular hemoglobin of 27 pg/cell. The white blood cell count was 7700/mm^3 and the platelet count was 430,000/mm^3. The prothrombin time was 12.9 seconds (1.1 times control) and the activated partial thromboplastin time was 22.6 seconds (0.8 times control).

Blood urea nitrogen, creatinine, calcium, phosphorus, and magnesium levels were normal. Total and direct bilirubin, total protein, and serum albumin were normal. Serum sodium was 135 mEq/l, potassium was 5.0 mEq/l, chloride was 104 mEq/l, CO_2 was 15 mEq/l, and glucose was 159 mg/dl. Uric acid, alkaline phosphatase, and alanine aminotransferase levels were normal. The aspartate aminotransferase level was elevated at 45 IU/l.

Cerebrospinal fluid (CSF) contained no white blood cells, 10 red blood cells/mm^3, a glucose level of 76 mg/dl, and a protein level of 19 mg/dl.

MANAGEMENT

The patient underwent emergent placement of a ventriculostomy catheter to manage increased intracranial pressure from the massive hydrocephalus. Decadron 0.4 mg/kg, phenytoin 20 mg/kg, and 500 mg of nafcillin were given intravenously. After that, decadron was given daily at the same dose, but the phenytoin was decreased to maintain an adequate serum level. Oxacillin 100 mg/kg/day was administered. The patient's level of alertness dramatically improved within 12 hours of ventriculostomy catheter placement. A magnetic resonance imaging (MRI) study obtained on day 3 postadmission showed decreased hydrocephalus and a paraventricular mass lesion. The patient received a craniotomy for tumor excision on day 4 postadmission, with frozen section of the biopsy indicating an anaplastic astrocytoma. He developed a mild left hemiparesis postoperatively with gradual resolution over the next several days. A postoperative MRI showed pneumocephalus, decreasing hydrocephalus, and a 2.5 cm residual tumor. The intraventricular drain was discontinued at 24 hours postoperative and weaning of decadron was begun on postoperative day 5. During this time interval, the nasolabial skin papules noted on the initial examination of the patient were biopsied, and the biopsy indicated angiofibromas. The presumptive diagnosis of tuberous sclerosis was made. An echocardiographic study did not demonstrate rhabdomyoma and ophthalmologic examination did not demonstrate retinal hamartomas. On postoperative day 10, the patient developed severe headache and lethargy, and mean pulse rate decreased from 80–60 beats/min. CT scan obtained at this time revealed normal ventricular size, but a ventriculoperitoneal shunt was placed because clinical findings suggested increased intracranial pressure. After placement of the ventriculoperitoneal shunt, the patient's neurologic status improved and he was discharged to home 5 days later. Final pathologic diagnosis of the intracranial tumor was subependymal giant cell astrocytoma.

DISCUSSION

Tuberous sclerosis is an inherited, congenital disorder that manifests, either at birth or develops in postnatal life, as tissue malformation involving multiple organs. The disease affects not only ectodermal but mesodermal and endodermal structures. The genetic pattern is one of autosomal dominance but is pleiotropic, affects multiple organs, and is extremely variable in expression, which supports the hypothesis that modifying genes are responsible for the variability in presentation. Severity of disease expression varies from individuals without clinical manifestations who are eventually diagnosed at necropsy to individuals with profound mental retardation, intractable seizures, and early death. The biochemical basis for the tissue malformations is unknown.

The tumors in the various organs are described as hemangiomas, fibromas, lipomyomas, or mixed tumors. The skin is frequently involved and characteristic lesions include facial sebaceous adenomas and the "shagreen patch." The shagreen patch represents thinning of the epithelium and hypertrophy of the connective tissue in the corium. It is often present in the area of skin overlying the posterior iliac crests.

In addition to cutaneous manifestations, there may be bone involvement with cystic lesions secondary to replacement by fibrous tissue growth seen radiographically. Renal tumors, usually mixed tumors of embryonic type, may also occur. Adenomas may develop in the pulmonary parenchyma and spontaneous pneumothorax has been described in several cases. Retinal phakomas (glial nodes that may become calcified) and retinal patches that have a rough surface free of blood vessels may be seen with the ophthalmoscope. Corneal and lens opacities may develop. In the heart, rhabdomyomas form tumors that may protrude into the chamber. Cardiac rhabdomyomas are the most frequent cause of fatalities in the infantile forms of the disease. Subendothelial lipomas or fibrolipomas and endocardial fibroelastosis also occur. Tumors may also arise in the thyroid, thymus, duodenum, liver, pancreas, or spleen.

A frequent finding in tuberous sclerosis is central nervous system involvement with characteristic lesions. White nodules of various sizes and with the consistency of cartilage can be found in the cortex, hence the name for which this disease is known. Frequently, there is a diminution of nerve cells and a proliferation of the glia. Giant cells with grotesque shapes, abnormal nuclei, and cytoplasmic vacuoles are found in the nodules as well as in the white matter. Additionally, small tumors are found in the walls of the lateral ventricle and frequently show proliferative and degenerative changes, marked gliosis, and a tendency to calcification and cyst formation. Paraventricular tumors, sometimes neoplastic as in the patient described, may develop and obstruct cerebrospinal fluid circulation and lead to hydrocephalus.

Treatment of the disease is primarily supportive and consists of anticonvulsant therapy for seizures and, as in this case, neurosurgical intervention for space-consuming lesions.

COMMENTARY

Brain tumors represent one of the few indications for which we administer large doses of steroids. Other indications such as spinal cord injury, asthma, and adrenal insufficiency remain on the list from which adult respiratory distress syndrome and sepsis have been dropped. As research on steroid moieties continues we expect better agents to be developed that will accomplish more specific therapeutic benefits with fewer side effects.

Suggested Reading

1. Warkany J. Hamartoses and adenomatoses. In: Warkay J, ed. Congenital malformations: notes and comments. Chicago: Year Book, 1971: 1260–1265.

Case 50

Randall P. Flick

The Johns Hopkins Hospital
Baltimore, Maryland, USA

HISTORY

A 6-year-old boy was admitted to an outside hospital with a 3-day history of rash consistent with varicella and a 1-day history of right hip pain and a refusal to bear weight. He had been started on oral acyclovir by his private pediatrician after the onset of the rash and fever 2 days prior to admission. In the emergency room the child was found to be alert, febrile to 38°C, and complaining of pain in his right hip. He was noted to have erythema and induration of both anterior thighs (right greater than left) and scrotum as well as diffuse skin lesions consistent with varicella. An aspiration of the right hip was done to rule out septic arthritis. Subsequently an intravenous line was placed, blood cultures were drawn, and the boy was started on intravenous nafcillin. The oral acyclovir was changed to intravenous acyclovir.

Following his admission the child did well until hospital day 2 when he became increasingly lethargic, hypotensive (lowest recorded blood pressure 78 mm Hg systolic), tachycardiac (heart rate 140–160 beats/min), and oliguric. He was transferred to the ICU where he was volume resuscitated and intubated when his Glasgow coma scale score reached a value of 7. A head CT scan showed no compression of the ventricles or cisterns. A lumbar puncture revealed an opening pressure of 44 cm H_2O. Blood cultures drawn on admission were positive for a Gram-positive cocci in chains at 48 hours growth. Transport was arranged to the Johns Hopkins Hospital PICU.

PHYSICAL EXAMINATION

On arrival at the PICU the child was intubated and mechanically ventilated. His Glasgow coma scale was 6, his temperature was 37.7°C, his pulse rate was 124 beats/min, and his blood pressure was 118/78 mm Hg. There were no focal neurologic findings. Examination of the head and neck were significant only for a bilateral chemosis, healing varicella, and the presence of a 5.5-mm oral endotracheal tube. There was no papilledema and the oropharynx was normal. The chest was clear and the heart rate was regular without murmurs, rubs, or gallops. The abdomen was soft with the liver and spleen being barely palpable at the respective costal margins. The scrotum was noticeably edematous and mildly erythematous without induration. Both anterior thighs were erythematous, indurated, and tender with the right being much more so than the left. No areas of fluctuance could be palpated. Distal pulses were 2+ and the capillary refill time was 2–3 seconds. Crusted lesions of varicella were distributed over the head, chest, abdomen, and extremities.

LABORATORY DATA

On admission to the referring hospital, his blood values were as follows: hematocrit 31%; platelets 186,000; and white blood cell (WBC) count 14,100 with 38% bands, 46% polymorphocytes, 7% lymphocytes, 5% monocytes, and 4% eosinophils. Other levels were: sodium 136 mEq/l; potassium 4.0 mEq/l; chloride 101 mEq/l; carbon dioxide 12 mEq/l; serum urea nitrogen 23 mEq/l; creatinine 0.8 mEq/l; and calcium 9.0 mEq/l. Radiographs of the right hip and chest were normal. Joint fluid findings were as follows: red blood cells (RBC) 36,000/mm³, WBC 39/mm³, and Gram stain was negative.

The patient's blood values at the time of admission to Johns Hopkins Hospital were: hematocrit 27.1%; platelets 143,000/mm³; and WBC 16,700/mm³ with 24% bands, 55% polymorphocytes, 1% eosinophils, 1% basophils, 8% lymphocytes, and 3% monocytes. Prothrombin time (PT) was 13.8 seconds and partial thromboplastin time (PTT) was 40.4 seconds. Blood gas levels were: fibrinogen 472 mg/dl; sodium 124 mEq/l; potassium 4.7 mEq/l; chloride 92 mEq/l; carbon dioxide 11 mEq/l; serum urea nitrogen 74 mg/dl; creatinine 4.8 mg/dl; glucose 92 mg/dl; total bilirubin 5.6 mg/dl; direct bilirubin 4.5 mg/dl; magnesium 1.9 mg/dl; calcium 6.7 mg/dl (ionized 0.88 mm/l); phosphorus 4.3 mg/dl; uric acid 10.6 mg/dl; total protein 4.7 mg/dl; albumin 2.1 mg/dl; ammonia (arterial) 28 mg/dl; lactate 0.9 mg/dl; aspartate transaminase (AST) 27 U/l; alanine transaminase (ALT) 44 U/l; alkaline phosphatase 212 U/l; amylase 3 U/l; creatinine kinase 60 U/l. Arterial blood gas values were: pH 7.32, pCO_2 24 mm Hg, pO_2 163 mm Hg (FiO_2 0.4). Urinalysis results were as follows: pH 5.0, specific gravity 1.011, positive dipstick for blood, microscopic with 2–3 RBC per high power field, 1–2 WBC per high power field, and rare cellular casts. Urine and serum were negative for toxicology.

MANAGEMENT

Following admission, the child demonstrated multiple organ system involvement with derangements in the hematologic (coagulation) as well as neurologic, renal, and hepatic systems. He was maintained on mechanical ventilation with mild hyperventilation because of a concern for increased intracranial pressure. His mental status improved over the ensuing 48–72 hours such that he was awake and sufficiently alert to allow for extubation on the fourth hospital day. A magnetic resonance imaging (MRI) and a lumbar puncture done to rule out acute or postinfectious encephalitis were found to be normal. The opening pressure was only slightly elevated at 22 cm H_2O. Acyclovir was discontinued on day 2 because of concern that the encephalopathy might have been a result of acyclovir toxicity given that there had been no dose adjustment in the light of marked elevations in blood urea nitrogen (BUN) and creatinine levels. Viral and bacterial cultures of the CSF showed no growth.

Renal function improved, with the creatinine returning to normal by the fourth hospital day. The PT and PTT (initially 1.2 and 1.5 times those of controls, respectively) normalized without specific therapy within 72 hours. The fibrinogen and fibrin split products remained within normal limits. Platelet counts were never less than the admission value of 143,000. Transaminase and alkaline phosphatase values remained normal. The bilirubin fell from 5.6 to 0.9 mg/dl over 3–4 days. Serum ammonia level, repeated on two occasions, was normal.

Ultrasound of the right thigh failed to show evidence of fascitis or myositis and the overlying cellulitis resolved over several days in response to antibiotics consisting of vancomycin and ceftriaxone. These were later changed to cefuroxime alone. No other cultures were positive other than the initial blood culture that was identified as group A β-hemolytic *Streptococcus*. Serum immunoglobulins and total hemolytic complement were normal.

Following a 14-day course of intravenous antibiotics the child recovered completely and was discharged to complete an additional 7 days of oral antibiotics at home.

DISCUSSION

A child presenting with the combination of fever, hypotension, hypocalcemia, and evidence of multiple organ dysfunction should be suspected of having toxic shock syndrome (TSS).

This child illustrates the relatively unusual case of TSS resulting from infection with group A *Streptococcus*. The case definition of classic TSS resulting from infection with a toxin-producing strain of *Staphylococcus aureus* includes those listed in Table 50.1.

In the late 1980s reports began appearing in the literature describing patients with a similar clinical presentation in association with infection with group A *Streptococcus*. These patients are similar to those with staphylococcal TSS in that they demonstrate multisystem involvement, fever, and hypotension associated with significant mortality. However, they differ in that rash and desquamation are often absent. More importantly, the patients usually have an easily identifiable source of infection that when cultured is positive for group A *Streptococcus*. Invariably the source is a soft tissue infection such as fascitis, myositis, or as in the case of this patient, cellulitis. Blood cultures were positive in slightly over half the patients reported by Stevens et al (1) in direct contrast to classic staphylococcal TSS in which blood cultures are usually negative. As in staphylococcal TSS the toxic streptococcal syndrome is the result of infection with an organism that is found to produce an exotoxin in approximately 80% of cases. In the case of a streptococcal source the toxin is usually pyrogenic exotoxin A. Strains producing this toxin have not been commonly seen since the first half of the century and are often associated with severe group A streptococcal infections.

Management of the child with group A streptococcal infection-associated TSS is similar to classic TSS in that it involves a diligent search for a source of infection, antibiotic therapy, and supportive care. An important difference

Table 50.1. Toxic Shock Syndrome Case Definition

Fever: Temperature ≥ 38.9°C

Rash: Diffuse macular erythroderma

Desquamation: 1–2 weeks after onset of illness, particularly of palms, soles, fingers, and toes

Hypotension: Systolic blood pressure ≤90 mm Hg for adults; < 5th percentile by age for children < 16 years of age; orthostatic drop in diastolic blood pressure ≥15 mm Hg from lying to sitting; orthostatic syncope or orthostatic dizziness

Involvement of three or more of the following organ systems:

1. Gastrointestinal—vomiting or diarrhea at onset of illness
2. Muscular—severe myalgia or creatinine phosphokinase level greater than twice the upper limit of normal for laboratory
3. Mucous membrane—vaginal, oropharyngeal, or conjunctival hyperemia
4. Renal—blood urea nitrogen or serum creatinine greater than twice the upper limit of normal; or ≥5 white blood cells per high power field in the absence of a urinary tract infection
5. Hepatic—total bilirubin, AST or ALT greater than twice the upper limit of normal for laboratory
6. Hematologic—platelets <100,000/mm^3
7. Central nervous system—disorientation or alterations in consciousness without focal neurologic signs when fever and hypotension are absent

Negative results on the following tests if obtained:

1. Blood, throat, or cerebrospinal fluid cultures; blood cultures may be positive for *Staphylococcus aureus*
2. Serologic tests for Rocky Mountain spotted fever, leptospirosis, or measles

Source: Centers for Disease Control. Case definitions for public health surveillance. MMWR 1990: 39(RR-13);38–39.

is the role of surgical management in these cases. Because they commonly involve soft tissue infections, many of which are deep, surgical drainage is often necessary to halt progression of the illness. Antibiotics alone are insufficient in those patients with fascitis, myositis, or other deep soft tissue infection. In the case of the patient we described, ultrasound was used to rule out deep soft tissue involvement. Mortality in the series of 20 adult patients reported by Stevens et al. was 30% in contrast to a case fatality rate of <5% in *Staphyloccocus*-associated TSS.

COMMENTARY

This is a case of a common disease (group A *Streptococcus*) presenting in an uncommon way—toxic shock syndrome. In addition to this point is the likelihood of the emergence of group A *Streptococcus* resistant to first line antibiotics, as is becoming the case with *Pneumococcus*. We must anticipate this event, for it will probably first appear in the PICU as a severe infection that is unresponsive to standard therapy.

Suggested Readings

1. Stevens DL, et al. Severe group A streptococcal infections associated with a toxic shock-like syndrome and scarlet fever toxin A. New Engl J Med 1989;321:1–7.
2. Chesney PJ, Davis JP. Toxic shock syndrome: Textbook of pediatric infectious diseases. 3rd ed. 1992, pp. 1277–1290.
3. Harnden A, Lennon D. Serious suppurative group A streptococcal infection in previously well children. Pediatr Infect Dis J 1988;7: 714–718.
4. Wong VK, Wright HT. Group A Streptococci as a cause of bacteremia in children. Am J Dis Child 1988;142:831–833.

Contents of Presentation/Diagnosis

Index

Page numbers followed by *t* or *f* indicate tables or figures, respectively.